REFERENCE

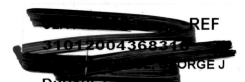
Georgia Law requires Library materials
to be returned or replacement costs paid.
Failure to comply with this law
is a misdemeanor. (O.C.G.A. 20-5-53)

D1063961

ADHD IN THE SCHOOLS

Also Available

ADHD Rating Scale–IV:
Checklists, Norms, and Clinical Interpretation
*George J. DuPaul, Thomas J. Power,
Arthur D. Anastopoulos, and Robert Reid*

Classroom Interventions for ADHD (video)
George J. DuPaul and Gary Stoner

Promoting Children's Health:
Integrating School, Family, and Community
*Thomas J. Power, George J. DuPaul,
Edward S. Shapiro, and Anne E. Kazak*

ADHD
in the Schools
Assessment and Intervention Strategies

THIRD EDITION

George J. DuPaul
Gary Stoner

Foreword by Robert Reid

THE GUILFORD PRESS
New York   London

© 2014 The Guilford Press
A Division of Guilford Publications, Inc.
72 Spring Street, New York, NY 10012
www.guilford.com

Printed in the United States of America

This book is printed on acid-free paper.

Last digit is print number: 9   8   7   6   5   4   3   2   1

The authors have checked with sources believed to be reliable in their efforts to provide
information that is complete and generally in accord with the standards of practice
that are accepted at the time of publication. However, in view of the possibility of
human error or changes in behavioral, mental health, or medical sciences, neither the
authors, nor the editors and publisher, nor any other party who has been involved in the
preparation or publication of this work warrants that the information contained herein
is in every respect accurate or complete, and they are not responsible for any errors
or omissions or the results obtained from the use of such information. Readers are
encouraged to confirm the information contained in this book with other sources.

Library of Congress Cataloging-in-Publication Data

DuPaul, George J.
   ADHD in the schools : assessment and intervention strategies / George J. DuPaul,
Gary Stoner.—Third edition.
      pages cm
   Includes bibliographical references and index.
   ISBN 978-1-4625-1671-1 (hardback)
   1. Attention-deficit-disordered children—Education—United States.   2. Attention-
deficit hyperactivity disorder—Diagnosis.   I. Stoner, Gary.   II. Title.
   LC4713.4.D87 2014
   371.93—dc23
                                                                2014006560

To the many students with ADHD, families, and teachers with whom we have worked over the course of our careers. We have learned a great deal from them, and we truly hope that learning is represented well enough in this text to be of help to others.

About the Authors

George J. DuPaul, PhD, is Professor of School Psychology at Lehigh University. He is a Fellow of Divisions 16 (School Psychology), 53 (Clinical Child and Adolescent Psychology), and 54 (Pediatric Psychology) of the American Psychological Association (APA) and is past president of the Society for the Study of School Psychology. Dr. DuPaul is a recipient of the APA Division 16 Senior Scientist Award and was named to the Children and Adults with ADHD Hall of Fame. His primary research interests are school-based assessment and treatment of disruptive behavior disorders, pediatric school psychology, and assessment and treatment of college students with ADHD. Dr. DuPaul's publications include over 190 journal articles and book chapters on assessment and treatment of ADHD, as well as the coauthored *ADHD Rating Scale–IV.*

Gary Stoner, PhD, is Professor in the Department of Psychology and Director of the Graduate Programs in School Psychology at the University of Rhode Island. He is a Fellow of the APA, past president of APA Division 16, and a member of the Society for the Study of School Psychology. Dr. Stoner's research interests include prevention and intervention with achievement and behavior problems, early school success, parent and teacher support, and professional issues in school psychology. He is past chair of the APA's Interdivisional Coalition for Psychology in Schools and Education and currently serves on the APA Commission on Accreditation.

Foreword

Attention-deficit/hyperactivity disorder (ADHD) is a problem that affects millions of students. In the United States, it is now the most commonly diagnosed psychological disorder of childhood. Worldwide prevalence is estimated at 5% among school-age children, but in the United States recent researchers have reported that over 10% of school-age students have been identified or considered as having ADHD.

ADHD is also a serious problem for our society. It is a chronic, lifelong disorder. Individuals with ADHD have an increased risk for a litany of serious problems. For children, risks include lower academic achievement and increased risk for learning disabilities, conduct disorder, or depression. Additionally, they are likely to encounter serious difficulty in social settings, which can result in social isolation. As children with ADHD enter adolescence, they are more likely than their peers to experience incarceration, contract a sexually transmitted disease, or be involved in multiple car accidents. While some symptoms may abate over time, the core problems remain through adulthood. Adults with ADHD are more likely than peers to be underemployed or unemployed.

In the United States, the direct cost of ADHD (e.g., medical costs, educational services) is estimated to be approximately $50 billion per year. Indirect costs (e.g., lost work time by family members) are difficult to quantify but may be even higher. In sum, ADHD poses clear individual, social, and economic concerns.

As one might expect, ADHD is quite possibly the most thoroughly studied psychological disorder in history. Searching an online database reveals that there are well over 10,000 scientific papers written on various aspects of ADHD. ADHD also has received a tremendous amount of attention in the media. Cover stories on ADHD appear regularly in national news magazines, and stories on ADHD appear frequently in broadcast media. However, even this amount of attention pales in comparison to the sources available on the Internet. Truly, there is an ocean of information on ADHD. Unfortunately, far too often, accounts of ADHD in the popular media or on the Internet are sensationalized or unrepresentative. The media often focus on dramatic first-person stories of success or failure. They chronicle an uplifting but atypical account of how a child overcame ADHD or, conversely, how the problems of ADHD led to other, much more serious problems. Websites hawk the latest "miracle cures," which—as regular as clockwork—will soon be replaced by the next nostrum. Other stories report on purported causes of ADHD.

Coverage commonly focuses on controversies. There is now a cottage industry of critics who focus on disputes—real or contrived—surrounding ADHD or the "uncertainties" of scientific knowledge —"uncertainties" that often are created from whole cloth by those with their own agendas. As a result, ADHD may seem shrouded in mystery; many people are unaware of exactly what ADHD is and how it affects individuals and ultimately society. Perhaps for this reason, there are numerous misconceptions about ADHD. Some of these misconceptions have attained mythic status, and are persistent, persuasive, and unrealistic. Unfortunately, these myths can have an effect on how ADHD is perceived and how educators respond to ADHD.

It is true that scientists do not totally understand the phenomenon of ADHD. This is partly because ADHD is a complex, multifaceted disorder. Children with ADHD are a highly heterogeneous group who can differ markedly even though they have the same diagnosis. Additionally, because different adults (e.g., parents, teachers) see a child in different environments that place different demands and expectations on the child, they may differ on their opinion of the child's problem.

The combination of information (and misinformation) overload and complexity poses a grave problem for educators, who are at the frontlines of ADHD treatment. Children and adolescents with ADHD spend over 1,000 hours annually in the schools. Other professionals (e.g., physicians, psychiatrists, psychologists) have only a minute fraction of the contact hours with individuals with ADHD that educators have. Success in school is crucial for these students, and it is an attainable goal. But it is not easily achieved, and requires educators to have solid, scientific information on crucial factors of ADHD that impact students' performance in the schools.

George J. DuPaul and Gary Stoner obviously are well aware of the critical need educators have for reliable information on this disorder. Based on my experience in the field, I can think of no individuals who are more qualified to provide this information. Both authors are widely hailed as among the preeminent scholars in the area of ADHD and the schools. Both have decades of practical experience working with the schools and in conducting research in assessment and treatment of students with ADHD. Both are keenly sensitive to the critical knowledge of ADHD that educators need to work successfully with these students. Most important, all of the information provided is based on the best, most up-to-date scientific evidence available, and is refreshingly free of bias or any outside agendas. It is quite obvious that the authors' only interest is in providing educators the most accurate information possible on the topic.

In this volume the authors have distilled the ocean of information into a manageable body that neither overwhelms potential readers nor skimps on critical information. They provide background knowledge along with an excellent treatment of controversies and fallacies around ADHD. Assessment and screening of ADHD and the schools' role in the process is discussed. A detailed section on interventions can inform educators on how best to address common problems posed by students with ADHD. Medication, one of the most contentious areas of ADHD treatment, is thoroughly covered in a highly balanced manner. The authors also provide an excellent section on working with parents of students with ADHD, which is a crucial factor in treatment.

All in all, this book, now in its third edition, remains an invaluable reference for educators. It is a volume no teacher who works with students with ADHD should be without. The authors are to be commended for yet again providing an invaluable resource.

ROBERT REID, PhD
University of Nebraska–Lincoln

Preface

Students who display inattentive and disruptive behavior present significant challenges to educational professionals. In fact, many children and adolescents who exhibit behavior control difficulties in classroom settings are diagnosed as having an attention-deficit/hyperactivity disorder (ADHD). Students with ADHD are at high risk for chronic academic achievement difficulties; the development of antisocial behavior; and problems in relationships with peers, parents, and teachers. Traditionally, this disorder has been identified and treated by clinic-based professionals (e.g., pediatricians, clinical psychologists) on an outpatient basis. Given that children and adolescents with ADHD experience some of their greatest difficulties in educational settings, it is important for school-based professionals to directly address the needs of students with this disorder. In addition, federal regulations governing special education eligibility have magnified the need for educators to receive training in assessing and treating students with ADHD in the schools. The purpose of this book is to assist school professionals in understanding and treating children and adolescents with ADHD.

When the first edition of this book was published in 1994, research and evaluation activities relating to children and adolescents with ADHD were primarily the realm of pediatricians, psychiatrists, and clinic-based psychologists; few school-based studies of the activities, functioning, and development of children with ADHD had been conducted. This situation has changed dramatically since then. We now see school-focused researchers, empirical investigations, and school-based issues regarding

ADHD becoming prevalent in the research literature and as topics at professional conferences. In this third edition, we have attempted to address the problems associated with ADHD from a school-based perspective, while recognizing the need for a team effort among parents, community-based professionals, and educators. Specifically, we have focused on how to (1) identify and assess students who might have ADHD; (2) develop and implement classroom-based intervention programs for these students; (3) identify and provide early intervention to young children at risk for ADHD; and (4) communicate with and assist physicians when psychotropic medications are employed to treat this disorder.

In this third edition, we have updated information in these major areas to address the understanding and management of ADHD in a comprehensive fashion for school-based professionals. In addition, we describe assessment and intervention strategies for college students with ADHD and provide expanded coverage of associated behavior disorders as well as assessment and treatment approaches for secondary school students with ADHD.

This book is intended to meet the needs of a variety of school-based practitioners, including school psychologists, guidance counselors, and administrators, as well as both general and special education teachers. Given that students with ADHD are found in nearly every school setting and experience a wide range of difficulties, there should be something of interest to all professional groups in this text. In addition, graduate students who are receiving training in a variety of school-based professions should find this book helpful in understanding this complex disorder. This is our attempt to contribute to continued forward movement of improved school-based practices, services, and supports for children and adolescents identified with ADHD. We sincerely hope readers find this volume to be useful in influencing both professional perspectives on ADHD in schools and the professional work of all those providing services to students with ADHD.

Acknowledgments

As was the case with the first and second editions, this book would not have reached fruition without the support and encouragement of a variety of people. We continue to owe a great deal to our former mentor and major professor, Dr. Mark Rapport of the University of Central Florida. His enthusiasm for the scientific study of ADHD combined with his emphasis on conducting investigations that are clinically and practically relevant provided us with an exemplar of the scientist-practitioner model in action. Furthermore, the high scientific and academic standards that he set for us and other graduate students have led, at least indirectly, to the completion of this book. We also continue to be inspired by the work of Dr. Russell A. Barkley of the Medical University of South Carolina. One of the true "giants" in the field of ADHD research, his support and guidance were critical to the preparation of the first edition of this text.

Next, we are grateful for the support and encouragement of our colleagues Drs. Arthur Anastopoulos, Christine Cole, John Hintze, Robin Hojnoski, Lee Kern, Patti Manz, William Matthews, Thomas Power, Edward Shapiro, Terri Shelton, Mark Shinn, and Lisa Weyandt. Our students at Lehigh University and the University of Rhode Island, too numerous to name, have also been supportive and patient throughout the time that we were preparing this book. Our continued success is directly related to the innovative ideas and challenges presented by our students. We specifically appreciate the assistance provided by

Sarah Cayless-Patches in double-checking and finalizing our reference section.

Great levels of patience and support were evidenced by our families, specifically our spouses, Judy Brown-DuPaul and Joyce Flanagan, respectively. Their willingness to tolerate "lost" evenings and weekends will not go unrewarded. We remain indebted to the editorial staff at The Guilford Press, most especially Natalie Graham, for continuing to support our work with the ideal blend of patience and prodding.

Contents

CHAPTER 1

Overview of ADHD

Amy, Age 4

Amy is a 4-year-old girl who lives with her mother, stepfather, and younger brother (age 2). She attends preschool four mornings per week at a local church. Her mother reports Amy was "a terror" as an infant. She was colicky, frequently cried, and demanded to be held "constantly." At about 11 months old, when she began walking, Amy's activity level increased and she "was always into everything." In fact, on one occasion when Amy was 2 years old, she was brought into the emergency room following ingestion of some cleaning fluids that she had found under the kitchen sink. Amy has been asked to leave several daycare and nursery school settings because of her high activity level, short attention span, and physical aggression toward peers. Although she is beginning to learn letters and numbers, it is very difficult for her mother or teacher to get her to sit still for any reading or learning activities. Amy's preference is to engage in rough-and-tumble activities and she can become quite defiant when asked to sit and complete more structured or quiet activities (e.g., drawing or coloring).

Greg, Age 7

Greg is a 7-year-old first grader in a general education classroom in a public elementary school. According to his parents, his physical and psychological development was "normal" until about age 3 when he first attended nursery school. His preschool and kindergarten teachers reported Greg to have a short attention span, to have difficulties staying seated during group activities, and to interrupt conversations frequently. These behaviors were evident increasingly at home as well. Currently, Greg is achieving at a level commensurate with his classmates in all academic areas. Unfortunately, he continues to evidence problems with inattention, impulsivity, and motor restlessness. These behaviors are displayed more frequently when Greg is supposed to be listening to the teacher or completing an independent task. His teacher is concerned that Greg may begin to exhibit academic problems if his attention and behavior do not improve.

Tommy, Age 9

Tommy is a fourth grader whose schooling occurs in a self-contained, special education classroom for children identified with emotional–behavior disorders in a public elementary school. His mother reports that Tommy has been a "handful" since infancy. During his preschool years, he was very active (e.g., climbing on furniture, running around excessively, and infrequently sitting still) and noncompliant with maternal commands. He has had chronic difficulties relating to other children: he has been both verbally and physically aggressive with his peers. As a result, he has few friends his own age and tends to play with younger children. Tommy has been placed in a class for students in need of social–emotional support since second grade because of his frequent disruptive activities (e.g., calling out without permission, swearing at the teacher, refusing to complete seatwork) and related problematic academic achievement. During the past year, Tommy's antisocial activities have increased in severity: he has been caught shoplifting on several occasions and has been suspended from school for vandalizing the boys' bathroom. Even in his highly structured classroom, Tommy has a great deal of difficulty attending to independent work and following classroom rules.

Lisa, Age 13

Lisa is a 13-year-old eighth grader who receives most of her instruction in general education classrooms. A psychoeducational evaluation conducted when she was 8 years old indicated a "specific learning disability" in math, for which she receives resource room instruction three class periods per week. In addition to problems with math skills, Lisa has exhibited significant difficulties with inattention since at least age 5. Specifically, she appears to daydream excessively and to "space out" when asked to complete effortful tasks either at home or at school. Her parents and teachers report that she "forgets" task instructions frequently, particularly if multiple steps are involved. At one time, it was presumed that her inattention problems were caused by her learning disability in math. This does not appear to be the case, however, because she is inattentive during most classes (i.e., not just during math instruction) and these behaviors predated her entry into elementary school. Lisa is neither impulsive nor overactive. In fact, she is "slow to respond" at times and appears reticent in social situations.

Roberto, Age 17

Roberto is a 17-year-old student who attends the 10th grade in a large urban high school. He was retained in grade twice during elementary school and has struggled academically throughout his academic career. Furthermore, his teachers described him as impatient, disruptive, restless, and lacking in motivation. As a result of his academic and behavior difficulties, Roberto has been provided with a variety of special education services, including placement in a learning support classroom, individual counseling, and, briefly, placement in an alternative school environment. Furthermore, school professionals have attempted to involve Roberto's family with community-based counseling services and have recommended consultation with his physician regarding psychotropic medication; these recommendations have been followed inconsistently over the years. Despite these services, Roberto's difficulties have worsened and have been compounded in recent years by his involvement in a local gang. He has been arrested on two occasions for shoplifting and vandalism and also is truant from school quite often. He has asked his parents to allow him to drop out of high school so that he can obtain a full-time job.

Jeff, Age 19

Jeff is a 19-year-old sophomore attending a private, liberal arts college. He was diagnosed with ADHD, combined type, when he was in elementary school owing to his frequent inattentiveness and impulsive behavior. Jeff's ADHD symptoms were controlled to some degree by the combination of stimulant medication and behavioral strategies implemented by his parents and classroom teachers. As a result, Jeff was able to obtain above-average grades in most academic areas, although he struggled with being prepared for class and studying for tests. He was provided with accommodations such as extra time on tests and reduced homework assignments. With support and extra time, Jeff was able to obtain competitive scores on the SAT, thus providing him with several options for college. His adjustment to college has been challenging given increased demands for independence and self-regulation. The student disabilities office provides Jeff with academic tutoring and coaching in organizational skills; he also continues to receive educational accommodations. Jeff has an overall grade point average (GPA) of 2.5 with variable performance across subject areas.

Although the six individuals described above are quite different, they share a common difficulty with attention, particularly to assigned schoolwork and household responsibilities. Furthermore, many children with attention problems, such as Amy, Greg, Tommy, and Roberto, display additional difficulties with impulsivity and overactivity. The current psychiatric term for children exhibiting extreme problems with inattention, impulsivity, and hyperactivity is *attention-deficit/hyperactivity disorder*, or ADHD[1] (American Psychiatric Association, 2013). As can be discerned from the above case descriptions, the term *ADHD* is applied to a heterogeneous group of students who are encountered in virtually every educational setting from preschool through college.

The purpose of this chapter is to provide a brief overview of ADHD. Specifically, we review information regarding the prevalence of this disorder, the school-related problems of children with ADHD, associated adjustment difficulties, methods of subtyping children with this disorder, possible causes of ADHD, the impact of situational factors on symptom severity, and the probable long-term outcomes for this population. This background material provides the context for later descriptions of school-based assessment and treatment strategies for ADHD.

PREVALENCE OF ADHD

Epidemiological (i.e., population survey) studies indicate that approximately 3–10% of children in the United States can be diagnosed with ADHD (Centers for Disease Control and Prevention [CDC], 2010; Froehlich et al., 2007) with a median estimate of 6.8% across multiple national surveys (Centers for Disease Control and Prevention, 2013). Because most general education classrooms include at least 20 students, it is estimated that one child in every classroom will have ADHD. As a result, children reported to evidence attention and behavior control problems are frequently referred to school psychologists and other education and mental health professionals. Boys with the disorder outnumber girls in both clinic-referred (approximately a 6:1 ratio) and community-based (approximately a 3:1 ratio) samples (Centers for Disease Control and Prevention, 2010, 2013; Froehlich et al., 2007). The higher clinic ratio for boys with this disorder may be a function in part of the greater prevalence of additional disruptive behaviors (e.g., noncompliance, conduct disturbance) among boys with ADHD (Gaub & Carlson, 1997). More than 50% of children diagnosed with ADHD receive psychotropic medication for this condition, while approximately 12% and 34% receive special education and mental health services, respectively (Pastor & Reuben, 2002). Thus, relative to other childhood conditions (e.g., autism and depression), ADHD is a "high-incidence" disorder that is

---

[1] Because multiple labels for attention-deficit/hyperactivity disorder have been used throughout the years and across disciplines, the term *ADHD* will be used in this text to promote simplicity. ADHD will be considered synonymous with other terms for the disorder, such as *hyperactivity* and *ADD*.

particularly prominent among males. In a manner similar to these other disorders, it typically requires the services of multiple community and education professionals to achieve positive developmental outcomes.

It should be noted that most ADHD research studies have focused on white males from middle-socioeconomic-status (SES) backgrounds. It is only in recent years that investigations have included more diverse samples in terms of sex, ethnicity, and SES. This is important because African American children are significantly more likely to exhibit ADHD symptoms based on teacher and parent report, yet these same children are only two-thirds as likely to be diagnosed and treated for ADHD as white children (Miller, Nigg, & Miller, 2009). On the one hand, the elevation of symptom reports may result in overidentification of African American children relative to population-based norms (Reid, DuPaul, Power, Anastopoulos, & Riccio, 1998). Alternatively, lower rates of diagnosis and treatment among African American children may be related to differences in parent beliefs about ADHD, greater exposure to socioenvironmental risk factors, and lack of access to treatment services (Miller et al., 2009). ADHD diagnoses are more prevalent for those with health insurance relative to those without insurance coverage (Centers for Disease Control and Prevention, 2013), so this may be an additional factor accounting for racial differences. Practitioners must be aware that social and cultural factors account, in part, for prevalence, diagnosis, and treatment patterns. Clearly, additional research regarding the role of culture, ethnicity, and SES is necessary to guide practitioners in the assessment and treatment of ADHD for children from diverse backgrounds.

SCHOOL-RELATED PROBLEMS OF CHILDREN WITH ADHD

Core Behavior Difficulties

The core characteristics (i.e., inattention and hyperactivity–impulsivity) of ADHD can lead to myriad difficulties for children in school settings. Specifically, because these children often have problems sustaining attention to effortful tasks, their completion of independent seatwork is quite inconsistent. Their performance on classwork also may be compromised by a lack of attention to task instructions. Other academic problems associated with attention problems include poor test performance; deficient study skills; disorganized notebooks, desks, and written reports; and a lack of attention to teacher lectures and/or group discussion. Children with ADHD often disrupt classroom activities, and thus disturb the learning of their classmates. For example, children with ADHD may exhibit impulsivity in a variety of ways, including frequent calling out without permission, talking with classmates at inappropriate times, and becoming angry when confronted with reprimands or frustrating tasks. Classwork and homework accuracy also may be affected deleteriously due to an impulsive, careless response style on these tasks.

By far the most ubiquitous classroom problem exhibited by children and adolescents with ADHD is a relatively high level of inattention or off-task behavior. In fact, comprehensive meta-analytic review found that, on average, students with ADHD are on-task about 75% of the time in contrast with an average of 88% on-task behavior by typically developing classmates. The effect size (1.40) associated with this group difference is large, meaning that there is a 1.4 standard deviation unit difference in the on-task behavior of these two groups (Kofler, Rapport, & Alderson, 2008). The on-task behavior of students with ADHD is also quite variable over time (Kofler et al., 2008) and is moderated by class activity and instructional context (Imeraj et al., 2013). Imeraj and colleagues (2013) found that elementary school students with ADHD exhibited significantly less time on-task relative to non-ADHD classmates during whole-group instruction and individual seatwork but not when the class was engaged with small-group work. Furthermore, significant on-task behavior differences were evident during highly academic subjects (i.e., math and language), as well as during transitions from one classroom activity to another but not during less academic subject periods (e.g., music, art). Thus, the inattention symptoms of ADHD seem to be sensitive to environmental context and activity; a finding that has clear implications for intervention as discussed in later chapters.

In-class problems related to high rates of physical activity include children leaving their seats without permission, playing with inappropriate objects (e.g., materials in desk that are unrelated to the task at hand), repetitive tapping of hands and feet, and fidgeting in their chairs. Although the latter behaviors may appear relatively benign, when they occur frequently they can serve as a significant disruption to classroom instruction.

Difficulties Associated with ADHD

Students with ADHD are at risk for significant difficulties in a variety of functional areas. It appears as though problems with inattention, impulsivity, and high rates of physical activity serve as a "magnet" for other difficulties that are, in some cases, more severe than the core deficits of ADHD. Of these difficulties, the three most frequent correlates of ADHD are academic underachievement, high rates of noncompliance and aggression, and disturbances in peer relationships.

Teachers and parents frequently report that children with ADHD underachieve academically compared with their classmates (Barkley, 2006; Weyandt, 2007). As stated previously, children with this disorder exhibit significantly lower rates of on-task behavior during instruction and independent work periods than those displayed by their peers (Platzman et al., 1992; Vile Junod, DuPaul, Jitendra, Volpe, & Lorah, 2006). Consequently, children with ADHD have fewer opportunities to respond to academic material and complete less independent work than their classmates (Pfiffner, Barkley, & DuPaul, 2006). Lower than expected rates of work completion may, in part, account for the association of ADHD with academic underachievement: up to 80% of children with this disorder have been found to exhibit academic performance problems (Cantwell & Baker, 1991). In fact, achievement test scores between students with ADHD and their non-ADHD peers differ by 0.71 standard deviation units (i.e., moderate to large effect size), with this gap continuing through college (Frazier, Youngstrom, Glutting, & Watkins, 2007). Furthermore, between 20 and 30% of children with ADHD are classified as having a learning disability due to deficits in the acquisition of specific academic skills (see Chapter 3 for details). Finally, the results of prospective follow-up studies of children with ADHD into adolescence and young adulthood indicate heightened risks for chronic academic failure as measured by higher rates of grade retention and dropping out of school relative to their peers (e.g., Barkley, Murphy, & Fischer, 2008).

The strong correlation between hyperactivity and aggression is well documented in the research literature (Barkley, 2006; Jensen, Martin, & Cantwell, 1997). Problems of aggression most frequently associated with ADHD include defiance or noncompliance with authority figure commands, poor temper control, and argumentativeness and verbal hostility, which presently comprise the psychiatric category of oppositional defiant disorder (American Psychiatric Association, 2013). Therefore, it is not surprising that oppositional defiant disorder is the most common codiagnosis with ADHD (i.e., associated or comorbid condition), as more than 40% of children with ADHD and 65% of teenagers with ADHD display significant oppositional defiant disorder-related behaviors (Barkley, 2006; Jensen et al., 1997). More serious antisocial behaviors (e.g., stealing, physical aggression, and truancy) are exhibited by 25% or more of students with ADHD, particularly at the secondary school level (Barkley et al., 2008).

Children who display aggression and ADHD-related difficulties are at greater risk for interpersonal conflict at home, in school, and with peers than are children who display ADHD alone (Johnston & Mash, 2001). Parents of children with ADHD report significantly greater stress than parents of typically developing children, with greater symptom severity associated with higher levels of parent stress (Theule, Wiener, Tannock, & Jenkins, 2013). Furthermore, the presence of parental depressive symptoms and/or co-occurring child conduct problems predicts greater levels of parent stress (Theule et al.). Not surprisingly, teachers report experiencing significant amounts of stress in interacting with students with ADHD, especially those who exhibit aggression along with ADHD symptoms (Greene, Beszterczey, Katzenstein, Park, & Goring, 2002). Finally, the combination of conduct problems and ADHD is strongly associated with the abuse of illicit drugs (Barkley et al., 2008; Biederman et al., 1997).

It is very difficult for many children with ADHD to initiate and maintain friendships with their classmates (Stormont, 2001). Studies employing sociometric measures have found uniformly high rates of peer rejection for children displaying ADHD-related behaviors (e.g., Hinshaw, Zupan, Simmel, Nigg, & Melnick, 1997; Hodgens, Cole, & Boldizar, 2000). The rate of peer rejection is particularly high for children displaying both aggression and ADHD. Typically, peer-rejection status is stable over time, reflecting the chronic nature of these children's interactional difficulties (Parker & Asher, 1987). The stability of peer-rejection status is particularly vexing because rejected status is a significant predictor of several problematic long-term outcomes for children with ADHD including delinquency, anxiety, and global impairment (Mrug et al., 2012). Of additional concern, approximately 22% of boys and 15% of girls with ADHD can be characterized as having a "social disability" representing social functioning that is 1.65 standard deviations below age and gender means on standardized measures of social functioning (Greene et al., 1996, 2002). Preliminary evidence also indicates that children with ADHD tend to be on the periphery of classroom social networks and to "hang out" together, thereby increasing the probability of disruptive behavior (Kelly, 2001). Not surprisingly, therefore, children with this disorder perceive peers and classmates to provide less frequent social support than do their non-ADHD counterparts (Demaray & Elliott, 2001).

Presumably, the disturbed peer relations of children with ADHD are due to inattentive and impulsive behaviors disrupting their social performance (Stormont, 2001). The most common performance deficits associated with this disorder include inappropriate attempts to join ongoing peer group activities (e.g., barging in on games in progress), poor conversational behaviors (e.g., frequent interruptions, paying minimal attention to what others are saying), employing aggressive "solutions" to interpersonal problems, and being prone to losing temper control when conflict or frustrations are encountered in social situations

(Barkley, 2006). A related concern in the social arena is that boys with ADHD are involved in team or individual sports for shorter time periods than their typically developing counterparts and are more likely than control children to exhibit aggression, display emotional reactivity, and be disqualified during team athletic activities (Johnson & Rosén, 2000). Surprisingly, children with ADHD often are able to articulate the proper social behaviors to be exhibited in specific situations, although there may be a tendency for them to propose aggressive solutions to interpersonal problems (Stormont, 2001). At present, the most prudent conclusion is that ADHD-related symptoms lead to social *performance* difficulties for these children, rather than to social *skills* deficits per se (see Chapter 8 for details).

Children with ADHD require more frequent medical and mental health care than their non-ADHD counterparts. For example, one study found that children with this disorder have more frequent primary care, pharmacy, and mental health service visits than do children without this disorder (Guevara, Lozano, Wickizer, Mell, & Gephart, 2001). As a result, health care costs for children with ADHD were more than double the costs for non-ADHD children (for a review, see Doshi et al., 2012). Costs for health care are even greater than for children with other chronic disorders such as asthma (Chan, Zhan, & Homer, 2002). The "true" costs for treating ADHD may actually be underestimated given that these children receive services in school and mental health settings (Chan et al., 2002). In fact, Pelham, Foster, and Robb (2007) estimated the total annual societal costs associated with ADHD to be $42.5 billion, with an average annual educational cost of $5,007 per student relative to non-ADHD peers above and beyond costs associated with general education (Robb et al., 2011). Thus, school professionals need to be cognizant of the greater need for health care in this population and attempt to help families access needed services in the community.

SUBTYPES OF ADHD

The current definition of ADHD includes a list of 18 behavioral symptoms divided into two sets (inattention and hyperactivity–impulsivity) of nine symptoms each (American Psychiatric Association, 2013). Given that the symptomatic profile will vary across individuals, children classified with ADHD are a heterogeneous group. In fact, there are at least 7,056 possible combinations of 12 out of 18 symptoms that could result in a diagnosis of ADHD. Broadening this inherent heterogeneity are the potential correlates of ADHD (i.e., academic underachievement, aggression, and peer relationship difficulties), as summarized previously. Therefore, attempts have been made to identify more homogeneous sub-types of ADHD to facilitate searches for causal factors, identify potential differences in long-term outcome, and, most important, aid in treatment planning (Barkley, 2006; Jensen et al., 1997; Willcutt et al., 2012).

There are three subtypes of ADHD according to DSM-5 (American Psychiatric Association, 2013), including combined presentation (ADHD-COMB), predominantly inattentive presentation (ADHD-IA), and predominantly hyperactive–impulsive presentation (ADHD-HI). Children with ADHD-COMB exhibit at least six of the nine inattention symptoms and at least six of the nine hyperactive–impulsive symptoms. Symptoms must have persisted for a minimum of 6 months, be inconsistent with an individual's developmental level, and directly impact social and academic activities. ADHD-IA is indicated for children who exhibit at least six inattention symptoms but fewer than six hyperactive–impulsive symptoms. Finally, children with ADHD-HI exhibit at least six hyperactive–impulsive symptoms but fewer than six inattention symptoms. A brief overview of each of the current subtypes is provided below, along with an exploration of the value of subtyping ADHD on the basis of the presence or absence of aggression or internalizing symptoms or on the basis of number of inattentive or hyperactive–impulsive symptoms.[2]

ADHD, Predominantly Inattentive Presentation

A previous American Psychiatric Association classification system (i.e., DSM-III; American Psychiatric Association, 1980) included two different subtypes of ADHD: attention-deficit disorder with hyperactivity (ADD+H) and attention-deficit disorder without hyperactivity (ADDnoH). The latter category included children who exhibited significant problems with inattention and impulsivity in the absence of frequent physical activity. When DSM-III was revised in 1987, this subtype was removed from the classification schema because of its minimal empirical underpinnings at the time.

Since the 1987 publication of DSM-III-R (American Psychiatric Association, 1987), a variety of research studies have been conducted that support the existence of an ADDnoH subtype (for a review, see Carlson & Mann, 2000). On the basis of this empirical evidence, this subtype was reintroduced to the psychiatric nomenclature with the publication of DSM-IV (American Psychiatric Association, 1994) and

---

[2]The advantages and disadvantages of subtyping children with learning disabilities versus those without learning disabilities are discussed in Chapter 3.

continues to be included in DSM-5 (American Psychiatric Association, 2013).

Children with ADHD, predominantly inattentive presentation (ADHD-IA), display significant problems with inattention in the absence of notable impulsivity and hyperactivity. There is initial evidence that children with ADHD-IA have greater problems with memory retrieval and perceptual–motor speed than their hyperactive–impulsive counterparts (Barkley, DuPaul, & McMurray, 1990). Furthermore, these children are described by parents and teachers as more "sluggish" cognitively, daydreamy, and socially withdrawn than children with ADHD-COMB (Hodgens et al., 2000; McBurnett, Pfiffner, & Frick, 2001). These and other findings have led some investigators to postulate a greater incidence of learning disabilities among this subtype relative to other children with the full syndrome of ADHD. For example, one investigation (Barkley, DuPaul, & McMurray, 1990) found a greater percentage of students with ADHD-IA (i.e., 53%) placed in classrooms for students with learning disabilities relative to those with ADHD-COMB (i.e., 34%). Furthermore, inattention symptoms are more likely to be associated with academic impairment than are hyperactive–impulsive symptoms (e.g., Bauermeister, Barkley, Bauermeister, Martinez, & McBurnett, 2012). Alternatively, there do not appear to be significant differences in neuropsychological or neurological functioning between children with ADHD-COMB relative to ADHD-IA (Willcutt et al., 2012).

In clinical samples, a smaller percentage (i.e., approximately 1.3%) of children have ADHD-IA relative to those with the full syndrome (e.g., Szatmari, Offord, & Boyle, 1989), while there may be a higher percentage of children with the inattentive presentation (4.4% vs. 2.2% for ADHD-COMB) in community samples (e.g., Froehlich et al., 2007). Furthermore, there is burgeoning evidence to indicate that such children should be identified separately from children with ADHD-COMB. These symptom presentations clearly differ with respect to associated difficulties, and perhaps in the areas of treatment response and long-term outcome (Willcutt et al., 2012). Barkley (2006) has argued that children with ADHD-IA also may differ from hyperactive–impulsive children in the qualitative nature of their attention deficits. Specifically, children with ADHD-COMB exhibit difficulties with sustained attention as a function of impaired delayed responding to the environment, while those with ADHD-IA are more likely to have problems with focused attention. Thus, different neural mechanisms may be involved, leading to discrepant behavioral response styles (Barkley, 2006). Furthermore, children with ADHD-IA who also display symptoms of sluggish cognitive tempo (e.g., confused, seems lost in a fog) exhibit outcomes such as social withdrawal and internalizing disorder symptoms that are not frequently found among children with ADHD-COMB (Bauermeister et al., 2012; Carlson & Mann, 2002). These important differences between symptom presentations have led researchers to suggest that ADHD-IA is a separate and distinct disorder from the combined type (Barkley, 2006: Milich, Balentine, & Lynam, 2001) and, at the very least, diagnostic criteria should include symptoms of sluggish cognitive tempo to allow more accurate identification of the inattentive subtype (Carlson & Mann, 2002).

There is also evidence of heterogeneity within the DSM-IV ADHD-IA subtype such that some children appear to be borderline ADHD-COMB (i.e., have four or five hyperactive–impulsive symptoms placing them just below the diagnostic threshold for combined presentation), while others have very few if any hyperactive–impulsive symptoms (Milich et al., 2001). It is possible that differences in hyperactive–impulsive symptom presentation may be associated with different impairments, outcomes, and treatment response.

In contrast to the ADHD-IA symptom presentation, children with the full syndrome of ADHD exhibit higher rates of impulsivity, overactivity, aggression, noncompliance, and peer rejection (Carlson & Mann, 2002). Furthermore, children with ADHD-COMB are more likely than their ADHD-IA counterparts to be diagnosed with other disruptive behavior disorders (e.g., oppositional defiant disorder and conduct disorder), be placed in classrooms for students with emotional disturbances, obtain a higher frequency of school suspensions, and receive psychotherapeutic intervention (Barkley, DuPaul, & McMurray, 1990; Faraone, Biederman, Weber, & Russell, 1998; Willcutt, Pennington, Chhabildas, Friedman, & Alexander, 1999). Although comparative long-term outcome studies have not been conducted, it is assumed that children with the full syndrome of ADHD are at greater risk for antisocial disturbance and behavioral adjustment difficulties. Little is known about the chronicity and longitudinal outcome of ADHD-IA in childhood, although one study found more than 60% of young children (4- to 6-year-olds) with this subtype continued to meet diagnostic criteria for at least one subtype of ADHD across 8 years (Lahey, Pelham, Loney, Lee, & Willcutt, 2005). A handful of studies have examined the differential response to psychostimulant medication (i.e., Ritalin, or methylphenidate [MPH]) between ADHD-COMB and ADHD-IA subtypes. These studies generally indicate a positive response to medication among most members of both subtypes, with lower doses found to be sufficient for a greater percentage of children with ADHD-IA (e.g., Barkley, DuPaul, & McMurray, 1991). To date, very few studies have compared response to nonpharmacological interventions among subtypes (for a review, see Willcutt et al., 2012).

ADHD, Predominantly Hyperactive–Impulsive Presentation

The predominantly hyperactive–impulsive type of ADHD (ADHD-HI) was introduced in DSM-IV (American Psychiatric Association, 1994). The field trials conducted prior to the publication of DSM-IV indicated that a small percentage of children with this disorder evidenced significant hyperactive–impulsive behaviors in the absence of inattentive symptoms (Lahey et al., 1994). The vast majority of these children were of preschool and early elementary school age, leading to speculation that the ADHD-HI subtype may be a precursor of ADHD-COMB. At least one study has confirmed this assumption, finding that nearly all young children (4- to 6-year-olds) in an ADHD-HI sample either remitted or shifted to ADHD-COMB across an 8-year assessment period (Lahey et al., 2005). In fact, minimal research has been conducted regarding the epidemiology, clinical characteristics, school performance, and treatment outcomes of the ADHD-HI subtype (Willcutt et al., 2012). There is scant evidence regarding prevalence of this subtype, with one study finding approximately 2% of children in a community sample to meet criteria for ADHD-HI (Froehlich et al., 2007). There is preliminary evidence that children with ADHD-HI are prone to the same comorbid disorders (i.e., oppositional defiant disorder and conduct disorder) as children with ADHD-COMB (Willcutt et al., 1999). Therefore, given the dearth of research on this presentation, the most prudent conclusion is that ADHD-HI represents a less severe form or an early manifestation of the combined presentation of ADHD (Lahey et al., 2005).

Limitations of the DSM Subtyping Approach

Although research has strongly supported the validity of DSM criteria for ADHD as a construct associated with significant functional impairment and documented the validity of the two symptom dimensions (i.e., inattentive and hyperactive–impulsive), evidence regarding the discriminant validity of ADHD subtypes has been mixed (Willcutt et al., 2012). Furthermore, Valo and Tannock (2010) found that DSM-IV subtype diagnoses are highly dependent on clinician decisions as to number of informants, type of assessment method, and ascertainment of symptom reports. Thus, subtype classification appears inherently variable (i.e., unreliable) as a function of differences in assessment methodology. Of additional concern, longitudinal studies have consistently shown instability of ADHD subtype membership over time. For example, Lahey and Willcutt (2010) found a significant percentage of children with each DSM subtype at an initial assessment (when children were between 4 and 6 years old) met criteria for each of the other subtypes at least once during a 9-year longitudinal study. In their comprehensive meta-analysis and review of the ADHD subtype literature, Willcutt and colleagues (2012) conclude that "nominal DSM-IV subtype categories are unstable due to both systematic and random changes over time" (p. 16). Thus, as discussed later in this chapter, it may be more appropriate to distinguish among children with ADHD on a continuous basis (i.e., number of inattentive and/or hyperactive–impulsive symptoms) than on a nominal basis (i.e., subtype categories). Although DSM-5 (American Psychiatric Association, 2013) did not adopt this continuous framework, the fact that DSM-IV ADHD "subtypes" were replaced with ADHD "presentations" represents the need to view diagnostic status as a snapshot in time (i.e., a presentation of symptoms) that may change over the course of development rather than children meeting criteria for nominal subtypes that appear to be inherently unstable.

ADHD with versus without Aggression

As stated previously, the term *aggressive* has been used to describe children who display higher than average rates of noncompliance, argumentativeness, defiance, and poor temper control. Many children displaying such behaviors meet the criteria for the classification of oppositional defiant disorder. Although there is a great deal of overlap or comorbidity between ADHD and oppositional defiant disorder (Barkley, 2006; see "Difficulties Associated with ADHD" section above), children with either disorder alone are distinct, especially with respect to long-term outcome, from those youngsters who are both hyperactive and aggressive (for a review, see Jensen et al., 1997).

Children with ADHD and aggression (i.e., oppositional defiant disorder or conduct disorder) exhibit greater frequencies of antisocial behaviors, such as lying, stealing, and fighting, than those who are hyperactive and not aggressive (Barkley, 2006). Children with ADHD plus externalizing disorder display poorer social skills than those with ADHD alone (Booster, DuPaul, Power, & Eiraldi, 2012). Thus, hyperactive–aggressive children are at higher risk for peer rejection than those displaying either ADHD or aggression in isolation. Greater levels of family dysfunction and parental psychopathology have been found among youngsters with both disorders as well (Jensen et al., 1997). Most important, children with both ADHD and aggression have the highest risk for problematic outcomes in adolescence and adulthood (e.g., greater prevalence of substance abuse) relative to any other subgroup of children with ADHD (Jensen et al., 1997).

Although these subtypes have not been found to exhibit different responses to psychostimulant medication (e.g., Barkley, McMurray, Edelbrock, & Robbins, 1989), there is considerable agreement among professionals that those children with ADHD *and* aggression will require more intensive and continuous professional service delivery to achieve favorable outcomes. The precursors to the combination of ADHD and aggression may hold some clues to the need for comprehensive multimodal treatment. A combination of within-child (i.e., irritable child temperament, shorter than average attention span, and high activity level) and environmental (i.e., coercive response style of family members, marital discord, and poor parental functioning) factors may lead to the coexistence of these disorders (Barkley, 2006). To the extent that these factors contribute to child maladjustment throughout development, the later the point of intervention, the greater the need for long-term, intensive, service delivery. The protracted and difficult nature of these behavior problems sometimes leads to children being placed in more restrictive placements outside of the public school and family environments.

ADHD with versus without Internalizing Disorder

Approximately 13–50% of children with ADHD exhibit symptoms of an anxiety or depressive disorder (Jensen et al., 1997). The presence of comorbid internalizing symptoms carries both positive and negative implications for children with ADHD. On the one hand, the association of internalizing symptoms with ADHD can serve as a protective factor wherein (1) hyperactive–impulsive behaviors are less severe than when internalizing symptoms are absent and (2) conduct disorder symptoms are less likely to be present (Pliszka, Carlson, & Swanson, 1999). Alternatively, the combination of ADHD and internalizing symptoms is associated with greater social impairment (as reported by teachers and parents) than ADHD alone (Karustis, Power, Rescorla, Eiraldi, & Gallagher, 2000). Furthermore, some studies have found a diminished effect of psychostimulant medication for children with ADHD and internalizing symptoms relative to children with ADHD without internalizing symptoms (e.g., DuPaul, Barkley, & McMurray, 1994). Thus, there may be important distinctions in clinical presentation, impairment, and treatment response between children with ADHD with and without internalizing symptoms, thereby supporting this as a viable subtyping scheme. This conclusion is tempered by the fact that what little research has been done in this area has (1) focused almost exclusively on anxiety rather than depressive disorders and (2) used a single-respondent (e.g., parent report) to assess internalizing symptomatology

(Booster et al., 2012). Nevertheless, at the very least, practitioners need to assess both externalizing and internalizing symptoms when evaluating children suspected of ADHD because such symptoms are likely to influence both the trajectory of children's difficulties and their response to certain interventions.

ADHD with Symptom Modifiers

As stated previously, ADHD subtype diagnoses appear unstable over time as children move from one subtype to another as a function of assessment period (Willcutt et al., 2012). Given this inherent instability of nominal (i.e., categorical) subtypes, Lahey and Willcutt (2010) recommend an alternative continuous method to address heterogeneity in the ADHD population. In their longitudinal study of 129 young children with ADHD and 130 comparison children followed over 9 years, Lahey and Willcutt found inattentive and hyperactive–impulsive symptom counts to be significant predictors of important indices of impairment including parent and teacher perceptions of need for treatment, interviewer ratings of child functioning, teacher ratings of peer disliking and ignoring, and reading and math achievement. Some areas of impairment were associated with inattentiveness alone (e.g., peer ignoring, math achievement), others were associated with hyperactivity–impulsivity alone (e.g., peer disliking, reading achievement), while the remaining areas were associated with counts of both symptom dimensions. Thus, Lahey and Willcutt recommend that rather than using nominal subtype classifications, practitioners should qualify the diagnosis of ADHD with counts for each symptom dimension (e.g., "Six symptoms of inattentiveness and five symptoms of hyperactivity–impulsivity were present at the time of assessment"). In this way, symptom presentation is documented dimensionally rather than categorically and it is clear that this is the current presentation of symptoms that may change over time. This is an intriguing recommendation that obviously requires more empirical study, but one that should be strongly considered by school-based practitioners.

In recognition of the importance of symptom counts and level of impairment in characterizing the severity of ADHD, DSM-5 includes three severity modifiers (i.e., mild, moderate, and severe; American Psychiatric Association, 2013). Mild ADHD is characterized by symptom counts at or near diagnostic thresholds along with relatively minor academic and/or social impairment. At the other extreme, severe ADHD is present when symptom counts are above the diagnostic threshold and major functional impairment is evident. Moderate ADHD represents symptom and impairment presentations that are between the two extremes of mild and severe ADHD.

POSSIBLE CAUSES OF ADHD

There is no apparent single "cause" of ADHD. Rather, ADHD symptomatology may result from a variety of causal mechanisms (Barkley, 2006; Nigg, 2006). Most of the research examining the etiology of ADHD is correlational. Thus, caution is warranted in attributing causal status to identified variables. Nevertheless, empirical data have been gathered regarding the potential causal contributions of a number of factors to ADHD (see Barkley, 2002; Nigg, 2006). Within-child variables, such as neurobiological factors and hereditary influences, have received the greatest attention in the literature (Barkley, 2006; Nigg, 2006). The contributions of these variables are summarized briefly below. Environmental influences (e.g., family stress, poor parental disciplinary practices) appear to modulate the severity of the disorder, but do not play as large a causal role as neurobiological variables (Barkley, 2006; Nigg, 2006).

Neurobiological Variables

Historically, neurobiological factors have received the greatest attention as etiological factors. The earliest hypotheses postulated that children with ADHD had structural brain damage that contributed to attention and behavior control difficulties (Barkley, 2006). There appear to be minor structural differences between the brains of individuals with ADHD and those of normal controls. Specifically, studies using both structural (e.g., magnetic resonance imaging [MRI]) and functional (e.g., positron emission tomography [PET]) imaging techniques have indicated important differences and possible abnormalities in the frontostriatal networks of the brain (for a review, see Nigg, 2006), as well as cerebellar regions, splenium of the corpus callosum, and right caudate (Valera, Faraone, Murray, & Seidman, 2007). Interestingly, one of the sections of the brain that has been studied in this regard is the prefrontal cortex, which purportedly is involved in the inhibition of behavior and mediating responses to environmental stimuli. In addition, the neurotransmitters, dopamine and norepinephrine, are presumed to be "less available" in certain regions of the brain (e.g., frontal cortex), thus contributing to ADHD symptomatology. This hypothesis has been based, in part, on the action of psychostimulants (e.g., Ritalin) in the brain wherein the availability of dopamine and norepinephrine is increased. Based on available evidence, it is presumed that these neurobiological differences are due to aberrations in normal brain development resulting from genetic, hormonal, and/or environmental factors (Nigg, 2006).

Hereditary Influences

There is consistent evidence that ADHD is a highly heritable disorder that runs in families (Waldman & Gizer, 2006). Evidence supporting the primary role of genetic factors has been obtained in a number of ways. First, there is a higher rate of concurrent and past ADHD symptoms in immediate family members of children with ADHD relative to their non-ADHD counterparts (e.g., Faraone et al., 1993). Furthermore, there is a higher incidence of ADHD among first-degree biological relatives relative to adoptive parents and siblings for children with ADHD who were adopted at an early age (e.g., Van der Oord, Boomsa, & Verhulst, 1994).

A second research strategy to investigate the heritability of ADHD symptoms has been to investigate symptom patterns in monozygotic (MZ) and dizygotic (DZ) twins. Specifically, the probability of one twin having ADHD given that the other twin has the disorder (referred to as a *concordance rate*) is significantly higher among MZ twin pairs than among DZ twin pairs (e.g., Levy, Hay, McStephen, Wood, & Waldman, 1997). Because MZ twins are genetically identical, while DZ twins share only 50% of their genes, it is presumed that higher concordance rates among MZ twins support a substantial role for hereditary (rather than environmental) factors in the expression of ADHD symptoms. In fact, twin studies allow behavioral genetic researchers to estimate the variance of ADHD symptoms that are accounted for by genetic, shared environment, and nonshared environment factors. Most of the variance is accounted for by genetic factors, as indicated by heritability estimates ranging from 60 to 90% (for a review, see Waldman & Gizer, 2006). A smaller but significant proportion of symptomatic variance (i.e., between 10 and 40%) is accounted for by nonshared environmental factors, while none of these studies support a significant role for shared environmental factors. Heritability estimates for ADHD are among the highest for any emotional or behavior disorder, exceeding estimates for schizophrenia and autism (Barkley, 2006).

Molecular genetic studies have provided initial support for the association of genes related to specific neurotransmitters and the phenotypic expression of ADHD symptoms (e.g., Barkley, Smith, Fischer, & Navia, 2006). Although it is likely that multiple genes related to both the dopaminergic and the noradrenergic systems are involved (Nigg, 2006), genes related to the dopaminergic system have received the greatest attention thus far (for a review, see Banaschewski, Becker, Scherag, Franke, & Coghill, 2010). For example, important differences in the dopamine transporter gene (*DAT1*) and the D4 dopamine receptor gene (*DRD4*) have been found in ADHD relative to non-ADHD samples (Waldman & Gizer, 2006). These are interesting findings given that dopamine is an important neurotransmitter in those parts of the brain (e.g., frontal cortex) that have been implicated in ADHD and that stimulant medications temporarily increase the availability of dopamine in the synaptic cleft. There is also growing consensus that the genetic roots of ADHD are related to multiple genes each of which may contribute a small percentage of the variance (Nigg, 2006) and that genetic contributions may be moderated by environmental experiences (Martel et al., 2011). Finally, it is important to note that genetic influences on ADHD are probabilistic, not deterministic. Heritability may reflect *liability* to disorder rather than genetic *determination* (Nigg, 2006).

Environmental Toxins

Over the years, a variety of environmental toxins have been hypothesized to account for ADHD symptoms. Some of the more popular theories have implicated nutritional factors, lead poisoning, and prenatal exposure to drugs or alcohol (Barkley, 2006). For example, Feingold (1975) argued that certain food additives (e.g., artificial food colorings, salicylates) led to childhood hyperactivity. Well-controlled studies that have examined this hypothesis, as well as similar assumptions about sugar, indicate that dietary factors play a minimal role in the genesis of ADHD (Barkley, 2006). More recently, investigators have found a significant relationship between maternal smoking (Milberger, Beiderman, Faraone, Chen, & Jones, 1996) or cigarette smoking (Mick, Biederman, Faraone, Sayer, & Kleinman, 2002) during pregnancy and later ADHD, as well as low birth weight and later ADHD (Mick, Biederman, Prince, Fischer, & Faraone, 2002). Presumably these environmental toxins and related factors may compromise brain development that then increases risk for ADHD. In his comprehensive review of etiological factors related to ADHD, Nigg (2006) estimated that prenatal exposure to alcohol and nicotine along with early childhood exposure to lead accounts for approximately 11% of the variance in later ADHD symptoms. If other environmental factors (e.g., low birth weight, low-level lead exposure, perinatal insults) are considered, approximately 35% of the variance in ADHD symptomology is accounted for.

Summary

The most prudent conclusion regarding the etiology of ADHD is that multiple neurobiological factors may predispose children to exhibiting higher rates of impulsivity and motor activity along with shorter than average attention spans compared with other children. The most promising evidence points to a hereditary influence and/or early exposure to a neurotoxin that may alter the size and functioning of prefrontal and striatal neural networks that serve as planning and organization centers of the brain (Nigg, 2006). Approximately 65% of the variance in ADHD symptoms is attributable to heritable effects (e.g., genetic main effects) and 35% of the variance is related to environmental factors, primarily early exposure to neurotoxins (see Figure 1.1). Furthermore, behavioral genetic studies have generally supported the notion of ADHD as a dimensional rather than a categorical disorder (e.g., Levy et al., 1997). Stated differently, everyone exhibits symptoms of this disorder on occasion. What sets children with ADHD apart from their nondiagnosed peers is that they may be genetically predisposed (through neurobiological differences) to exhibit these behaviors at a significantly higher rate than others of the same age and gender.

Several caveats should be kept in mind about etiological conclusions. First, research in this area has been fraught with methodological difficulties that reduce confidence in interpreting results (Nigg, 2006). Second, despite the fact that within-child variables appear to be the primary causal factors, this finding does not denigrate the role of the environment in the maintenance of ADHD symptoms. For instance, as

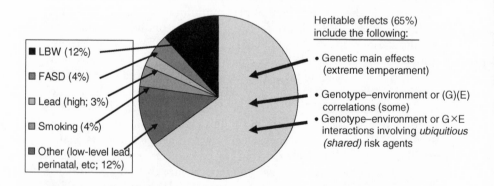

FIGURE 1.1. Schematic depiction of likely etiological influences on emergence of ADHD. LBW, low birth weight; lead (high), exposure to lead levels of 10 µg/dl or higher; FASD, fetal alcohol spectrum disorders. From Nigg (2006, p. 309). Copyright 2006 by The Guilford Press. Reprinted by permission.

discussed in Chapters 4, 5, and 6, interventions that involve the manipulation of environmental conditions can be quite effective in enhancing the functioning of children with this disorder. Third, at present, there is no known connection between the "cause" of an individual's ADHD and treatment planning. As such, determination of etiology is minimally related to enhancing successful outcomes. Perhaps as the use of advanced assessment technologies, particularly in the realm of molecular genetics, becomes more widespread, clinically useful information about the etiology of ADHD will be forthcoming.

THE IMPACT OF SITUATIONAL FACTORS ON ADHD SYMPTOM SEVERITY

Although neurobiological variables are hypothesized to be the primary causes for ADHD, the role of environmental factors in setting the occasion for or reducing the probability of ADHD-related behaviors remains important for professional service delivery. Both antecedent and consequent stimuli are critical in determining the severity of attention problems, impulsivity, and behavior control. In fact, the development of classroom interventions for children with ADHD is enhanced by (1) determining the behavioral function of ADHD-related behaviors and (2) implementing strategies that are linked directly to behavior function (DuPaul & Ervin, 1996; see also Chapters 2, 4, and 5). For example, if one determines that a child's inattentive disruptive behavior reliably results in access to teacher attention, then the classroom intervention should provide access to teacher attention contingent on nondisruptive behavior. The prevailing assumption is that although environmental factors affect the behavior of all children, the performance of children with attention and behavior control problems is much more sensitive to these events.

Important antecedent and/or setting events that affect the probability of ADHD-related behaviors occurring include the type of commands or instructions a child is given, the degree to which a child is supervised during independent work, the number of children present during instruction (Barkley, 2006), and the presentation of academic tasks that are perceived as difficult or aversive.

Teachers often state that children with attention and behavior control problems are able to complete work more accurately if they interact "one-to-one" with a "supervisor" (e.g., teacher, aide, peer). When asked to attend to seatwork or instruction in group settings, however, students with ADHD encounter frequent difficulties (Barkley, 2006). In a similar fashion, when independent work is closely supervised, children with

ADHD are able to produce a greater quantity and a higher quality of output relative to minimal supervision situations. Children with ADHD also are more likely to complete tasks that are stimulating and interesting to them, as well as those that are within their range of skills (i.e., work that is at the instructional level). Furthermore, there is preliminary evidence that children with this disorder behave more appropriately when given a choice among several tasks rather than told to complete one specific assignment (e.g., Dunlap et al., 1994).

Children with ADHD are more likely to attend to commands that are given in a straightforward, declarative manner (e.g., "Get back to work") than those delivered as a question or as a request for a favor ("Will you please get back to work?") (Anastopoulos, Smith, & Wein, 1998). Furthermore, instructions are more likely to be followed when they are delivered once potential distractors (e.g., toys, television) have been removed and the student has made eye contact with the instructor. Finally, compliance with instructions is enhanced by continuing to supervise the child during the initial minute or so after giving the command (Barkley, 1997b). Thus, the antecedent conditions that will promote better behavior control and academic performance include provision of effective commands along with supervision of the child's work on a one-to-one basis.

A variety of factors affect the degree to which consequences control the behavior of children with ADHD. These include the latency between behavior and its consequences, the frequency of reinforcement, how salient or "motivating" the consequences are to the child, and the manner in which verbal reprimands are delivered (Pfiffner et al., 2006). Children with ADHD perform akin to their classmates under conditions of relatively immediate and frequent reinforcement (Pfiffner et al., 2006). This is particularly the case when the type of reinforcement is highly salient and meaningful to the child. Unfortunately, reinforcement is delayed and infrequent in most general education classrooms. Furthermore, the typical reinforcers (e.g., grades and teacher praise) provided in schools are usually on the low end of the saliency continuum.

Verbal reprimands are commonly used by teachers to reduce students' disruptive behaviors (White, 1975). Usually, reprimands are delivered in a loud voice in front of the class, while the teacher exhibits nonverbal cues (e.g., frown, ruddy complexion) that indicate anger with the perpetrating student(s). Alternatively, an impressive body of research indicates that reprimands are more likely to reduce behavior when delivered privately to the child, relatively immediately following a transgression, and with a minimum of discussion and affect (e.g., Pfiffner & O'Leary, 1987). The latter factors are particularly important when attempting to reduce the disruptive behavior of an inattentive student.

ADHD as a Disorder of Impaired Delayed Responding

The crucial role that the interaction of within-child biological factors and environmental events play in determining the severity of ADHD symptoms has led to changes in the conceptualization of the deficits underlying this disorder. In particular, the central feature of ADHD may be impairment in delayed responding (i.e., behavioral inhibition) rather than a deficit in attention per se (Barkley, 1997a, 2006). Many important settings (e.g., classroom) and abilities (e.g., internalization of speech) require the capacity to delay responding to the environment. Thus, deficits in delayed responding lead to the exhibition of ADHD symptoms in multiple settings and deleteriously affect the development of rule-governed behavior.

Barkley (1997a) has articulated a theoretical model of ADHD as a disorder of behavioral inhibition wherein impaired delayed responding to the environment compromises the development of four critical executive functions. The latter includes working memory, self-regulation of affect–motivation–arousal, internalization of speech, and behavioral analysis/synthesis. Impairments in the development of these executive functions in turn lead to myriad problems in cognitive, academic, and social functioning. This theoretical model makes intuitive sense, is consistent with the literature on this disorder (for a review, see Barkley, 1997a), and has clear implications for practice.

Interventions for this disorder must include changes in within-child variables (e.g., temporary change in brain functioning through stimulant medication) and/or changes in antecedent and consequent stimuli to increase the probability of delayed responding, thereby leading to attentive, productive behavior (Barkley, 1997a). Unfortunately, most classrooms are structured in a manner that provides delayed and infrequent reinforcement under the assumption that students become "internally motivated" to conform with rules and complete academic tasks. These are precisely the conditions most likely to lead to inattentive disruptive behaviors (i.e., impaired response inhibition) in children with ADHD. Thus, the challenge to education professionals is to incorporate environmental stimuli known to enhance student success into all classrooms where impulsive inattentive students are being taught (see Chapters 4, 5, and 6).

LONG-TERM OUTCOME OF CHILDREN WITH ADHD

For many years it was assumed, particularly by members of the lay community, that children with ADHD would "outgrow" their behavior control difficulties upon reaching adolescence or early adulthood. Unfortunately, this assumption has not been borne out by longitudinal investigations of the disorder (see Barkley, Murphy, & Fischer, 2008). As children with ADHD progress into their teenage years, the *absolute* frequency and intensity of their symptoms decline (Barkley, 2006). That is, they improve with respect to attention, impulsivity, and especially overactivity as compared with their own behavior during preschool and elementary school years. Of course, their peers are exhibiting similar improvements in behavior control, thereby contributing to an ongoing discrepancy between adolescents with ADHD and their classmates. In fact, 70–85% of children with ADHD will continue to exhibit significant deficits in inattention and impulsivity *relative* to their age-mates during their adolescence (Barkley et al., 2008; Biederman et al., 1996).

In addition to continued ADHD symptomatology, teenagers with ADHD display adjustment problems in a variety of areas of functioning. First, over 60% of adolescents with this disorder have been found to exhibit frequent defiance and noncompliance with authority figures and rules (e.g., Barkley, Fischer, Edelbrock, & Smallish, 1990; Biederman et al., 1997). Furthermore, more than 40% of teens with ADHD display significant antisocial behaviors such as physical fighting, stealing, and vandalism (e.g., Barkley, Fischer, et al., 1990; Gittelman, Mannuzza, Shenker, & Bonagura, 1985). When compared with their non-ADHD classmates, adolescents with this disorder are at higher risk for grade retentions, school suspensions, dropping out of school, and substance abuse. Children with ADHD may engage in significantly higher levels of nicotine use in adolescence and experience higher rates of alcohol and drug use disorders as adults (Charach, Yeung, Climans, & Lillie, 2011). The risk for drug or alcohol use seems to be attributable to the presence of significant conduct problems in addition to ADHD-related behaviors (e.g., Biederman et al., 1997; Gittelman et al., 1985), although this relationship appears to be moderated by parental monitoring (e.g., high parental monitoring may mitigate risks associated with ADHD and conduct problems; Molina et al., 2012). Thus, for a large percentage of children with ADHD, it is unrealistic to assume that they will "outgrow" experiencing problems in daily living simply as a function of maturation.

Several prospective longitudinal investigations have followed children with ADHD into adulthood. In general, these have found that over 50% of children with ADHD will continue to evidence symptoms of the disorder, especially with respect to inattention and impulsivity, into adulthood, especially when parent report rather than self-report data are used (Barkley, Fischer, Smallish, & Fletcher, 2002). Problems of academic achievement and antisocial behavior that were noted for adolescents with this disorder continue to be the highest risks for this group in adulthood. Almost a third of these adults will have dropped out of high school, with only 5% completing a university degree program as compared with over 40% of control group subjects (Barkley et al., 2008). In particular, inattention symptom severity is a significant predictor of long-term educational achievement including risk for dropping out of high school (Pingault et al., 2011). Approximately 25% or more of these children will develop chronic patterns of antisocial behavior that persist into adulthood and that are associated with other adjustment problems (e.g., substance abuse, interpersonal difficulties, occupational instability). Older adolescents and young adults with ADHD are more likely than their non-ADHD counterparts to receive speeding tickets and to experience car accidents as the driver (Barkley, Guevremont, Anastopoulos, DuPaul, & Shelton, 1993; Barkley, Murphy, DuPaul, & Bush, 2002). In addition, children with ADHD followed into adulthood have a significantly higher risk for sexually transmitted disease, head injury, and emergency department admissions (Olazagasti et al., 2013). Negative outcomes related to risky behavior appear to be moderated by the presence of conduct disorder and those individuals with ADHD alone do not appear to be at higher risk relative to the general population (Olazagasti et al., 2013). Finally, girls with ADHD are at significant risk not only for continued ADHD symptomatology and related impairment, but may also be at higher risk for self-injury and suicide attempts as older adolescents and young adults (Hinshaw et al., 2012). On a positive note, approximately one-third of children followed into adulthood are seen as symptom-free and relatively well adjusted (Barkley, 2006). Yet this childhood disorder carries risks for long-term outcome that are quite high relative to the non-ADHD population.

Investigators have searched for childhood variables that can reliably predict the adolescent and adult outcomes of individuals with ADHD. Minimal specific predictors have been identified beyond those variables (e.g., intelligence test scores, SES) that are predictive of outcome for the general population. Nevertheless, there are two classes of predictors that are noteworthy for practitioners to consider in their work. First, an early onset of antisocial behaviors, especially lying, stealing, and fighting, is predictive of later antisocial outcome and perhaps continued ADHD (Barkley, 2006; Biederman et al., 1996). *Early onset* is defined as prior to the ages of 8–10 years old. Second, being rejected by one's peers in childhood is predictive of continued interpersonal adjustment problems in later years (Barkley, 2006; Parker & Asher, 1987). Therefore, at the present time, the combination of the child's cognitive ability, the child's level of aggressiveness and peer rejection, family stability, psychosocial adversity, and childrearing practices represents the best predictive scheme (Barkley, 2006; Biederman et al., 1996).

Given the protracted nature of the disorder and the attendant long-term risks for a large percentage of children with ADHD, there is clear consensus that multiple treatment modalities are necessary throughout a child's school-age years (Barkley, 2006). Thus, rather than attempting to "cure" the disorder, school professionals and parents should help children "compensate" for their behavior control problems. Furthermore, it is assumed that ADHD is a disorder that lies at the interface of a child's neurobiology (e.g., genetic differences leading to differences in brain structure and function) and the environment (i.e., situational factors), wherein a child is predisposed to engage in higher frequencies of disinhibited and highly active behavior relative to peers, especially under certain environmental circumstances. Therefore, treatment may entail modifications to school and home environments, as well as attempts to change within-child variables through the use of psychotropic medication. With these perspectives in mind, our emphasis throughout this book is to promote methods to create and maintain "prosthetic environments" (Barkley, 2006) that allow children with ADHD to succeed academically, emotionally, and socially. To achieve these outcomes a concerted effort must be made by school professionals, parents, and other health practitioners over the course of multiple school years.

OVERVIEW OF SUBSEQUENT CHAPTERS

The purpose of this book is to provide education and health care professionals with a guide to the assessment and treatment of students with ADHD in school settings. An attempt has been made to identify evaluation and intervention techniques that have a sound empirical basis and are practical for real-world application. In this third edition of our text, we have updated and expanded our coverage of assessment and intervention strategies that can be effectively used in school settings across the developmental spectrum.

A model for the school-based screening and assessment of ADHD is presented in Chapter 2. It is proposed that the evaluation of students who might exhibit ADHD-related behaviors involves the use of multiple assessment techniques across home and school settings. The purpose of assessment is not simply to arrive at a diagnosis, but, more important, to guide the development of an effective treatment plan. Assessment of ADHD in the context of a multi-tiered, data-based decision-making model is emphasized.

The relationship between ADHD and comorbid disorders is examined in detail in Chapter 3. Although ADHD is not a learning disability per se, a significant minority of children with attention and behavior control problems display academic skills deficits. Furthermore, ADHD may be associated with externalizing (e.g., oppositional defiant disorder) and internalizing (e.g., depression) disorders. Suggestions are offered for making differential diagnostic and special education eligibility decisions for students with ADHD.

ADHD is a disorder with an early onset, with symptoms typically exhibited during the preschool and early elementary school years. Thus, in Chapter 4, we outline methods for identifying young children who might be at risk for ADHD, as well as strategies to minimize the severity of associated disruptive behaviors (e.g., aggression and defiance) and promote early school success. Given that ADHD can be chronic and is associated with poor school outcomes, early identification and intervention may be critical in enhancing the long-term success of children with this disorder.

One of the most effective intervention approaches for ADHD is the manipulation of antecedent and consequent events in the classroom environment. In Chapter 5, behaviorally based methods that have been found to enhance behavior control, academic performance, and social behavior are described. We propose a data-based, problem-solving model for the development of academic and behavioral interventions that can be implemented with integrity, particularly in elementary school settings. The important connection between data derived from functional and curriculum-based assessments and intervention design is emphasized in the discussion of these techniques.

ADHD is a chronic disorder associated with impairment across secondary and postsecondary education settings. For this edition, we provide a new chapter focused on intervention and support strategies for students in middle school, high school, and college (Chapter 6). In particular, treatment is directed not only to reduce symptoms and enhance general areas of functioning but to promote self-regulation and organization skills. Specific challenges in working with students at the secondary and postsecondary level are addressed.

The most widely studied and cost-effective treatment for ADHD is the prescription of psychotropic medications, primarily stimulants such as Ritalin (MPH). These medications can lead to improvements in on-task behavior, impulsivity, social behavior, compliance, and academic productivity in as many as 70–80% of children with ADHD. Descriptions of the specific medications (including nonstimulants), behavioral effects, adverse side effects, and dose–response factors are provided in Chapter 7. Furthermore, methods for school-based practitioners to aid physicians in evaluating medication response are delineated.

Multiple interventions across settings frequently are necessary to ameliorate ADHD symptomatology. Thus, medication and school-based behavioral interventions may be supplemented by social skills training, parent education, and/or behavioral family therapy. These treatments are described in Chapter 8. Furthermore, suggestions are provided on how to advise parents regarding proposed treatments for ADHD that have minimal or lack empirical support.

A team approach to treatment of ADHD is crucial to successful outcome. Communication among professionals and parents is discussed in detail in Chapter 9. All too often miscommunication between school and home or school-based professionals and community-based professionals (e.g., physicians) results in inefficient service delivery. Methods to foster appropriate communication among treatment team members are delineated in this chapter as well. Professional guidelines (e.g., American Academy of Pediatrics, 2011) for assessment and treatment of ADHD are discussed.

Potential future directions for school-based programming and research on ADHD are discussed in Chapter 10. For example, greater attention to vocational counseling/programming is clearly needed for children with this disorder. In addition, specific strategies to promote success for college students with ADHD are necessary. The suggestions offered in this book are merely a starting point with an obvious need to develop school-based strategies that lead to more successful outcomes for students exhibiting ADHD-related difficulties from early childhood to young adulthood.

CHAPTER 2

Assessment of ADHD in School Settings

Multiple assessment techniques typically are employed across home and school settings in the comprehensive evaluation of children who may have ADHD (American Academy of Pediatrics, 2011; Barkley, 2006). Although the diagnostic criteria for this disorder have been developed and published primarily by physicians (i.e., American Psychiatric Association, 2013), school professionals must be knowledgeable regarding appropriate evaluation procedures for several reasons. First, general education teachers rate symptoms of ADHD (e.g., distracted from tasks, short attention span, careless errors, excessive movement, and rushes through assignments) among the most common problem behaviors of children and adolescents (Harrison, Vannest, Davis, & Reynolds, 2012). Thus, school psychologists must be in a position to conduct an assessment of ADHD themselves, or, at least, to be cognizant of community-based professionals who could provide an appropriate evaluation. Second, school psychologists have direct access to sources of information and data (e.g., teachers, observations of child behavior in natural settings) crucial to the differential diagnosis of ADHD. Third, ADHD is prevalent among certain populations (e.g., children with learning disabilities) frequently served by school psychologists (Barkley, 2006). Finally, children with ADHD may be eligible for special education services under the "other health impairment" category of the Individuals with Disabilities Education Improvement Act (IDEIA; Public Law 108-446). Thus, school psychologists will be called upon to help determine whether referred children are eligible for such services under this category.

The purpose of the present chapter is to describe a school-based assessment approach in the evaluation of ADHD that incorporates those techniques having the greatest empirical support in the literature. Proper use of this evaluation methodology assumes that the professional conducting the assessment will have received appropriate training in the use of the DSM-5 (American Psychiatric Association, 2013) classification system as well as in clinical assessment techniques. First, DSM-5 criteria for ADHD are reviewed in the context of a school-based assessment paradigm and their limitations for this purpose are delineated (American Psychiatric Association, 2013). Second, a behavioral assessment approach to the evaluation of ADHD is described, one that incorporates multiple sources of data collected across school and home settings. Finally, the specific steps of the assessment process are detailed in the context of an educational decision-making paradigm based on the model proposed by Salvia and Ysseldyke (1998), as well as in the context of a response-to-intervention (RTI) service delivery framework. The stages of the ADHD evaluation described include screening, multimethod assessment, interpretation of obtained results to reach a diagnostic decision, development of a treatment plan based on assessment data, and ongoing evaluation of the success of the intervention program.

THE USE OF DIAGNOSTIC CRITERIA IN THE SCHOOL-BASED ASSESSMENT OF ADHD

Current Definition of ADHD

ADHD has been defined and conceptualized in a variety of ways over the past century, thus leading to confusion among professionals regarding proper diagnosis and evaluation procedures (Barkley, 2006). In recent decades, there is a consistent consensus that ADHD is characterized by the display of developmentally inappropriate frequencies of inattention and/or hyperactivity–impulsivity (American Psychiatric Association, 2013). These two dimensions of behaviors lead to impairment in functioning wherein the child with ADHD demonstrates difficulties with delaying responding to the environment, developing self-control, and maintaining consistent work performance over the course of time (American Psychiatric Association, 2013; Barkley, 2006).

The behaviors, or "symptoms," comprising ADHD according to DSM-5 criteria (American Psychiatric Association, 2013) include difficulties with inattention (e.g., often has difficulty sustaining attention in tasks or play activities) and hyperactivity–impulsivity (e.g., often has difficulty waiting his or her turn). To be considered symptoms of ADHD, some of the behaviors must have been initially exhibited in childhood (i.e., prior to age 12) and must be chronically displayed across two or more settings (American Psychiatric Association, 2013). A child must be reported to exhibit at least six of the nine inattention symptoms and/or at least six of the nine hyperactive–impulsive behaviors. The ADHD diagnosis is usually determined by establishing the developmental deviance and pervasiveness of symptoms. At the same time, it is equally important to rule out alternative causes for the child's inattention, impulsivity, and motor restlessness. These may include poor academic instruction and management practices; gross neurological, sensory, motor, or language impairment; mental retardation; or severe emotional disturbance (Barkley, 2006).

As described in Chapter 1, there are three presentations of ADHD. The combined presentation describes children who exhibit at least six inattention and at least six hyperactive–impulsive symptoms for a minimum of 6 months. This is the "classic" variant of ADHD that has been studied widely in the literature and is the most problematic presentation. ADHD, predominantly inattentive presentation (previous terms have included *undifferentiated attention deficit disorder* and *attention deficit disorder without hyperactivity*), is diagnosed in those children exhibiting at least six of the nine inattention symptoms and fewer than six hyperactive–impulsive behaviors. Finally, ADHD, predominantly hyperactive–impulsive presentation, is diagnosed for those children who display at least six of the nine hyperactive–impulsive symptoms but fewer than six inattention symptoms.

Advantages of the DSM Approach

Although the diagnostic criteria for ADHD have been developed in the context of a medical model for child behavior problems, there are several reasons why these criteria are useful in educational settings. First, the symptom list describes a set of problem behaviors that reliably covary in some children. The diagnosis (i.e., constellation of covarying behaviors) can be used to predict the relative success of possible interventions, to predict the risk for concurrent or future behavioral difficulties, and to suggest possible controlling variables (Barlow, 1981). Second, the use of DSM criteria structures the assessment in a standardized fashion, thus potentially increasing interprofessional agreement regarding diagnostic status. Third, such criteria guide the selection of competing hypotheses (i.e., other disorders or problems) that could potentially account for apparent symptoms of ADHD. Conclusions based on differential diagnosis may increase the chances of planning a successful intervention program in the classroom. For instance, if a child's attention problems were related to an anxiety disorder as opposed to ADHD, initial treatment strategies would be quite different.

Fourth, another advantage of the use of DSM criteria in the assessment protocol is that discussions of these symptom lists may indicate which problem behaviors should serve as targets for intervention. For example, those symptoms that are most frequently endorsed or are deemed most important by parents and teachers might become the initial focus of treatment. Last, incorporating agreed-upon diagnostic criteria into the evaluation (i.e., using a common language) will ultimately enhance communication with other mental health (e.g., clinical child psychologists) or medical professionals regarding the child's psychological status, thus fostering a team approach to treatment.

Limitations of the DSM Approach

Although DSM criteria are important components of the evaluation process, several limitations of this approach must be considered. First, the criteria for ADHD were developed in the context of a medical model, thus implying that the location of the "problem" is within the child. The characterization of the child as having a disorder could diminish attempts to assess environmental variables that may play a role in causing or maintaining the problem behaviors. Second, the use of a psychiatric classification system promotes a search for pathology that could, under certain conditions, result in overidentification of children with behavior disorders (i.e., identification of "false positives"). These circumstances suggest the need for a multimethod assessment approach wherein objective measures (e.g., behavioral observations) supplement the use of more subjective assessment techniques, such as a diagnostic interview (Achenbach & McConaughy, 1996). Third, the use of a psychiatric classification system and the resulting receipt of a diagnostic label may compromise a child's self-esteem if others come to view him or her as "disordered." Although frequently a topic of professional discussion, the possible iatrogenic effects of being diagnosed with ADHD have not been empirically investigated to date. A fourth important limitation of the DSM approach is that the psychometric properties (e.g., reliability, validity) of the various diagnostic criteria are not well established (Gresham & Gansle, 1992). Finally, there is some debate as to whether children's emotion and behavior problems should be conceptualized as diagnostic categories (i.e., one either has or does not have a disorder) or as dimensions (i.e., behavior of all individuals lie on a continuum); most empirical evidence strongly suggests that ADHD is a dimensional construct (Coghill & Sonuga-Barke, 2012).

Several skills are necessary to ensure the proper use of the DSM classification paradigm (adapted from Barlow, 1981). First, the school psychologist should have enough familiarity with child psychopathology to know which problem behaviors typically covary (e.g., inattention, impulsivity, and overactivity). Second, a working knowledge of current

DSM criteria for most childhood disorders, not just ADHD, is necessary. This requires not only familiarity with symptom lists, but also criteria with respect to age of onset and minimum duration of problem behaviors. Finally, the psychologist must have had training in the use of a comprehensive assessment protocol to determine which symptoms are present in a specific student's repertoire.

ADHD is best viewed as a result of a "poor fit" between the biological endowment and characteristics of the child and the environment, such as the structure and prevailing contingencies in the classroom. In this context, diagnostic criteria provide suggestions about problem behavior covariation, controlling variables, and effective interventions based on what is known about ADHD in general (Barlow, 1981). Therefore, discussions of DSM criteria are supplemented with multiple assessment methods conducted across settings to determine the specific problem behaviors, controlling variables, and possible intervention strategies that are applicable for an individual student. The diagnosis of ADHD is but one step in the process of designing and evaluating interventions to promote greater classroom success.

OVERVIEW OF ASSESSMENT METHODS

Typically, a behavioral assessment approach is employed in the evaluation of ADHD wherein multiple methods of data collection are utilized across informants and settings (see Anastopoulos & Shelton, 2001; Barkley, 2006; Pelham, Fabiano, & Massetti, 2005). In particular, emphasis is placed upon obtaining reliable information regarding a child's behavior from parents and teachers as well as from firsthand observations of student performance. Therefore, the major components of the evaluation include interviews with the child's parent(s) and teacher(s), questionnaires completed by parents and teachers, and observations of child behavior across multiple settings and under varied task conditions. Although many of these same procedures are used when evaluating adolescents, some modifications (e.g., inclusion of self-report measures) are necessary to maintain the reliability and validity of the assessment data (see "Developmental Considerations" section below).

Each evaluation technique is discussed in detail in the context of the stages of the assessment process in the next section. Interviews with the parent(s), teacher(s), and child are conducted to determine the presence or absence of various DSM symptoms, as well as to identify historical and/or current factors possibly serving to maintain identified problem behaviors. Behavior rating scales completed by the student's parent(s) and teacher(s) provide data that establish the severity of ADHD-related behaviors relative to a normative sample. To supplement parent and teacher report, several direct measures of student behavior are used. The child's behavior is observed across settings (e.g., classroom and playground) on several occasions to establish the frequency and/or duration of various target behaviors. Behavioral frequencies are usually compared to those displayed by several of the student's classmates to determine the deviance of the referred child's behavior. Finally, the products of the child's behavior (e.g., academic productivity and accuracy, quality of desk organization) can be collected and/or examined. Although each of these techniques is limited in some manner, when used in a multimodal assessment package a system of "checks and balances" develops such that the drawbacks of any single measure are balanced by data obtained through other means (Anastopoulos & Shelton, 2001; Barkley, 2006).

Several assessment techniques typically employed by school psychologists have limited utility in the diagnostic evaluation of ADHD. Typically, the results of cognitive, neuropsychological, and educational tests are not helpful in determining whether a child has ADHD or not. To date, no individually administered test or group of tests has demonstrated an acceptable degree of ecological validity to be helpful in the diagnostic process (Barkley, 1991, 2006). For example, although students with ADHD obtain Full Scale IQ scores that are, on average, 0.61 standard deviation units below typically developing peers (Frazier, Demaree, & Youngstrom, 2004), the test most frequently employed by school psychologists (i.e., Wechsler Intelligence Scale for Children–IV [WISC-IV; Wechsler, 2003]) has not been found to reliably discriminate children with ADHD from those with other disorders including learning disabilities (e.g., Barkley, DuPaul, & McMurray, 1990). More important, scores on the Working Memory Index (previously called "Freedom from Distractiblity") are not reliable diagnostic indicators of ADHD (Anastopoulos, Spisto, & Maher, 1994). Poor performance on this index may be due to a variety of possible causes, including memory difficulties or performance anxiety. Furthermore, children with ADHD often display appropriate levels of attention and behavioral control under task conditions that are highly structured and involve one-to-one interaction with a novel adult, as is typically found in most testing situations (Barkley, 2006). Thus, although individually administered tests may be helpful in determining the child's intellectual and educational status, they are not necessary components of the diagnostic evaluation of ADHD.

Standardized measures of sustained attention and impulse control have been incorporated routinely into the diagnostic evaluation of ADHD (Anastopoulos & Shelton, 2001; Barkley, 2006). Purportedly, these tests provide objective data that are less influenced by factors (e.g., parental psychopathology) that may bias parent and teacher reports

(Gordon, 1986). One of the more popular standardized measures is the Continuous Performance Test (CPT; Rosvold, Mirsky, Sarason, Bransome, & Beck, 1956) and its variants, including the Gordon Vigilance Task (Gordon, 1983) and the Conners Continuous Performance Test (Conners, 2000).

Although scores on CPTs appear to discriminate between children with ADHD and their typically developing counterparts at a *group* level, the utility of these measures in assessing *individual* children is limited by several factors. First, several investigations have failed to obtain significant correlations between criterion measures (e.g., teacher ratings) and scores on various CPTs (e.g., Epstein et al., 2003). Second, when the effects of age, sex, and receptive vocabulary skills are partialed-out, scores on these measures have failed to discriminate among children with ADHD, children with conduct disorder, children with anxiety disorder, and their typically developing peers (Werry, Elkind, & Reeves, 1987) or those with reading disorders (McGee, Clark, & Symons, 2000). Even when significant correlations are obtained between CPT scores and criterion measures, these typically are of low magnitude (i.e., between absolute values of 0.21 and 0.50), suggesting that the results of clinic-based tasks account for minimal variance of criterion indices (Barkley, 1991, 2006). Furthermore, CPT scores, either alone or in combination, have been found to result in classification decisions that are frequently discrepant with a diagnosis of ADHD based on parent interview and behavior rating scale data (DuPaul, Anastopoulos, Shelton, Guevremont, & Metevia, 1992). Finally, even when clinically significant scores are obtained on CPTs, the degree to which these scores are specific to ADHD and aid in differential diagnosis is questionable (e.g., McGee et al., 2000). Therefore, the most prudent conclusion, at present, is that the use of laboratory-based instruments in the evaluation of ADHD is limited by rather suspect ecological validity (Anastopoulos & Shelton, 2001; Pelham et al., 2005; Rapport, Chung, Shore, Denney, & Isaacs, 2000).

Measures that typically are used by school psychologists to assess a student's emotional functioning are not useful in evaluating whether a child has ADHD. Projective techniques, such as the Thematic Apperception Test (Murray, 1943), are based on a theoretical assumption that problem behaviors are caused by underlying emotional difficulties. This assumption has no empirical support, at least in relation to the behaviors comprising ADHD. Furthermore, projective tests have been criticized for their questionable levels of reliability and validity (Gregory, 1996).

Self-report questionnaires completed by children and adolescents have become increasingly popular in recent years (e.g., Conners, 2008). A number of psychometrically sound self-report checklists are available, including the Youth Self-Report (YSR; Achenbach & Rescorla, 2001), the Youth Inventory–4 (Gadow et al., 2002), and the Self-Report of Personality for the Behavior Assessment System for Children–2 (BASC-2; Reynolds & Kamphaus, 2004). Given long-standing concerns that children with disruptive behavior disorders are typically poor reporters of their own behavior (Landau, Milich, & Widiger, 1991) and may overestimate their academic and social competence (i.e., positive illusory bias; e.g., Ohan & Johnston, 2011), self-report ratings, particularly of disruptive behavior, academic functioning, and social skills, should be interpreted with caution. Alternatively, growing evidence suggests adolescents with behavior disorders may be able to provide information that may aid in both diagnostic (Conners, 2008) and treatment (Smith, Pelham, Gnagy, Molina, & Evans, 2000) decisions. Also, self-report data are important to collect when evaluating adolescents who may be diagnosed with ADHD to allow assessment of covert areas of functioning (e.g., depressive symptoms) and to engender student cooperation with the evaluation and treatment process (see "Developmental Considerations" section below).

STAGES OF ASSESSMENT OF ADHD

Services for students with learning and/or behavioral difficulties currently are delivered in the context of a three-tiered RTI model (Burns, Deno, & Jimerson, 2007). Universal services and instruction for all students are provided at Tier 1, while Tier 2 services and instruction are provided in small groups or on an individual basis for students at risk of learning and/or behavioral difficulties. Finally, at Tier 3 individualized, intensive supports and instruction are provided for those students who do not respond sufficiently to Tier 2 intervention. Our model for the assessment of students suspected of ADHD should be implemented for those at-risk students who do not exhibit a sufficiently positive response at Tier 2 (i.e., students who are being considered for Tier 3 intervention). In this way, the assessment of ADHD is not only focused on making an accurate diagnosis but also on identifying interventions that may be helpful at Tier 3.

Following teacher report of attention and behavior control difficulties despite the implementation of Tier 2 interventions and supports, the school-based evaluation of ADHD is conducted in five stages (DuPaul, 1992; see Figure 2.1). These stages are based on the educational decision-making model originally proposed by Salvia and Ysseldyke (1998). First, teacher ratings are obtained and a brief interview is conducted with the teacher to screen for the severity and frequency of possible ADHD

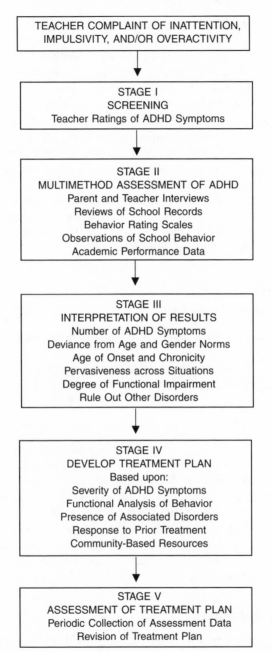

FIGURE 2.1. Five stages of the school-based assessment of ADHD.

symptoms. Second, if the findings of this screening are significant, then multiple assessment methods are used across sources and settings to document the child's functioning among a number of areas. Third, the evaluation results are interpreted such that classification and diagnostic decisions can be made. Fourth, a treatment plan is developed based on the obtained assessment data. Last, the child's school behavior and academic performance are assessed on an ongoing basis to determine the success of and the need for changes in the intervention program.

These stages of assessment are discussed in detail below. Initially, for each phase of the assessment, a series of questions to be addressed are identified, based in part on guidelines for behavioral assessment provided by Barrios and Hartmann (1986). Next, the process of assessment during each stage of the evaluation is delineated. Finally, the manner in which specific techniques are used to answer the assessment questions at each phase of the evaluation is reviewed.

Stage I: Screening

Questions to Be Addressed

The screening process is designed to answer the following questions:

1. Does this student have a problem related to possible ADHD?
2. Is further assessment of ADHD required?

Screening Process

Screening for possible ADHD should be conducted whenever a teacher reports a lack of response to Tier 2 intervention due to a student's difficulties paying attention during instruction, inconsistent completion of independent tasks, inability to remain seated at appropriate times, or display of impulsive disruptive behavior. A brief interview with the teacher is conducted to specify the behavioral concerns and to identify environmental factors that may be eliciting and/or maintaining the child's problem behaviors. Teacher ratings of the frequency of ADHD symptoms are then obtained.

Screening Techniques

The initial interview with the teacher should address the frequency, intensity, and/or duration of specific problem behaviors. The role of various environmental factors (e.g., task parameters, method of instruction, behaviors of classmates) also should be explored to establish antecedent and consequent events for the problem behaviors. To establish whether the problem behaviors may be related to ADHD, both the presence or absence of the 18 DSM-5 (American Psychiatric Association, 2013) symptoms of this disorder should be determined, as should the chronicity of the apparent ADHD-related behaviors. If six or more inattention symptoms and/or six or more hyperactive–impulsive symptoms are reported to occur frequently, then further assessment of ADHD is warranted. Even if fewer than six symptoms in each dimension are reported, further assessment of ADHD may be warranted, especially for students at the secondary level.

The most efficient screening method is for the teacher to complete a DSM-based rating scale (e.g., ADHD Rating Scale–IV; DuPaul, Power, Anastopoulos, & Reid, 1998) regarding the child's typical behavior over the course of the school year. The teacher indicates on a 4-point Likert scale the frequency of the 18 behavioral symptoms of ADHD directly adapted from DSM-5 (American Psychiatric Association, 2013). As with the teacher interview, if six or more of the items in either the inattention or hyperactivity–impulsivity domains are rated as occurring "often" or "very often," then further assessment of possible ADHD is warranted. If a lesser number of items are endorsed in this frequency range, this does not rule out further assessment of ADHD but does necessitate strong consideration of other explanations (e.g., learning disabilities) for teacher concerns.

Stage II: Multimethod Assessment of ADHD

Questions to Be Addressed

Data from multiple assessment techniques are gathered to answer the following questions:

1. What is the extent and nature of the ADHD-related problems?
2. What are the frequency, duration, and/or intensity of the problem behaviors?
3. What environmental factors maintain these problems?
4. In what settings do the ADHD-related behaviors occur and for how long have these been exhibited?

Assessment Process

If the initial screening results are indicative of possible ADHD, then a more comprehensive evaluation of the child's overall functioning is warranted. Initially, the child's parent(s) and teacher(s) are interviewed to specify problem behaviors, identify possible antecedent and consequent events for these behaviors, and explore the causal role of various historical variables. A review of archival data (e.g., school records) is completed to provide additional historical data. Thus, the initial phase of the evaluation process is designed to identify specific problem behaviors, environmental factors, and historical variables that require further assessment.

The student's parent(s) and teacher(s) complete several questionnaires to provide more specific data regarding the frequency and/or severity of problem behaviors. These ratings help to establish the developmental deviance of ADHD-related behaviors relative to normative data, as well as to identify whether such behaviors are evident across settings and caretakers. Furthermore, parent and teacher ratings provide unique data, above and beyond information from diagnostic interviews, regarding child behavior across settings (Vaughn & Hoza, 2013). The specific questionnaires utilized will vary as a function of the target behaviors to be assessed and the age of the child, as discussed later in this chapter.

The final phase of the formal evaluation of ADHD is composed of direct observations of child behavior across settings and the collection of academic and social performance data. These techniques can provide crucial information regarding the frequency and duration of target behaviors, whether specific antecedent and consequent events serve to elicit or maintain the problem behaviors, and the degree to which the ADHD-related behaviors compromise the child's social and academic functioning. From an intervention design perspective, the most critical activity is to gather data in the context of a functional behavioral assessment (DuPaul & Ervin, 1996).

Assessment Techniques

Teacher Interview. The teacher should be asked to describe the student's difficulties in specific behavioral terms in the context of a problem identification interview as described by Bergan and Kratochwill (1990). Furthermore, current DSM diagnostic criteria for a variety of child behavior disorders should be reviewed with the teacher. In addition to ADHD, the presence or absence of behaviors associated with oppositional defiant disorder, conduct disorder, generalized anxiety disorder, separation anxiety disorder, and depression should be ascertained. It is important to review this set of problems for two reasons. First, apparent symptoms of ADHD may actually be manifestations of another disorder. For instance, a child who has a mood disorder may exhibit problems with concentration. Thus, the diagnosis of ADHD is arrived at by ruling out competing hypotheses (i.e., disorders) for the problem behaviors. A second reason to review these diagnostic criteria is that many children with ADHD also exhibit symptoms of other disorders. The most frequent associated diagnosis is oppositional defiant disorder; approximately 40–65% of children with ADHD exhibit symptoms of this disorder (Barkley, 2006). Furthermore, the combination of ADHD and other behavior or emotional disorders implicates the need for multiple interventions, as discussed later.

While ascertaining the presence or absence of each of the behavioral symptoms, the teacher also is asked to provide specific examples of those behaviors indicated to be present as well as to estimate their frequency. The typical antecedent (e.g., type of instruction) and consequent (e.g., teacher response to child misbehavior) events surrounding each problematic behavior should also be identified because these may be serving to maintain and/or exacerbate behavioral difficulties. Current management techniques and their relative degree of success then should be discussed.

It is imperative that information regarding the quality of the child's academic performance and peer relationships be gathered. Some children with ADHD may exhibit significant academic skills deficits beyond task completion difficulties. Of course, an academic skills assessment (e.g., curriculum-based measurement) would be warranted in such situations. Teacher observations regarding the child's social interaction style and acceptance by peers are helpful in determining whether intervention in this area is necessary. Many children with ADHD will exhibit a controlling, aggressive interaction pattern with others, resulting in low acceptance or overt rejection by their classmates (Stormont, 2001). Teacher interview data are used to identify possible social skills deficits that could be targeted for further assessment and intervention, as well as to delineate those settings and/or times of the school day where social relationship difficulties are most likely to be exhibited.

Review of School Record. The student's school record should be reviewed to obtain data that may be helpful in pinpointing the onset and course of classroom ADHD-related difficulties. For instance, teachers often grade the quality of a child's work habits and conduct on report cards. Not surprisingly, most students with ADHD are found to obtain below-average rankings in these areas across grade levels. These below-average grades are often supplemented with teacher comments regarding poor task completion, high degrees of restlessness, or frequent talking to peers without permission. The specific grade level where such grades and comments first appear is important to note so that it can be cross-referenced with the age of onset of ADHD as reported by the parents.

A more structured approach to reviewing school records is provided by the School Archival Records Search (SARS; Walker, Block-Pedego, Todis, & Severson, 1998). The SARS provides a standardized format for gathering information regarding 11 variables that are predictive of behavior disorders and/or school dropout. Variables include number of different schools attended, days absent, low achievement, grades retained, academic/behavioral referrals, current individualized education plan, nonregular classroom placement, receiving supplemental instruction, referral for outside services, negative narrative comments, and school discipline contacts. These individual variables load on to three factors: Disruption, Needs Assistance, and Low Achievement. Walker and colleagues (1998) have established cut points for each individual variable and factor score that are predictive of school difficulties. As might be expected, children with behavior disorders (presumably including ADHD) are more likely to receive positive scores (i.e., below established cut points) for Disruption and Low Achievement. The primary advantage of the SARS is that it pinpoints key predictor variables in a standardized structured fashion, thereby providing a reliable account of a student's past academic and behavioral history.

Parent Interview. A brief (i.e., 30–45 minutes) interview with the student's parent(s) should be conducted either in person or by telephone. Although discussion of the child's past and current functioning across a variety of areas (e.g., medical history) is possible, the most important lines of questioning are as follows. First, the presence and frequency of behavior control difficulties at home should be identified. This is best accomplished by reviewing current DSM diagnostic criteria for ADHD and related disruptive behavior disorders (oppositional defiant disorder, conduct disorder) with the parent. In addition, the presence of symptoms associated with internalizing disorders (e.g., anxiety disorders) that could be causally related to a child's inattention and hyperactivity–impulsivity should be identified. As with the teacher interview, a review of DSM criteria will aid in ruling out the presence of other disorders that may be causally related to the exhibition of ADHD symptoms.

A second area of discussion for the parent interview is information regarding the child's early childhood development. It is important to pinpoint the onset of the ADHD-related behaviors as well as to gather information about their chronicity over time. The early childhood behavior of children with ADHD typically is characterized as highly active and difficult to control (e.g., DuPaul, McGoey, Eckert, & VanBrakle, 2001). In some cases, however, the child's behavior is not seen as problematic until school entry, when independent task demands increase. This is particularly the case when the parents have little previous experience with children (e.g., the child being assessed is an only or oldest child) and/or have unrealistic expectations regarding child behavior.

A third area of investigation is the child's family history of behavioral, emotional, and learning problems. Although this may be uncomfortable for a parent and professionals to discuss, it is important for two reasons. First, research indicates that ADHD may have a genetic or familial component (Nigg, 2006), and thus tends to run in families. The presence of ADHD in the family increases the odds that the identified child has ADHD as well. Second, in about a third of cases, the child's mother may be depressed or have a history of depression (Barkley, 2006). There also is a greater incidence of paternal antisocial behavior in the families of children with ADHD (Barkley, 2006). The presence of such difficulties in the family has direct implications for treatment: home-based interventions for ADHD are more likely to be successful when implemented following amelioration of parental psychopathology and problems related to family functioning. For example, depressed mothers of children with behavior disorders evidence a higher failure rate in response to training in behavior modification strategies relative to mothers who are not depressed (Patterson & Chamberlain, 1994).

Parent Ratings. One or both parents should complete several questionnaires to determine the developmental deviance of the child's ADHD-related behaviors, as well as to establish the pervasiveness of problem behaviors across settings. Several general, or "broadband," behavior rating scales with adequate normative data and sound psychometric properties (for a review, see Barkley, 2006; Pelham et al., 2005) can serve this purpose well. Chief among these questionnaires are the Child Behavior Checklist (CBCL; Achenbach & Rescorla, 2001), the BASC-2, and the Conners 3rd Edition (Conners–3; Conners, 2008).

Each of these behavior rating scales have specific advantages that should be considered when selecting measures. Specifically, the CBCL and the BASC-2 contain large item pools, and hence provide wide coverage of both internalizing and externalizing disturbances. This broad coverage facilitates differential diagnosis because competing hypotheses (e.g., presence of other disorders) for the exhibition of ADHD symptoms can be explored. Because the item pool and factor structure of the parent and teacher versions of these scales are quite similar, cross-informant agreement can be specifically examined. This information may be invaluable given that parent and teacher agreement (i.e., about the child's cross-situational exhibition of symptoms) is important in making an ADHD diagnosis. Alternatively, the Conners–3 provides extensive coverage of externalizing symptoms while still being relatively brief. The latter scale is particularly advantageous in situations where parents may be reluctant to spend extensive time completing question-naires.

In addition to one of the broadband rating scales, the parent(s) should complete two "narrowband" questionnaires containing items more specific to ADHD-related behaviors: a DSM-based rating scale (e.g., the ADHD Rating Scale–IV) and the Home Situations Question-naire (HSQ; Barkley, 1990). The ADHD Rating Scale–IV provides information regarding the frequency of occurrence of each of the 18 symptoms of this disorder in the home setting. The number of items rated as occurring "often" or "very often" is tallied. Scores on the Inat-tention and Hyperactive–Impulsive factors can be compared to norma-tive data to determine the developmental deviance of ADHD symptom-atology (DuPaul, Power, et al., 1998). Parental responses on the HSQ allow determination of the number of home settings in which behavior problems are exhibited by the child. In addition, the severity of behavior problems within each situation is rated on a 1 (mild) to 9 (severe) Lik-ert scale. The revised version of the HSQ (HSQ-R; DuPaul & Barkley, 1992) provides more specific information regarding the pervasiveness of attention problems across home situations. Thus, the HSQ will be helpful in determining the situational specificity and severity of conduct problems, whereas the HSQ-R provides data regarding these same vari-ables for attentional difficulties, which may be particularly helpful if the child is suspected of having the predominantly inattentive or inattentive (restrictive) presentation. For example, a child who is reported to display attentional difficulties in one or two situations may be less likely to have ADHD, predominantly inattentive presentation, than a child whose attentional difficulties are evident across many situations.

Many children with ADHD symptoms will exhibit significant dif-ficulties with homework completion and study skills. When parents or teachers report homework problems, additional assessment is necessary to determine which homework-related behaviors need to be addressed. Initially, the parent could be asked to complete either the Homework Problem Checklist (Anesko, Schoiock, Ramirez, & Levine, 1987) or the Homework Performance Questionnaire (Power, Karustis, & Hab-boushe, 2001). These measures provide data regarding the frequency or severity of various problems (e.g., the child denies having a homework assignment, fails to complete homework) related to homework. Parent responses on these questionnaires can lead to further inquiry as to the specific problems that may be present at each step of the homework completion process.

The Impairment Rating Scale (IRS; Fabiano et al., 1999) can be used to determine the degree to which parents perceive a child's ADHD symptoms to cause impairment in functioning. The IRS contains seven items related to various areas of functioning (e.g., the child's relationships with siblings) that could be affected by ADHD symptoms.

Teacher Ratings. As is the case with parent questionnaires, there is a plethora of well-standardized, broadband teacher rating scales available. The three most prominent of these questionnaires are the TRF (Achenbach & Rescorla, 2001), the BASC-2, and the Conners–3. As mentioned previously, these broadband measures have many advantages, including a wide coverage of possible problem areas and extensive standardization samples facilitating normative comparisons by gender and age.

In conjunction with one of these broadband rating scales, inclusion of two or more additional measures should be considered. First, if the teacher has not already done so during the screening process, a narrow-band measure of ADHD symptoms, like the ADHD Rating Scale–IV should be used to determine the specific frequency of ADHD-related behaviors from the teacher's perspective. Second, the School Situations Questionnaire (SSQ; Barkley, 1990) and/or the School Situations Questionnaire–Revised (SSQ-R; DuPaul & Barkley, 1992) should be completed. The SSQ and the SSQ-R provide information regarding the pervasiveness across situations and severity level of conduct and attention problems, respectively.

In many cases, students referred for a diagnostic evaluation also are reported to evidence peer relationship and academic performance difficulties. Thus, teacher perceptions of student functioning in these areas should be assessed as well. There are several psychometrically sound social skills questionnaires that are available, with the most prominent and widely researched instrument being the Social Skills Improvement System (SSIS; Gresham & Elliott, 2008). Where indicated, teacher ratings of social competence should be supplemented by peer nominations and/or ratings as the latter provide information beyond teacher ratings that are important in assessing children's social competence (Kwon, Kim, & Sheridan, 2012). Teacher ratings of academic achievement difficulties can be obtained through use of the Academic Performance Rating Scale (DuPaul, Rapport, & Perriello, 1991) or the Academic Competency Evaluation Scale (DiPerna & Elliott, 2000). Ratings on one of the latter questionnaires may indicate the need for further assessment of academic skills deficits. Finally, a teacher version of the IRS is available to determine teacher perceptions of the degree to which ADHD symptoms impair functioning. The IRS contains six items related to potential areas of impairment of school functioning.

Assessment of Executive Functioning. Typically, ADHD is associated with compromised executive functioning particularly in the areas of planning, organization, and impulse control. In a comprehensive meta-analysis, Frazier and colleagues (2004) found small (0.15) to large (1.00) effect size differences between children with ADHD and non-ADHD controls for many common neuropsychological tests that assess executive function (e.g., Stop Signal Task—Verbruggen, Logan, & Steven, 2008; Wisconsin Card Sorting Test—Heaton, Chelune, Talley, Kay, & Curtiss, 1993). Thus, at a group level, measures of executive function can discriminate individuals with ADHD from typically developing peers. Furthermore, executive functioning assessed in childhood may predict, in part, longer-term academic and behavioral outcomes (Miller, Nevado-Montenegro, & Hinshaw, 2012). Alternatively, as discussed previously in this chapter, these measures may not provide sufficient predictive power to ascertain diagnostic status at an individual level due to false negative findings (Lambek et al., 2011). Furthermore, the degree to which executive function measures discriminate those with ADHD from children with other psychopathological disorders remains to be demonstrated. Yet, if time and resources are available, direct testing (e.g., continuous performance test) and indirect (e.g., teacher ratings on the Behavioral Rating Inventory of Executive Function [Gioia, Isquith, Guy, & Kenworthy, 2000]) observations can be included in a comprehensive assessment protocol.

Direct Observations of Behavior. Interview and rating scale data are subject to several limitations, including the inherent biases of those answering the interview questions and completing the questionnaires (Barkley, 2006). Thus, these data should be supplemented with assessment of child behavior that is potentially less subject to such biases. Direct observation of student behavior on several occasions and across settings and situations is one of the best methods to achieve this goal. In many cases, direct observations will provide the most fruitful data when conducted during independent seatwork situations. Typically, observation sessions are 10–30 minutes in length and are repeated across several days to establish a consistent estimate of behavioral frequency. Furthermore, observations are conducted on a repeated basis in several situations (e.g., math work time, language arts instruction) in the classroom, as well as in other school settings such as the playground and cafeteria. The latter provides the opportunity to observe interactions between the referred child and his or her peers.

Several behavior observation coding systems have been developed for use in determining the frequencies of various ADHD-related behaviors during classroom task periods (for a review, see Barkley, 2006; Platzman et al., 1992). These include the ADHD Behavior Coding System (Barkley, 1998; Barkley, Fischer, Newby, & Breen, 1988), the Hyperactive Behavior Code (Jacob, O'Leary, & Rosenblad, 1978), the Classroom Observation Code (Abikoff, Gittelman-Klein, & Klein, 1977), the Behavior Observation of Students in Schools (BOSS; Shapiro, 2011b), and the ADHD School Observation Code (ADHD SOC; Gadow, Sprafkin, & Nolan, 1996). Each of these systems requires observers to classify behaviors into a variety of categories (e.g., off-task, fidgets) using interval recording procedures. Regardless of the coding system used, the two goals of this phase of the assessment process are to (1) establish the frequency of inattentive, impulsive, and/or restless behaviors relative to classmates; and (2) obtain stable unbiased estimates of these frequencies by conducting observations on several occasions in the same classroom setting.

Platzman and colleagues (1992) reviewed the various observational methods that have been developed to aid in the assessment of ADHD. Several of their findings are noteworthy for practitioners. First, they found that observations conducted in the classroom provided data that were better at discriminating children with ADHD from controls than were observations conducted in clinic analog settings. This finding further attests to the need for school-based practitioners to be involved in ADHD evaluations. Second, three categories of behavior were found to consistently discriminate between ADHD and non-ADHD samples: off-task behavior, excessive gross motor activity, and negative vocalizations (e.g., refusal to obey commands). Thus, observation systems that include these categories of behavior are most likely to provide sensitive diagnostic data. Third, they found very few studies that included female participants. Because a smaller percentage of girls with ADHD are defiant and aggressive (Barkley, 2006), certain observation categories (e.g., negative vocalization) may be less discriminatory between girls with and without ADHD. As a result, practitioners may need to emphasize differences in off-task behavior when evaluating girls suspected of having this disorder.

Because normative data based on large representative samples are lacking for most of these observation codes, the behavior of the referred student should be compared with one or two classmates who have been identified as "typical" or "average" by the classroom teacher. In this fashion, each child would be evaluated relative to a classroom-based standard of behavior. Statistically significant differences between students with ADHD and comparison peers have been found even after one or two relatively brief (i.e., 20-minute) observations. Group differences are particularly evident for frequency of passive engaged behavior (e.g., listening to teacher instruction) and for various forms of off-task behavior (i.e., vocal, motor, and passive), with no apparent differences in active engaged time (e.g., working on written task; Vile Junod et al., 2006).

In addition to coding the child's behavior during task situations, it is sometimes helpful to collect supplemental observation data. For instance, teacher behaviors (e.g., prompts, reprimands, feedback) could be coded as possible antecedent and/or consequent events for child behavior. Such data are critical to determining the function of the challenging behavior, and therefore are important for treatment planning purposes. The specific teacher or classmate behaviors to be observed might be identified in the course of the teacher interview discussed previously. For example, the BOSS includes teacher-directed instruction (i.e., instances when the teacher is directly teaching the whole group, a small group, or an individual student) that is coded on a momentary time sampling basis at the start of every fifth interval. Another option is to code teacher behaviors such as positive attention and/or negative reprimands on an interval recording basis simultaneous with observations of child behavior. Such recording makes it possible to determine the percentage of observation intervals where specific teacher and child behaviors have occurred contiguously. For example, one might find that teacher positive attention occurred during a very low percentage of intervals where the child was on-task, while negative reprimands from the teacher were quite frequent when the child was off-task. In such cases, it might be hypothesized that teacher attention is reinforcing off-task rather than on-task behavior. Suggestions for modifications in teacher behavior (e.g., increasing positive attention to on-task behavior) can be generated readily from observations of this type.

Assessment of Academic Functioning. Students with ADHD score, on average, about 0.71 standard deviation units below their typically developing peers on standardized achievement tests (Frazier et al., 2007). Furthermore, teacher ratings indicate significantly lower academic performance, compromised day-to-day performance on classroom tasks, and inconsistent homework completion and quality relative to that of their classmates (Barkley, 2006; McConaughy, Volpe, Antshel, Gordon, & Eiraldi, 2011). It is helpful to obtain relatively direct measurements of academic behavior prior to intervention, as changes in scholastic status can be considered one of the more socially valid outcomes of treatment. Important academic behaviors to assess include the completion and accuracy of independent classwork, completion and accuracy of homework, acquisition of skills being taught in the curriculum, and organizational skills.

Completion and accuracy rates on assigned work should be calculated. First, the amount of written work (i.e., percentage of items) completed relative to the amount of work assigned (Rapport, DuPaul, Stoner, & Jones, 1986) or relative to "typical" classmates during observation sessions should be calculated. Second, the percentage of items completed correctly (i.e., academic efficiency score; Rapport et al., 1986) is calculated to determine task accuracy. In many cases, students with ADHD will complete significantly less work or complete tasks in a less accurate fashion due to their problems with inattention and/or carelessness. Such data are relatively straightforward to collect in conjunction with observations of the student's classroom behavior, discussed previously. The teacher should collect data regarding homework completion and accuracy over a short time interval (e.g., 2–3 weeks) contemporaneous with the ADHD evaluation. Parents also can be asked to record the frequency of completion of various steps in the homework process over a similar time period. Furthermore, items indicated to be problematic on the Homework Problem Checklist can be used to generate possible targets for intervention.

Brief probes of a child's acquisition of skills being taught in the curriculum (i.e., curriculum-based measurement [CBM]; Shinn, 1998) can be very helpful in at least two ways. First, CBM data can pinpoint the instructional level of a child within a given subject area. It is possible that a child's attention and behavior difficulties may result from the frustration of being asked to do academic work that is beyond the child's capabilities. Stated differently, it is possible that the child is being instructed at a *frustrational* rather than at an *instructional* level. It also could be that a child is consistently being asked to complete work that is too easy (e.g., mastery-level material), resulting in attentional problems. Second, because CBM probes are relatively brief (2–3 minutes), these data can be collected periodically once instructional changes are made, thus providing valuable information regarding intervention effects on skill acquisition.

Finally, the organization of the child's desk (i.e., neatness and preparedness) can be examined directly on a regular basis over a short time interval (e.g., 2–3 weeks) and compared with classmates' desks (Atkins, Pelham, & Licht, 1985). A frequent complaint of teachers is that children with ADHD have unorganized, messy desks, with a resultant loss of task and text materials. Here too information may be gleaned that helps to pinpoint the source(s) of a student's academic difficulties, as well as to identify potential foci for instructional support.

Assessment of Social Functioning. As discussed in Chapter 1, children and adolescents with ADHD frequently experience impaired relationships with peers that are characterized by aggression and/or peer rejection. In turn, being rejected by peers may significantly increase risks for problematic long-term outcomes such as delinquency, anxiety, and global impairment (Mrug et al., 2012). Thus, it is critical to determine whether students with ADHD are experiencing social and peer relationship difficulties, as well as ascertain the specific nature of these difficulties so that they can be targeted for intervention.

Typically, social functioning is assessed through parent and teacher ratings on standardized questionnaires such as the SSIS. These ratings can provide important information about (1) the degree to which social behaviors are deviant from age and gender norms and (2) the extent to which problematic behaviors are evident across home and school settings. In this way, significant impairment can be defined based on a specific standard score (e.g., score > 65) or percentile (e.g., score > 93rd percentile) threshold on parent and/or teacher ratings. Although not always feasible and acceptable, peer nominations (e.g., "Who do you like to play with the most?") and ratings provide additional, critical information about a student's social behaviors and peer status. For example, Kwon and colleagues (2012) found that peer nominations and ratings contributed significant variance in predicting student social status and positive school functioning (e.g., academic competence) above and beyond teacher ratings of social behaviors. Furthermore, Kwon and colleagues showed the value of collecting teacher and peer ratings of contextually relevant social behaviors (e.g., "offers to help other kids when they need it," "is a leader when he or she is with other kids") beyond general ratings of social competence. Contextually relevant social behavior assessment can provide data that directly translate into specific behavioral objectives for peer relationship interventions.

If peer relationship difficulties are identified, then observations of the child's interpersonal behaviors should be conducted in the settings of concern. An observation system that has been found useful for collecting data regarding social behaviors in lunchroom and playground settings is the ADHD SOC. Typically, children with ADHD exhibit higher than average frequencies of aggressive and negative behaviors (Barkley, 2006). In most cases, their rates of positive social behavior are not substantially different from their normal counterparts (Stormont, 2001). Results of these types of observations can be used not only to document the type and severity of peer relationship difficulties but also to target specific behaviors for intervention.

Stage III: Interpretation of Results (Diagnosis/Classification)

Questions to Be Addressed

Data from the multimethod assessment are used to determine the diagnostic status of the referred child by reviewing the following questions:

1. Does the child exhibit a significant number of behavioral symptoms of ADHD according to parent and teacher report?
2. Does the child exhibit ADHD symptoms at a frequency that is significantly greater than that demonstrated by children of the same gender and chronological age?
3. At what age did the child begin demonstrating significant ADHD-related behaviors, and are these behaviors chronic and evident across many situations?
4. Is the child's functioning at school, at home, and/or with peers significantly impaired?
5. Are there other possible problems (e.g., learning disabilities) or factors (e.g., teacher intolerance for active behavior) that could account for the reported display of ADHD symptoms?

Interpretation Process and Procedures

The data obtained with the previously described techniques can be used to address interpretation questions. Although each of the assessment techniques has limitations, the advantage of using a multimethod approach is that each of their strengths and weaknesses will be balanced out as part of the larger evaluation package. The overriding goals are to derive accurate data regarding the frequency and severity of ADHD-related behaviors across caregivers and settings, as well as to determine possible causes for these difficulties. To the extent that these goals are achieved, relative confidence can be placed in conclusions drawn as a result of the assessment. The interpretation of evaluation data is discussed relative to each of the major assessment questions.

Number of ADHD Symptoms? The number of ADHD symptoms is determined based on parent and teacher interview data in conjunction with ADHD Rating Scale–IV results. When caregivers and teachers report six or more inattention symptoms or six or more hyperactive–impulsive symptoms (particularly during the interviews), this is considered diagnostically significant for one of the three presentations of ADHD according to DSM-5 guidelines (American Psychiatric Association, 2013). Specifically, to receive a diagnosis of ADHD, combined presentation, the child should be reported to evidence at least six of the nine inattention symptoms *and* six of the nine hyperactive–impulsive behaviors. For a diagnosis of ADHD, predominantly inattentive presentation, six of the nine inattention symptoms must be reported combined with fewer than six hyperactive–impulsive behaviors. Finally, a diagnosis of ADHD, predominantly hyperactive–impulsive presentation, would be warranted for children who are reported to exhibit at least six hyperactive–impulsive symptoms and a maximum of five inattention symptoms.

Frequency of ADHD-Related Behaviors? The parent and teacher questionnaires discussed previously all contain at least one factor related to ADHD (e.g., labeled "Hyperactivity," "Attention Problems," "Overactive–Restless"). When a child's score on factors related to ADHD is greater than 2 standard deviations above the mean for his or her gender and chronological age, this result is considered significant for ADHD (Barkley, 2006). Scores on these same factors that are between 1.5 and 2 standard deviations above the mean are considered to be in the borderline significant (i.e., mild) range for ADHD. Thus, children receiving scores in the upper 2–7% of ADHD symptoms for their age and gender may be identified as having ADHD (depending on other assessment findings).

When determining whether scores are diagnostically significant, it also is important to consider the child's ethnicity. Parent and teacher ratings of ADHD symptoms may vary across ethnic groups, with African American children receiving significantly higher scores than European American and Hispanic children (DuPaul, Power, et al., 1998; Reid et al., 1998). Although ethnic group differences are partially accounted for by SES, even when the effects of the latter are removed systematic differences remain. In fact, ADHD symptom reports for African American children are, on average, 0.45 standard deviation units above ratings for European American children (Miller et al., 2009). These group differences could potentially result in overidentification of ADHD among African American children; however, data suggest that ethnic-minority children may be significantly less likely to be diagnosed with this disorder than white children. In fact, African American and Hispanic children are 69% and 50% less likely, respectively, to be diagnosed with ADHD compared with white children (Morgan, Staff, Hillemeier, Farkas, & Maczuga, 2013). Given the potential impact of race and ethnicity on diagnostic findings, practitioners must be especially cautious when evaluating children from different cultural backgrounds and should rely on multiple measures when assessing ADHD symptoms. Furthermore, it is imperative to use rating scales that include normative data that are representative of the U.S. population in terms of ethnic diversity.

Behavioral observation data are used to determine the frequencies of ADHD-related behaviors displayed by the referred student as compared to his or her classmates. If a large enough sample of observations is collected, the difference in behavioral frequencies between the referred and the nonreferred students could be tested statistically using a *t*-test, for example. The child with ADHD should be exhibiting inattentive, impulsive, and/or restless behaviors at a significantly higher frequency than classmates. When similar rates of behavior are observed across referred and nonreferred students, then other lines of investigation (e.g., inadequate methods of behavior management) may need to be pursued.

Age of Onset and Chronicity of Problem Behaviors? Parent report of the onset of ADHD symptoms is obtained during the interview. Typically, the age of onset is reported to be when the child begins formal schooling (i.e., kindergarten or first grade) or earlier. The consistency of ADHD-related behaviors across grades or time can be confirmed through inspection of the child's previous report cards in the school record. The onset of at least some ADHD symptoms should be reported to be prior to age 12 and these must be occurring on a daily basis for at least 6 months (American Psychiatric Association, 2013).

Are Problem Behaviors Occurring across Situations? At a general level, if both the parent(s) and teacher(s) are reporting significant display of ADHD-related behaviors across home and school environments, then this criterion is met. The pervasiveness of inattentive behaviors and/or conduct problems across situations *within* home and school environments can be determined using the original and revised versions of the HSQ and the SSQ. A finding of attention or conduct problems being reported in 50% or more of identified situations is considered significant (Barkley, 1990). In addition, if scores on these rating scales are 1.5–2.0 standard deviations above the mean using normative data (see Barkley, 1990), a more stringent criterion is reached.

To the degree that significant ADHD-related behaviors are reported to occur across home and school settings, relative confidence can be placed in the conclusion that within-child variables (i.e., presence of ADHD) account for the behavioral control difficulties to a large degree. When inconsistencies between parent and teacher report are obtained, which is typical (Wolraich et al., 2004), confidence in the diagnosis of ADHD is reduced. In general, teacher ratings are given more credence because the school is the more problematic setting for most children with ADHD and teachers have greater exposure to children within a specific age range.

Functional Impairment? The degree to which the child's academic, social, and emotional functioning is impaired is determined through examination of all of the measures discussed previously. The most frequently encountered signs of impairment associated with ADHD are academic achievement below expectations for the child and poor acceptance by peers (American Psychiatric Association, 2013; Barkley, 2006).

Thus, a child with ADHD would be expected to produce less complete and less accurate schoolwork than classmates based on observational data and teacher ratings. Furthermore, ratings for the child on scales of social competence and peer relationships would be below average for his or her age and gender. Observational data may confirm the latter, as the child may exhibit high rates of aggressive behavior on the playground or may be ignored by classmates during free-play periods.

Other Factors Accounting for ADHD-Like Behavior? The ADHD diagnosis is usually arrived at by establishing the developmental deviance and pervasiveness of symptoms by addressing the previous questions. At the same time, it is crucial to consider alternative causes for the child's inattention, impulsivity, and motor restlessness. One possibility is that these behaviors are secondary to the frustrations encountered due to a child's academic difficulties. If, for instance, the child begins to exhibit ADHD symptoms later in childhood after several years of learning difficulties or only exhibits problem behaviors during academic instruction in his or her weaker subjects, then this possibility must be entertained strongly. Alternatively, if ADHD symptoms began early in life and are pervasive across settings, then a more plausible conclusion is that the child has both ADHD and a learning disability (see Chapter 3 for additional details).

A second possibility is that the child is encountering emotional and/or adjustment difficulties that have led to inattentive, impulsive, and/or restless behaviors. If this were the case, then interview and questionnaire data would indicate significant symptoms of an alternative disorder (e.g., anxiety disorder, conduct disorder) or a difficult situation (e.g., recent parental divorce) in addition to or in lieu of ADHD symptoms. Furthermore, the symptoms of emotional disturbance would predate the onset of ADHD-related behaviors. The latter would be of relatively recent onset and would probably not be exhibited on a chronic and cross-situational basis. In the case of adjustment problems, there typically will be a clear onset of symptoms in relation to an identifiable event or set of events of importance to the child/family. The practitioner should carefully consider differential diagnostic guidelines as per DSM-5 (American Psychiatric Association, 2013).

Poor or inconsistent academic instruction and/or behavior management practices are other possible causes of apparent ADHD symptoms. This hypothesis should be explored whenever assessment data are inconsistent across sources and settings—for example, parents and teachers disagree about the severity and frequency of ADHD symptoms. This is particularly true when there are discrepancies among several teachers regarding the presence or absence of ADHD symptoms. If the latter are reported by a single teacher in the absence of a developmental history of ADHD-related difficulties and other data supporting the diagnosis of ADHD, then closer inspection of instructional and management variables is necessary. Rather than classifying the problem behaviors as resulting from "within-child" variables (i.e., ADHD), it may be that faulty teaching practices warrant modification.

Once a diagnostic decision is reached, the findings and resultant treatment recommendations must be communicated to the student's teachers and parents, as well as to any community-based professionals (e.g., pediatrician) who may be working with the child. Typically, a written report is generated and results and recommendations are orally reviewed with pertinent school personnel and parents. Issues and procedures related to communication of assessment results are discussed in greater detail in Chapter 9.

Stage IV: Designing the Treatment Plan

Questions to Be Addressed

The following questions should be addressed when designing an intervention program for students with ADHD:

1. What are the student's strengths and weaknesses (e.g., motivation and skills)?
2. What are the behavioral objectives for intervention?
3. What are the possible functions for the child's ADHD-related behaviors?
4. What are the optimum intervention strategies?
5. What additional resources are available to address the child's ADHD-related problems?

Intervention Planning Process and Procedures

The assessment process does not conclude with a diagnosis, for the diagnosis is just one step in the process of determining which intervention strategies are most likely to be successful. Thus, the assessment data are used to generate an appropriate treatment plan. The intervention strategies that have the greatest research support in the treatment of ADHD are the prescription of psychostimulant medication (e.g., MPH) and behavior modification procedures (Barkley, 2006; Fabiano et al., 2009; MTA Cooperative Group, 1999; Pelham & Fabiano, 2008). The specifics of these interventions are reviewed in greater detail in Chapters 4–7; further information regarding these interventions can be obtained through comprehensive literature reviews (e.g., Barkley, 2006; Pelham & Fabiano, 2008).

Interventions for ADHD typically are designed to impact target behaviors across academic and social domains. Because ADHD symptoms are, by definition, exhibited across settings, then treatment strategies must be outlined for multiple caretakers (e.g., parents and teachers) to be used across a number of situations. Although an explicit goal of the intervention program is to decrease the frequency of various ADHD-related behaviors (e.g., inattention to task materials), the primary emphasis is on enhancing competencies in a number of areas and improving behavioral, academic, and social functioning. Thus, treatment targets are behaviors that should increase in frequency as a function of treatment, such as completion of independent work, compliance with teacher directives, accuracy of academic responding, and positive interactions with peers. Behavioral objectives must be designed on an individual basis using data from direct observations of classroom behavior, as well as the results of parent and teacher ratings. Assessment results also will identify behavioral competencies (e.g., adequate peer relations) that possibly could aid in the amelioration of the child's deficits. Those behaviors occurring at the lowest frequencies and/or deemed most crucial to classroom functioning by the teacher usually serve as initial intervention targets.

Several factors are considered in the process of choosing appropriate interventions for an individual child with ADHD. First, the severity of the child's ADHD should be categorized into one of four levels (i.e., borderline, mild, moderate, severe) based on the number of symptoms reported on parent and teacher ratings, as well as the degree of functional impairment evidenced (American Psychiatric Association, 2013). The greater the severity of ADHD symptoms, the more likely a referral to a physician for a medication assessment will be warranted.

In general, the treatment of first resort will be the implementation of a behaviorally based intervention involving changes in antecedent conditions and/or application of positive reinforcement techniques designed to increase task-related attention and completion of assigned work (American Academy of Pediatrics, 2011; DuPaul & Stoner, 2010). Observation results will aid in this process by providing baseline data and helping to identify antecedent and consequent events that could be manipulated as part of the intervention.

In fact, a second important factor to consider in designing psychosocial interventions for children with ADHD is the function that their ADHD-related behaviors serve (DuPaul & Ervin, 1996; also see Chapters 4 and 5 for more details). The most likely function for ADHD-related behavior is to avoid or escape effortful tasks, such as independent seatwork or homework. A second possible function is to gain adult or peer attention. A frequent consequent event for ADHD-related behavior is a verbal reprimand from the teacher, as well as nonverbal (e.g., smiles) and verbal reactions (e.g., laughter) from the student's classmates. An additional possible function is for ADHD-related behavior to result in access to an object or activity that appears more reinforcing than the stimuli that the child is expected to attend to. For example, when presented with a set of written math problems to complete, the student begins playing with a toy that he keeps in his desk. Finally, ADHD-related behavior may result in sensory stimulation, such as accessing pleasant thoughts (e.g., daydreaming).

The specific function that is operational for a child's behavior in the classroom setting can be determined through descriptive assessment, experimental analysis, or both (Gresham, Watson, & Skinner, 2001; Watson & Steege, 2003). Most typically, teacher interview and behavior observation data are used to develop a working hypothesis as to the function(s) of a particular behavior. Rarely are full-scale experimental analyses conducted in classroom settings (Ervin, Ehrhardt, & Poling, 2001). Interventions are then designed to promote functionally equivalent behavior (e.g., vis-à-vis the hypothesized function) through changes in antecedent and/or consequent conditions (see Chapter 5).

In addition to behavioral function, specific settings where intervention procedures are to be implemented are identified based on observation data or the use of a scatter plot (Touchette, MacDonald, & Langer, 1985). For example, a student with ADHD may exhibit the lowest frequencies of desired behaviors in classroom rather than in playground settings. Furthermore, task-related attention and work completion rates may be different across academic subject areas. Initial interventions may be designed to increase attention and work completion frequencies during instruction in those academic areas where the child exhibits the greatest ADHD-related difficulties and in the classroom setting only. As progress is achieved, target behaviors in other academic settings may be addressed.

A third factor to consider in developing treatment strategies is the presence of additional behavior or learning disorders. For example, many children with ADHD also are oppositional and defiant in response to authority figure commands (American Psychiatric Association, 2013). Noncompliant and aggressive behaviors would then become additional targets of the classroom intervention program. A referral to a community-based professional (e.g., clinical child psychologist) may be necessary so that parents could receive education in appropriate behavior management strategies at home.

An additional consideration in designing the treatment plan is a child's response to previous interventions. If, for example, a Tier 2 behavioral program has been implemented in a general education class-room, yet the child continues to exhibit a high frequency of ADHD-related behaviors, then other treatment modalities (e.g., prescription of stimulant medication or provision of special education services at Tier 3) may need to be recommended. As is the case for most children with special needs, the preference is for placement and treatments considered to be least restrictive. In fact, most children with ADHD are placed primarily within general education settings (Pastor & Reuben, 2002; Pfiffner et al., 2006). Thus, in an RTI framework, response to Tier 1 and/or 2 interventions should be the major criterion in determining whether a child's behavior control problems are severe enough to warrant special education eligibility at Tier 3 (see Chapter 3 for further discussion of this issue).

A final factor to consider is the availability of treatment resources in the community. For instance, this availability will determine whether the child and his or her family are referred to a community-based professional, such as a clinical child psychologist, or whether home-based interventions are to be designed by the school psychologist. When both parents and teachers are actively involved in the treatment process (e.g., through implementation of behavior modification strategies), there is a greater probability of success. In some cases, parents will be referred for training in behavior management strategies when such services are available. Another option is for school-based practitioners to provide conjoint behavior consultation services wherein caregiver(s) and teacher(s) serve as consultees jointly working with a consultant to identify problem(s) and needs, delineate environmental circumstances triggering and/or reinforcing challenging behavior, develop interventions to implement in home and school settings, and adjust intervention strategies based on process and outcome evaluation data (Sheridan & Kratochwill, 2008).

Stage V: Program/Intervention Evaluation

Questions to Be Addressed

Once the intervention program is designed and implemented, ongoing assessment is conducted to answer the following questions:

1. Are changes occurring in the target behaviors and collateral areas of functioning?
2. Are intervention procedures being implemented as prescribed?
3. Are the treatment changes socially valid and clinically significant?
4. Are target behaviors normalized?

Intervention Evaluation Process

The assessment of the child with ADHD does not conclude with the diagnosis, but continues on an ongoing basis as intervention procedures are implemented. In this context, the initial evaluation data not only contribute to diagnostic decisions but also serve as baseline or preintervention measures. If outcome assessment data are not collected once treatment begins, one can never be sure that the intervention is successful or whether it requires adjustments. Single-subject design methodology should be employed to evaluate treatment-related changes in target behaviors (DuPaul & Stoner, 2010). More details regarding the use of single-subject methodology to evaluate behavioral change can be obtained by consulting several excellent texts on this topic (e.g., Kazdin, 1992; Kratochwill & Levin, 1992; Riley-Tillman & Burns, 2009).

Throughout the treatment process, the student serves as his or her own "control," and behavioral change is evaluated in comparison with baseline or nonintervention conditions. This process requires the repeated acquisition of assessment data across settings and caretakers at various points in the intervention program. In addition, treatment integrity is evaluated to ensure the accurate application (e.g., treatment adherence) of the prescribed intervention. If the intervention is implemented as designed and reliable behavior change occurs, then one can assume that the treatment is working as planned. If not, then changes to either the intervention or the manner in which it is implemented by teachers or parents must be made. Thus, ongoing assessment is crucial to the treatment process and the two are inexorably linked.

Intervention Evaluation Techniques

In most cases, narrowband assessment techniques such as direct observations of behavior and academic performance data, discussed previously, are used to evaluate treatment-related change. Such data contribute to addressing whether behavioral changes are occurring as planned in association with the intervention. For example, direct observations and performance data are collected on a daily or weekly basis in the context of a single-case research design such as a reversal or multiple baseline across settings design (Kazdin, 2011). Changes in the mean, intercept, and trend of the data are used to determine whether the intervention has led to increases in task-related attention, compliance with classroom rules, and academic productivity and accuracy (see Chapter 5 for a specific example of the evaluation of a classroom intervention program). Analyses can also include nonparametric statistical analyses to detect statistically reliable change (Levin, Ferron, & Kratochwill, 2012), as well as calculation of effect size to determine magnitude of treatment-induced change (Burns & Wagner, 2008). Occasionally, interobserver agreement is assessed by having a classroom aide, teacher, or other observer present when data are collected. Interobserver agreement should be assessed at least several times per treatment phase to ensure that observation and performance data are reliable.

Several additional assessment techniques are used to determine whether reliable behavior change has occurred as a function of the intervention. First, teacher ratings on the CBCL, BASC-2, or Conners–3 are collected at several points, including prior to the intervention, during the treatment phase, following the return to baseline phase (if applicable), and approximately 1 month after the formal intervention has ceased. Thus, general behavior ratings are obtained at least once per treatment phase. Even though these ratings were collected during the initial evaluation, it is important to obtain them on an additional occasion prior to treatment implementation, as "practice effects" on these measures have been found (Barkley, 2006). A second administration of teacher ratings during baseline would reduce the possibility of attributing change to the treatment when it was actually due to a regression to the mean artifact. Teacher ratings that contain fewer items, such as the ADHD Rating Scale–IV, can be collected on a weekly basis throughout all treatment phases. Typically, the means of the various teacher ratings are compared across phases to determine whether the teacher perceives any treatment-induced improvements in performance and behavior control.

One alternative to repeated administrations of teacher rating scales is the use of daily behavior report cards (DBRCs) that contain several items assessing the specific behaviors (e.g., attention to assigned work) targeted for intervention (Chafouleas, Riley-Tillman, & Sugai, 2007; Volpe & Fabiano, 2013). DBRCs not only serve as an effective home–school communication system (see Chapter 5 for details on using DBRCs as an intervention) but also can provide valuable progress monitoring data. Specifically, DBRCs can be administered on a continuous basis both prior to and following intervention to determine whether treatment leads to changes in target behaviors. DBRCs are also more time efficient and easier to complete for teachers than are most standardized rating scales.

A second assessment component necessary to document treatment-related change is a method to determine whether the intervention has been implemented as prescribed (Gresham, Gansle, Noell, Cohen, & Rosenblum, 1993; Noell et al., 2005; Perepletchikova, Treat, & Kazdin, 2007). If medication effects are being assessed, then pill counts are conducted on a regular basis (e.g., weekly) to ensure that the medicine has been administered. Alternatively, when a parent or teacher is carrying out the intervention (e.g., classroom-based token reinforcement program), treatment adherence is more difficult to determine. Ideally, direct observations of teacher behavior would be conducted occasionally throughout treatment to assess whether the intervention steps are being carried out as planned. Of course, there would then be no way to ensure that treatment integrity was intact during intervention sessions where an observer was not present. In such cases, observations of teacher behavior would be supplemented by checklists outlining the intervention steps. The teacher or treatment agent would be expected to complete the checklist every time the intervention was being implemented in an effort to promote adherence. Such checklists also could be completed by someone other than the treatment agent (e.g., classroom aide) on a regular basis. Another option is to audiotape intervention sessions for later review regarding implementation integrity (Power, DuPaul, Shapiro, & Kazak, 2003). Without at least occasional treatment integrity checks, one cannot be sure that the intervention is being applied as designed.

Although it is important to demonstrate that an intervention has led to reliable changes in the student's behavior and performance, it is crucial to determine whether such changes are socially valid and clinically meaningful. For example, a mean increase in the percentage of on-task behavior from 50 to 65% during independent work may be statistically significant, but the end result is that the student still spends too much time off-task and is not any more productive academically. Interventions that lead to behavior changes that do not meaningfully impact on the student's classroom performance are usually abandoned quite readily by the child's teacher.

The clinical significance and social validity of behavioral change can be assessed in a variety of ways (Kazdin, 2000; Schwarz & Baer, 1991). First, students, teachers, and/or parents could complete consumer satisfaction ratings at the conclusion of treatment or at various points during the intervention. Each participant's views on specific components of the intervention could be obtained in this manner. A second related technique is to have the teacher complete treatment acceptability ratings of various possible intervention strategies (Finn & Sladeczek, 2001). The acceptability of interventions may actually be assessed prior to treatment as an aid in the consultation and treatment design process (Sheridan & Kratochwill, 2008).

A third way of determining the clinical significance of an intervention is to assess whether it has led to the "normalization" of behavior. Stated differently, does the intervention enhance the student's attention span, academic productivity, and social behaviors to the point where his or her performance and behavior in the classroom is indistinguishable from those of his or her peers? This particular outcome can be evaluated by collecting concurrent assessment data on one or more classmates during various points in the intervention. In this way, the treated child's performance can be compared directly with that of his or her typically developing counterparts. If ethical or practical considerations preclude the assessment of normal classmates, several statistical procedures can be used to determine whether clinically meaningful change has occurred. For example, if normative data are available for a specific measure, then a reliable change index (Jacobsen & Truax, 1991) can be calculated to evaluate whether the treatment has led to statistically reliable improvements in behavior. Furthermore, Jacobsen and Truax (1991) have provided several formulas for determining whether an intervention has led to normalization of performance. For example, MPH (Ritalin) has been found to "normalize" the task-related attention and academic productivity of a large percentage of children with ADHD who participated in a 6-week medication trial (DuPaul & Rapport, 1993; see Chapter 7 for details). Although normalization of classroom performance is not always possible, it is one of the more important considerations in determining the value of obtained treatment effects.

DEVELOPMENTAL CONSIDERATIONS IN THE ASSESSMENT OF ADHD

Developmental factors may alter the content and, to some degree, the process of conducting an ADHD evaluation, especially when the referred student is a preschooler or an adolescent (Anastopoulos & Shelton, 2001). We address issues related to the identification of young children at risk for ADHD in Chapter 4. With regard to assessing ADHD in adolescents, there are several reasons why evaluation procedures may differ relative to assessment of children. First, for adolescents who are at least 17 years old, the symptom thresholds are five in each symptom category (i.e., inattention and hyperactivity–impulsivity) rather than six (American Psychiatric Association, 2013). This lowered symptom threshold reflects the possible diminution of symptoms across development. Second, the overall functioning of the teenager with ADHD can be more impaired than during the childhood years, given a higher risk for conduct disturbance or antisocial behavior (Barkley et al., 2008) and academic underachievement (Barkley et al., 2008; Frazier et al., 2007). In addition, several empirical investigations have indicated a higher frequency of substance abuse (e.g., Sihvoia et al., 2011) among adolescents with ADHD, although this relationship may be moderated by gender and presence of antisocial behavior problems (e.g., stealing, vandalism). Thus, in addition to the core deficits of ADHD, teenagers with this disorder may exhibit a variety of behavioral and/or emotional distur-bances, and therefore procedures designed to screen for these associated difficulties must be incorporated into the evaluation of adolescents with ADHD.

When evaluating an adolescent referred for ADHD-related difficul-ties, it is very important that a reliable history of the problem behaviors is obtained because, by definition, ADHD symptoms should be evident prior to the age of 12. Because the reliability of historical information provided by parents is often quite low, even for younger children, care should be taken to obtain "reliability checks" of parental verbal reports (Cantwell, 1986). Alternatively, Sibley, Pelham, and colleagues (2012) found parent retrospective reports to be correlated with actual child-hood measures of ADHD. In addition to parent report, information about the child's history should be gathered from the student's school record, including report cards, previous psychological evaluations, and disciplinary history.

A third factor to consider in the assessment of adolescents suspected of having ADHD is the input of the students themselves. The teenager's perception of current adjustment difficulties must be obtained in addi-tion to parent and teacher reports. Adolescent self-report of ADHD symptoms has been found to correlate with clinician ratings (Adler et al., 2012), although the association of self-report with ratings from par-ents and teachers is equivocal across studies (see Barkley, Fischer, et al., 2002; Connors, Connolly, & Toplak, 2012; Sibley, Pelham, et al., 2012). Regardless of the relationship between self-report and other measures, the former may provide critical information (e.g., presence of depressive symptoms) not available from other sources. Moreover, adolescents are likely to agree more fully with the results of evaluations in which their own opinions were given greater attention, and hence may be more will-ing to participate with treatment recommendations (DuPaul, Guevre-mont, & Barkley, 1991). Thus, the major change to the ADHD evalu-ation when assessing an adolescent is the inclusion at the multimethod assessment stage of several self-report measures, such as a diagnostic interview with the student and the completion of behavior rating scales. The student may also play a more active role in the formulation, imple-mentation, and assessment of the treatment plan. At the very least, self-report and consumer satisfaction data should be obtained from the stu-dent during the treatment evaluation stage on an ongoing basis.

The content of the ADHD evaluation is somewhat different when assessing an adolescent, relative to assessment of younger children. First, as mentioned previously, a diagnostic interview with the student should be conducted that incorporates DSM criteria for the same disor-ders reviewed with the adolescent's parent and teacher. Second, various self-report questionnaires are completed by the student, including the Conners–3 Self-Report (Conners, 2008), YSR version of the CBCL, Self-Report of Personality for the BASC-2, and Youth Inventory–4. Normative data are available for all of these measures. Given the higher risk of affective or emotional disturbance among adolescents with ADHD relative to their normal counterparts, it is often necessary to include questionnaires tapping internalizing symptomatology, such as the Reynolds Adolescent Depression Scale–Second Edition (Reynolds, 2002).

A final change in the ADHD evaluation is the inclusion of behavior ratings from multiple teachers. The interpretation of the resultant ratings can be problematic given the limited sample of student behavior that each teacher observes. It is often helpful to obtain ratings from several individuals, including nonteachers (e.g., guidance counselor) with whom the teenager has the greatest amount of contact. Rather than relying on the analysis of any single teacher rating (as with younger children), consistencies among the resultant profiles (e.g., elevations on factors related to ADHD) are used to document the pervasiveness or lack thereof of behavioral control difficulties across settings. Further details regarding the content of ADHD evaluations with adolescents are available (Anastopoulos & Shelton, 2001; Barkley, 2006; Sibley, Pelham, et al., 2012).

IMPLEMENTATION OF THE ASSESSMENT MODEL

The assessment model proposed in this chapter represents what we believe to be a comprehensive evaluation process for identifying students with ADHD and designing classroom interventions for this population. As such, it is an idealized model that must be adapted for practical application at the local level. Some assessment components or processes (e.g., parent interview) may be less feasible for some school personnel. Therefore, changes to the assessment model may be necessary. It is positive to note, however, that most school psychologists report using a multi-informant, multisetting, multimethod approach to assessment of ADHD as articulated in our model (Demaray, Schaefer, & DeLong, 2003).

As an example of a local adaptation of this assessment model, the Carroll County (Maryland) Public Schools have developed ADHD procedural guidelines for teachers and school psychologists (Carroll County Public Schools, 1997). These guidelines structure the ADHD identification and treatment process into four, rather than five, stages: screening, multimodal assessment of ADHD, interpretation of results, and treatment. Although the screening stage is virtually identical to the content and process of this stage as described in this chapter, some adaptations have been made to the multimethod assessment protocol. For example, parents are asked to complete a questionnaire rather than an interview that outlines current behavioral concerns as well as developmental, medical, and family histories. Nevertheless, this second stage of the Carroll County guidelines includes the core components of the multimethod protocol proposed in this chapter, such as parent and teacher behavior questionnaires, direct observation, and review of school records.

Although our assessment model may include some components that are impractical for some school districts, it is possible to adapt this process to meet the needs and practical limitations of a local school district. The overall objective would be to retain core features of this model. First, the assessment process should utilize a data-based problem-solving model wherein psychometrically sound measures are used to make identification and treatment decisions. Second, a triage system should be used in the context of an RTI framework wherein students are screened to determine who will require more involved assessment and/or treatment, particularly at Tier 3. Third, the input of multiple respondents using more than one type of measure should be sought to obtain a comprehensive picture of a child's home and school functioning. As is the case for evaluating learning disabilities, practitioners should never rely on a single instrument or questionnaire to make ADHD identification decisions. In similar fashion, professionals from a variety of educational and medical disciplines may be involved in collecting and interpreting assessment data. Thus, a team approach to the assessment and intervention development/evaluation process is optimal (Dang, Warrington, Tung, Baker, & Pan, 2007). Fourth, assessment data (e.g., functional behavioral assessment and/or curriculum-based assessment) that are useful for treatment planning should be collected routinely. Last, some subset of assessment measures should be collected periodically to determine the success of intervention plans and to guide ongoing changes in treatment.

CASE EXAMPLES

Case Example 1

Arthur was a 7-year-old second grader referred to the school psychologist by his general education teacher due to problems completing independent seatwork, talking without permission, and noncompliance with school rules. The teacher indicated that the quality of Arthur's academic work was similar to that of his classmates when she worked with him individually. Alternatively, due to his inconsistent completion of assigned work and frequent inattention during tests, Arthur was reported to achieve below his presumed potential. Given his difficulties, several Tier

2 interventions (daily report card, classwide contingency management system) were implemented. Despite some initial intervention success, Arthur's behavioral difficulties persisted.

After briefly discussing the case, the school psychologist asked the teacher to complete a screening instrument (i.e., the ADHD Rating Scale–IV). Arthur's ratings were beyond the 93rd percentile for the total score as well as the Inattention and Hyperactive–Impulsive factor scores. Also, six inattention and six hyperactive–impulsive symptoms (using DSM-5 criteria; American Psychiatric Association, 2013) were reported to occur "often" or "very often." Based on this screening information, the nature of the referral, and Arthur's minimal response to Tier 2 interventions, a multimethod assessment of ADHD appeared warranted.

As a first step in the assessment process, an interview with Arthur's classroom teacher was conducted. In the course of the interview, it was reported that he displayed frequent problems with inattention, impulsivity, overactivity, and noncompliance across most school settings and classroom activities. These problems were most evident when independent seatwork was assigned and when the teacher was instructing the whole class or small groups. There did not appear to be any differences in this behavior across academic subject areas. Arthur was reported to evidence six of the nine inattention symptoms and seven of the nine hyperactive–impulsive symptoms of ADHD on a frequent basis. These symptoms had been exhibited on a daily basis over the past 6 months (i.e., since the beginning of the school year). Furthermore, a significant number (i.e., five out of eight) of symptoms of oppositional defiant disorder were reported to occur on a frequent basis. The latter included noncompliance with teacher commands, frequent losses of temper, and deliberate annoyance of others. Problems associated with other disorders (e.g., conduct disorder, depression) were not reported to occur frequently.

As a result of his attention and behavior problems, Arthur was not achieving at a level commensurate with his classmates in either mathematics or reading skills. Nevertheless, his teacher did not feel that he had learning problems in either subject area. She reported that when she worked with him on an individual basis, he was able to demonstrate adequate knowledge in both skill areas (e.g., he was able to read high-interest material). When he was asked to complete independent work, particularly material that did not capture his interest, he was not able to demonstrate his abilities due to a lack of work completion.

Arthur had few friends in the classroom and was rejected by many of his peers. He did not follow the rules of games and frequently was verbally and physically aggressive in unstructured settings (e.g., on the playground). His teacher felt that many of his disruptive behaviors (e.g., talking out in the classroom) were an attempt to elicit attention from his peers. Unfortunately, these efforts to promote peer interaction resulted in further ostracism by his classmates.

The teacher reported a great deal of frustration in trying to manage Arthur's behavior. Her interventions had included ignoring his disruptive behavior, making public reprimands to get back on task, sending notes to his parents following misbehavior, giving him a reward (e.g., access to classroom computer) for a week of appropriate behavior, and reducing the number of items he is expected to complete for seatwork. None of these strategies resulted in consistent behavioral improvement.

Arthur's report cards from previous school years were reviewed. The written comments of his kindergarten and first-grade teachers indicated that he displayed similar problems with behavior control, albeit less severe, as reported by his current teacher. A pattern of attention and behavior control problems beginning at an early age and occurring across school years was evident.

Arthur's mother was interviewed briefly by telephone. She corroborated the teacher's report of significant problems with inattention, impulsivity, and overactivity. In fact, nearly all of the symptoms of ADHD were reported to occur on a frequent basis at home. These had been evident since he was 3 years old and attended a nursery school program. She reported that Arthur was very defiant and uncooperative at home, especially in response to maternal commands. He did not sustain his attention to most household chores unless he was interested in completing them. A majority of the symptoms of oppositional defiant disorder were indicated to be present. No further DSM-5 (American Psychiatric Association, 2013) symptomatology was reported. He did not have a history of significant medical difficulties or developmental delays. Arthur's father was reported to have had similar attention and behavior problems as a child, but was now a successful businessman. No other significant problems were reported for immediate family members. Finally, she stated that she was very interested in receiving help in managing Arthur's behavior, as the stress level in the household was directly related to the degree to which he behaved in an appropriate manner. Previous attempts at intervention, including family therapy, had failed.

Maternal responses on the CBCL resulted in significant elevations on three subscales: Attention Problems, Aggression, and Delinquent. T-scores on these scales were above 67, or greater than the 95th percentile. All remaining subscales were below the 93rd percentile (i.e., in the normal range). Ratings on the ADHD Rating Scale–IV were two standard deviations above the mean for the total score and both subscales.

Arthur's attention problems were reported to occur in almost all home situations identified on the HSQ-R and their average severity was 2 standard deviations above the mean.

Teacher ratings were consistent with those provided by Arthur's mother. On the Teacher Report Form of the CBCL, significant elevations were obtained on the Attention Problems and Aggression subscales. T-scores were above 70, or greater than the 98th percentile for both dimensions. Remaining subscale scores were in the normal range. On the SSQ-R, Arthur was reported to exhibit attention problems in every school setting at a severity level that was 2 standard deviations above the mean. Teacher ratings on the SSIS resulted in a below-average score (T-score of 85) for social skills. Finally, ratings on the Academic Performance Rating Scale were in the clinically significant range (i.e., 1.5 standard deviations below the mean) for the Academic Productivity factor only.

Arthur's behavior was observed on several occasions in both the classroom and on the playground. Classroom observations (using the BOSS) were conducted for 20 minutes on three occasions (once during math seatwork, twice while working on a phonics worksheet). Arthur was noted to display high rates of off-task verbal and motor behaviors. Specifically, he displayed off-task verbal behavior during an average of 20% of the observation intervals, while exhibiting off-task motor behavior approximately 15% of the time. In contrast, randomly selected classmates were observed to exhibit off-task verbal behavior only 4% of the time and were engaged in off-task motor behavior during less than 8% of the observation intervals. Arthur's playground behavior was observed on two occasions using the ADHD SOC. He was noted to be more verbally and physically aggressive than randomly selected classmates. Thus, direct observations were consistent with both parent and teacher report of significant behavior control difficulties.

Academic performance data were collected in conjunction with observations of Arthur's behavior during independent seatwork. He completed an average of 60% of the work assigned over these three occasions. This is in contrast to an average completion rate of 95% for his classmates. On a positive note, the accuracy of his work was uniformly high (i.e., $M = 93\%$ correct). This corroborates the teacher's contention that Arthur's abilities were commensurate with those of his classmates, but that he simply did not finish the assigned work.

The next step in the evaluation process was to interpret the results. Arthur's teacher and mother independently reported at least six inattention and six hyperactive–impulsive symptoms to be evident on a frequent basis. According to his mother, he began exhibiting ADHD-related difficulties at the age of 3 with no diminishment of severity. Thus, these symptoms were evident at an early age and were displayed across several years. Maternal and teacher ratings indicated Arthur's problems with inattention, impulsivity, and overactivity were more frequent and severe than those of the vast majority of other boys his age. This was corroborated by direct observations of his classroom behavior. Furthermore, attention problems were reported to be pervasive across numerous school and home situations. Finally, Arthur's ADHD-related behaviors had compromised his peer relationships and academic performance to a significant degree.

Although Arthur also was reported to display a significant number of oppositional defiant disorder symptoms, the presence of the latter could not fully account for his attention difficulties. It was particularly noteworthy that his symptoms of ADHD predated the onset of his problems with noncompliance and defiance. Specifically, the former were reported to occur as early as age 3, while the latter were not evident until Arthur was 6 years old. There were no indications of any emotional or learning difficulties that could account for his ADHD symptoms. Thus, he was determined to have both ADHD, combined presentation, and oppositional defiant disorder.

Arthur's teacher was interviewed regarding the antecedents and consequences surrounding his off-task disruptive behavior in the classroom. In addition, the school psychologist recorded the frequency of antecedent (e.g., task presentation) and consequent (e.g., peer laughter) events during various classroom situations. Interview and observation data indicated that Arthur's disruptive behavior was most likely to occur when he was asked to complete independent seatwork and that this behavior was followed by frequent teacher reminders for him to focus on his work. It appeared that the function of his off-task behavior was to avoid and escape classwork.

Several Tier 3 interventions were implemented based on this evaluation. First, the school psychologist and teacher designed a classroom intervention program that included modifying task demands, token reinforcement, response cost, and a home–school communication program (see Chapter 5 for details of classroom programming). These interventions were designed to reduce Arthur's desire to avoid work by enhancing the positive aspects of the latter while providing greater motivation for him to complete assigned tasks. Second, referrals were made to a clinical child psychologist and Arthur's pediatrician for provision of parent education and a medication assessment, respectively. Parent education was necessary due to his high level of defiance and inattention at home. A medication assessment was recommended due to the severity of Arthur's ADHD and the high likelihood of continued impairment in functioning in a number of key areas. The chronicity and severity of his behavior problems may require special education programming, which Arthur's family would like to avoid if possible. The probability of special education placement may be reduced if Arthur is a positive responder to medication. Finally, a peer relationship intervention was designed to address Arthur's playground behavior. Specifically, a peer-mediated procedure was used wherein several of his classmates were trained to prompt and reinforce appropriate social behavior. It was felt that this combination of interventions would be necessary over the long term given the chronicity and severity of Arthur's ADHD.

The school psychologist periodically assessed Arthur's classroom performance to evaluate his progress and to determine whether changes were warranted in his intervention program. Teacher ratings and classroom observations were obtained on at least a weekly basis during the initial stages of implementing the multicomponent behavioral intervention. Adjustments were made to the timing and frequency of reinforcement as a result. These same measures were used on a daily basis over several weeks of evaluating three different doses of MPH (i.e., 5 mg, 10 mg, 15 mg). Over the course of the school year, these measures were periodically readministered to ascertain whether further adjustments in behavioral procedures or medication dosage were necessary.

Case Example 2

Keesha was a 10-year-old African American girl participating in a fifth-grade general education classroom in an urban school setting. She had experienced some difficulties with reading and math throughout her school years, although she had never been referred for special education services. Her current teachers became concerned that she might have ADHD because she frequently had difficulties concentrating on her work, often forgot class materials and assignments, and frequently appeared distracted. Teacher ratings on the Inattention subscale of the ADHD Rating Scale–IV were above the 85th percentile, indicating a need for further assessment of possible ADHD.

Parent and teacher ratings on the BASC-2 resulted in clinically significant scores in the Inattention and Anxiety domains, with only borderline ratings of hyperactivity–impulsivity and conduct problems. Her mother's and teacher's responses to diagnostic interview questions revealed that although Keesha exhibited seven of the nine inattention symptoms of ADHD, she only exhibited three hyperactive–impulsive symptoms. Furthermore, her inattention problems were relatively recent (i.e., began occurring at the beginning of the school year). Keesha also was reported by both her mother and her teacher to exhibit symptoms of generalized anxiety disorder (e.g., excessive concerns regarding the quality of her social and academic performance) that appeared to be worsening as the school year went on. Keesha's mother and teacher did not report significant symptoms of oppositional defiant disorders or conduct disorder.

The school psychologist observed Keesha's behavior during reading and math class activities (e.g., teacher-led instruction, independent seatwork, small-group work). Keesha displayed off-task behavior (e.g., looking away from task or activity, talking with classmates) during approximately 15% of the observation intervals, whereas her classmates exhibited similar behavior during only 6% of those intervals. Keesha also was noted to complete far less written seatwork than her peers.

An interview with Keesha revealed that she "felt stupid" and frequently felt frustrated by her inability to read material at the same pace as her classmates. She recognized that she often did not get her work done and stated that she was worried that she would not pass fifth grade. She also indicated a concern about her mother's health as the latter had been ill frequently during the current school year. Finally, Keesha reported that she did not have many friends and that she felt embarrassed when she had to speak in front of a group of her peers. Self-report ratings of anxiety symptoms also were elevated.

Given that Keesha's attention problems were relatively recent, were not associated with many hyperactive–impulsive symptoms, and appeared to be associated with significant anxiety disorder symptoms, the school assessment team concluded that she probably did not have ADHD. The school psychologist suggested that she receive individual counseling at school for her anxiety symptoms and that further evaluation by a clinical psychologist might be necessary. Furthermore, because of her chronic academic difficulties and lack of response to Tier 1 and 2 instructional interventions, assessment of possible learning disabilities should be conducted by the school team.

INVOLVEMENT OF SCHOOL PROFESSIONALS IN THE ASSESSMENT PROCESS

Over the years, there has been controversy as to the role of school professionals in the diagnostic assessment of ADHD. For example, legislation in several states have limited school-based identification of students with ADHD, particularly for the purpose of referring them for possible medication treatment. Opponents of schools being involved in the diagnostic process point out that ADHD is a "medical diagnosis," given its inclusion in DSM-5 (American Psychiatric Association, 2013), and therefore evaluations of this disorder should be conducted by medical professionals.

Yet when one examines the assessment methods that are empirically supported for identification of ADHD, it is clear that school psychologists and other educational professionals have the training and expertise to be involved in this process. In fact, a survey study indicates that school psychologists were as likely to use empirically supported assessment methods as clinical psychologists (Handler & DuPaul, 2002). School psychologists also have more opportunities—to conduct observations in classroom and playground settings than do other professionals. Furthermore, very few medical professionals have that same background, expertise, and opportunities—at least as far as administration of rating scales and behavioral observations is concerned. Also, the mere inclusion of ADHD in DSM-5 (American Psychiatric Association, 2013) does not delegate the responsibility for making this diagnosis solely to medical professionals, as diagnostic criteria for intellectual and learning disabilities (entities that are assessed routinely by school psychologists) also are included in the DSM. Finally, because children with ADHD arguably experience their greatest difficulties in school settings, for school professionals not to be involved in identification is tantamount to malpractice.

To be clear, we are not advocating for school psychologists and other educators to be the only professionals identifying children with ADHD. On the contrary, we strongly believe that the diagnosis and treatment of students with this disorder requires collaboration among parents, school professionals, physicians, and other community-based professionals (e.g., clinical psychologists). A comprehensive assessment of ADHD requires the collection of reliable and valid data regarding child functioning across settings. All too often, community-based evaluations of children suspected of having ADHD do not include detailed information from the school. Alternatively, school-based evaluations may neglect parental input. Thus, school-based professionals should seek to collaborate with others, such that school-based data can be communicated in a systematic fashion to physicians and clinical psychologists so that informed diagnostic decisions are made (see Chapter 9).

SUMMARY

The school-based evaluation of ADHD comprises multiple assessment techniques utilized across a variety of settings and sources of information. The evaluation must be considered in the context of a three-tiered RTI framework wherein response to Tier 1 and Tier 2 interventions is assessed prior to considering ADHD. Following a teacher referral for possible ADHD and a lack of response to Tier 2 interventions, five stages of assessment are conducted: (1) screening for ADHD symptoms, (2) multimethod assessment, (3) interpretation of results to reach a classification decision, (4) development of the treatment plan, and (5) ongoing assessment of the intervention program. The goal of the evaluation is not simply to arrive at a diagnosis of ADHD, but to determine an intervention plan at Tier 2 or 3 that is likely to succeed based on the information gathered. The use of a behavioral assessment approach incorporating parent and teacher interviews, parent and teacher rating scales, direct observations of behavior, and academic performance data is the optimal methodology for addressing both goals of the evaluation process. Importantly, assessment data are collected on an ongoing basis throughout treatment to determine the efficacy and/or limitations of the intervention program.

CHAPTER 3

ADHD and Comorbidity

Practical Considerations
for School-Based Professionals

Children and adolescents with ADHD frequently present with significant co-occurring problems, including academic underachievement, conduct problems, anxiety symptoms, and depression, as well as intra- and interpersonal difficulties. The technical term used in psychiatry and psychology to describe the co-occurrence of two or more disorders is *comorbidity*. Comorbidity, or multiple disorders/problems, may be experienced either concurrently or developmentally (e.g., one problem, followed by another, over time). The term *comorbidity* also may be used to describe familial comorbidity, for example, to describe the co-occurrence of a child diagnosed with ADHD, as well as his or her parent being so diagnosed (Pliszka, 2011).

In a review of ADHD and psychiatric comorbidity, Spencer, Biederman, and Mick (2007) reported that oppositional defiant disorder or conduct disorder co-occur in approximately 30–50% of children and adolescents diagnosed with ADHD. They further reported findings of comorbid depression occurring in the range of 29–45% over the lifetime of individuals with ADHD. Jarrett and Ollendick (2008) report that anxiety disorders occur in about 25% of cases of ADHD. Data for two other issues of concern derived from Spencer and colleagues (2007) are that learning disabilities occur in about 25% of cases of ADHD, and that youth with ADHD are at significantly higher risk for substance use and abuse (e.g., tobacco, alcohol, and drugs) as compared with nonidentified peers.

The co-occurrence of problems with ADHD such as those noted previously presents a variety of challenges for education and mental health professionals, chief among them assessment and diagnostic challenges, and treatment or support challenges. For example, the process of differential diagnosis is complicated by co-occurring problems, and leads to questions such as "Might one of these problems (e.g., ADHD) be causing the other (e.g., learning disabilities) or vice versa, and if so, are the presenting problems the result of one disorder or two?" From a treatment perspective, practitioners are faced with deciding how to sequence interventions, or how to concurrently treat multiple problems. Another reason that treatment becomes more complex with co-occurring problems is that functional impairment typically increases with comorbidity (see, e.g., Crawford, Kaplan, & Dewey, 2006; Connor & Doerfler, 2008).

In this chapter, we present an overview of ADHD and comorbid problems, and discuss issues relevant to professional practice in schools that arise as a function of comorbidity. After examining relationships between ADHD and learning problems, we consider ADHD and other externalizing problems, ADHD and internalizing problems, and ADHD and adjustment problems. We then delineate a number of assessment and treatment issues, and end with a discussion of ADHD and special education in schools.

As already noted, children with ADHD frequently present with significant co-occurring problems. For example, children with ADHD underachieve academically (Barkley, 2006; Forness & Kavale, 2001). Within classroom settings, these children often exhibit significantly lower rates of on-task behavior during instruction and independent work periods than those displayed by their classmates (Abikoff et al., 1977). As a result, children with ADHD have fewer opportunities to respond during academic instruction and complete less independent work relative to their peers (Pfiffner & DuPaul, in press). The latter may, at least partially, account for the association of ADHD with academic underachievement; up to 80% of children with this disorder have been found to exhibit learning and/or achievement problems (e.g., Cantwell & Baker, 1991; Frick et al., 1991; Pastor & Reuben, 2002). Furthermore, the results of prospective follow-up studies of children with ADHD into adolescence (Barkley et al., 2008) indicate some of the greatest risks for this population are chronic academic underachievement and higher rates of dropping out of school.

Given the association between ADHD and academic underachievement, it is important for school psychologists and other education professionals to be aware of the potential for learning difficulties among children diagnosed with or suspected of having ADHD. In addition, where warranted, it is incumbent upon these professionals to design and implement effective prevention and intervention strategies to enhance academic functioning.

ASSOCIATION OF ADHD
WITH ACADEMIC UNDERACHIEVEMENT

One of the most common and potentially debilitating difficulties exhibited by children with ADHD is chronic academic underachievement relative to their intellectual capabilities (Barkley, in press). The clear majority of students with this disorder obtain lower academic grades than expected across one or more subject areas. Furthermore, these children typically obtain significantly lower standardized achievement test scores than do comparable groups of typical children (Barkley, DuPaul, & McMurray, 1990; Cantwell & Satterfield, 1978). Problems with academic performance are differentially associated with ADHD even among groups of children with other psychological disorders. For example, children with ADHD have been found to receive the poorest teacher ratings of academic competence on the Child Behavior Checklist (CBCL; Achenbach & Rescorla, 2001) among clinic-referred groups of children (McConaughy, Achenbach, & Gent, 1988). This academic underachievement presumably is due to the exhibition of the core symptoms (i.e., inattention, impulsivity, and motor restlessness) of ADHD in classroom settings, although this is a matter of some debate, as discussed in the next section.

The chronic achievement difficulties exhibited by many children with ADHD increase their risk for poor scholastic outcome, as measured by a number of variables. Approximately 40% or more of children with ADHD are placed in special education programs for students with learning disabilities or behavior disorders (Barkley, 2006). Furthermore, about one-third of children with ADHD in research samples have been retained in at least one grade before reaching high school (Barkley et al., 2008). School suspensions and expulsions occur at a higher than average frequency for students with ADHD, although this may be due, at least partially, to the higher rate of conduct disorder among children with attention deficits (Barkley, Fischer, et al., 1990). Moreover, the high school dropout rate is higher (i.e., about 10%) among students with this disorder relative to the general population (Barkley et al., 2008). The academic performance difficulties associated with ADHD may even persist into adulthood, as follow-up studies indicate that only about 20% of adults with a childhood history of the disorder are continuing their education at age 21 as opposed to about 50% of normal samples (Weiss & Hechtman, 1986, 1993). The educational problems and outcomes associated with this disorder thereby increase the risk of experiencing significant vocational and social difficulties in adulthood (Barkley, Fischer, et al., 1990; Weiss & Hechtman, 1986, 1993; Whalen, Jamner, Henker, Delfino, & Lozano, 2002).

Association between ADHD and Academic Problems: Empirical Evidence

One factor that has obfuscated conclusions about the association between ADHD and learning problems is the confusion between academic *skills* deficits (i.e., learning disabilities) and academic *performance* deficits. The former presumes a lack of *ability* to learn a specific subject matter, at least as the material is currently taught. As such, the student may show deficiencies in the actual skills being taught even under conditions of individual instruction. Alternatively, a deficit in academic *performance* would be defined as an instance where a student possesses the necessary skills but does not demonstrate this knowledge on a consistent basis under typical classroom conditions (e.g., by producing accurate independent seatwork). In the case of the child with ADHD, a lack of attention to academic materials may lead to poor performance on assigned tasks even though the child may possess the requisite skills to complete the assignment correctly. Furthermore, inattention and behavioral control difficulties could compromise the student's *availability* for and engagement in learning activities (e.g., missing important teacher lecture points due to inattention), and thus lead to greater levels of academic underachievement (Silver, 1990). The academic performance of children with ADHD also may be deficient due to their inefficient and inconsistent problem-solving abilities (Douglas, 1980). Unfortunately, much of the work that has investigated the relationship between ADHD and academic problems has not clearly differentiated between academic skills deficits and performance difficulties.

Empirical investigations of the association between ADHD and academic problems primarily have employed correlational designs. Very few studies have been conducted that have used research designs allowing for attributions of causality (e.g., ADHD causes learning disabilities or vice versa). In contrast, much research has examined the prevalence of academic problems in populations of children with ADHD. Most of these studies defined academic problems as learning disabilities, although there have been great inconsistencies in the definition of this construct across studies. Nevertheless, the term *learning disabilities* will be used here when discussing this literature given the preference for this label by the authors of the studies reviewed. Although substantial numbers of children with ADHD have been found to evidence learning disabilities relative to the normal population, the prevalence rates vary greatly between studies and the association between the two disorders is decidedly less than perfect.

Studies of Causal Relations between ADHD and Learning Disabilities

One informative set of longitudinal studies (Fergusson & Horwood, 1995; Fergusson, Horwood, & Lynskey, 1993; Fergusson, Lynskey, & Horwood, 1997) has been conducted in New Zealand with a sample of over 700 children, and has demonstrated clear linkages between ADHD behaviors in elementary and middle school (based on maternal and teacher ratings) and later levels of academic achievement (middle school through age 18). Specifically, structural equation models demonstrated that early high levels of ADHD behaviors were associated with concurrent and later lower levels of academic achievement.

Rapport, Scanlan, and Denney (1999) attempted to replicate the findings of Fergusson and colleagues (1993) by assessing ADHD symptoms and scholastic achievement in an ethnically diverse sample of 325 Hawaiian schoolchildren. These investigators confirmed the relationship between early ADHD symptoms (based on teacher ratings) and later academic achievement (based on a group-administered achievement test). Further analyses indicated that the influence of ADHD behaviors on scholastic status was mediated by both cognitive (e.g., memory) and behavioral (e.g., classroom deportment) variables.

Although structural equation modeling techniques do not allow direct tests of causality, they do provide measures of relative influence among variables. It is clear from the studies reviewed that ADHD-related behavior (e.g., inattentiveness and impulsivity) directly influences academic achievement in a negative fashion, with higher levels of ADHD symptoms associated with inferior scholastic performance. In fact, inattentiveness may play an even stronger role in influencing reading achievement than do other factors (e.g., family SES) purported to have an effect on reading (Rowe & Rowe, 1992). It is important to note, however, that the relationship between achievement and ADHD is most likely bidirectional, although this assumption was not supported by Fergusson and Horwood's (1993) study.

More Recent Perspectives on the Relationship between ADHD and Learning Difficulties

Researchers continue to investigate, speculate, and write about the relationship between attention deficits and learning difficulties. We discuss some of this work here, and note from the outset that the basic conclusions to be drawn today remain consistent with those of previous work, as delineated in the following section of this chapter. Pastor and Reuben (2002) conducted the largest study examining the prevalence rates of ADHD and learning disabilities, and their co-occurrence. Here, researchers from the National Center for Health Statistics reported pertinent results from the National Health Interview Survey conducted in 1997–1998. Data were gathered for more than 8,600 children between the ages of 6 and 11 within more than 78,000 households determined to be representative of the U.S. population. From the data collected, the researchers generated national estimates of the prevalence of ADHD, the prevalence of learning disabilities, and the prevalence of the co-occurrence of these childhood disorders. A primary finding of the study was that in 1997–1998 over 2.6 million children 6–11 years of age were reported to have ever had a diagnosis of ADHD or learning disabilities. Three percent of children 6–11 years had been diagnosed with ADHD only, 4% with only learning disabilities, and 4% for children with both conditions. These same researchers reported very similar statistics for a sample of 23,000 children with ADHD who were studied between the years 2004 and 2006 (Pastor & Reuben, 2008).

These estimates are consistent with previous ones for prevalence of ADHD in the population of U.S. children (Barkley, 1990, 1998, 2006). Also consistent with previous research were findings that boys were three times more likely than girls to be diagnosed with ADHD (Pastor & Reuben, 2002, 2008). Of further interest, children with a sole diagnosis of learning disabilities were five times more likely to be participating in special education services relative to children with a sole diagnosis of ADHD. This finding is consistent with our previous discussion suggesting that some, but not all, children diagnosed with ADHD will experience significant learning problems warranting special education services. However, in comparing children with ADHD alone, children with learning disabilities alone, and children with both diagnoses, children with co-occurring ADHD and learning disabilities were reported to have the highest rates of prescription drug use and use of mental health services during the previous year (Pastor & Reuben, 2008). By comparison, usage rates of these two supports were next highest for children with ADHD, and lowest among the three groups for children with learning disabilities alone.

On a related prevalence topic, but with more of an educational service delivery focus, Forness and colleagues (Forness & Kavale, 2001; Forness, Kavale, Sweeney, & Crenshaw, 1999) report that children with ADHD represent more than 40% of children in special education programs in the category of emotional disturbance. Furthermore, children with ADHD make up approximately 25% of the population of children receiving special education services for learning disabilities. These researchers go on to suggest that careful diagnosis of the presence or absence of comorbidities such as learning disabilities and conduct disorder is a crucial component to determining appropriate service delivery mechanisms and school-based interventions.

In a similar manner, other prominent researchers in the area agree with the importance of careful diagnosis (Barkley, in press; Shaywitz, Fletcher, & Shaywitz, 1995; Shaywitz & Shaywitz, 1991), while making the case that ADHD and learning disabilities are distinct disorders with different underlying causes. In positing ADHD as a disorder of disinhibition and self-control, with neuropsychological underpinnings, Barkley (1997a) suggests from his review of available research that ADHD involves demonstrated inhibitory and executive function deficits not found among children with learning disabilities. Similarly, Shaywitz and colleagues (1995) basically view learning disabilities as having their foundation in cognitive factors, but view ADHD as having behavioral foundations. They too recognize and underscore the importance of determining the occurrence of one, the other, or both in a given child who is struggling in the classroom with problems of learning and attention.

Summary

Despite the limitations noted, available empirical evidence indicates a consistent relationship between ADHD and significant academic skills deficits (i.e., learning disabilities). At least one out of every three or four children with ADHD is likely to have a specific learning disabilities (for a review, see DuPaul, Gormley, & Laracy, 2013). Furthermore, the majority of children with ADHD will be seen as underachieving academically, presumably due to inconsistent completion of assignments and/or low levels of accuracy on seatwork and tests. Nearly 40% of students with learning disabilities will display significant symptoms of ADHD as well. Thus, there is a great deal of overlap between the two disorders. It is important to note, however, that the association between ADHD and learning disability is not perfect and that they are not one and the same disorder. In fact, most children with ADHD do *not* have learning disabilities and most students with learning disabilities do *not* meet diagnostic criteria for ADHD. Nevertheless, the fact that a significant minority of children in each group can be identified with both disorders must be considered when planning school-based assessment and intervention procedures, as discussed later in the chapter.

It is unclear whether ADHD "causes" or leads to learning disabilities in some children or vice versa. No study to date has been conducted that adequately addresses this issue. It is perhaps a task that is nonachievable. Investigations employing structural equation modeling have shed some light on this question, however. These indicate that ADHD-related behaviors, specifically inattentiveness and hyperactivity–impulsivity, exert a strong negative influence on academic achievement. This relationship may be reciprocal (i.e., level of reading achievement may influence classroom inattentiveness); however, the effect of ADHD on achievement appears to be more clear-cut. In fact, the results of one study (Rowe & Rowe, 1992) indicate that inattentiveness is one of the most prominent factors determining reading achievement.

Although the direction of causality is presently unknown, it is clear that many children with ADHD have academic skills deficits that must be addressed. It has been speculated that certain ADHD presentations may be associated with a greater likelihood of learning problems. For instance, some studies have investigated whether children with ADHD, predominately inattentive presentation, are at higher risk for learning disabilities than children with ADHD, combined presentation. In general, these studies have not found significant differences in the prevalence of learning disabilities between ADHD presentations (Lahey & Carlson, 1992). Conversely, certain subtypes of children with learning disabilities may be at higher risk for behavior control problems, including ADHD. Specifically, Rourke (1988) has identified children with nonverbal learning deficits to be at higher risk for such difficulties. In fact, future research into the association between ADHD and learning disabilities should divide samples into known presentations or subtypes of each disorder rather than grouping children into two heterogeneous samples. The former procedure may provide the best opportunity to identify which children with ADHD are at greatest risk for learning deficits and vice versa.

ASSESSMENT GUIDELINES: ADHD AND ACADEMIC PERFORMANCE DEFICITS

As previously noted, the academic achievement difficulties of children with ADHD can be divided into two categories: academic performance deficits and academic skills deficits. Thus, the school-based assessment of students referred for attention problems must include measures of academic achievement that tap potential performance and skills deficits. The assessment of ADHD is detailed in Chapter 2. The following section is intended to delineate evaluation procedures relevant to the academic functioning of referred children. First, methods to screen for academic skills deficits among children who might have ADHD are discussed. In similar fashion, procedures to screen students with academic skills difficulties (i.e., learning disabilities) for ADHD are covered. Next, because the most frequent achievement problem exhibited by children with ADHD is inconsistent academic performance (e.g., work completion), techniques to assess possible performance deficits are detailed. Finally, methods to determine whether a child's attention problems are due to a lack of academic skills, ADHD, or both are delineated. A case study is presented to further explicate this challenging discrimination.

Screening Procedures

Whenever a child is referred due to attention and behavior control problems possibly related to ADHD, several procedures should be incorporated into the evaluation to screen for academic skills deficits. First, questions related to academic difficulties should be incorporated into the parent and teacher interviews (see Chapter 2; see also Barkley, 1990, 1998, 2006, in press). In particular, the child's teacher should be asked to provide information regarding possible difficulties in each subject matter area. Second, teacher ratings of academic achievement difficulties should be obtained through use of the Academic Performance Rating Scale (APRS; DuPaul, Rapport, & Perriello, 1991) or the Academic Competence Evaluate Scale (ACES; DiPerna & Elliott, 2000). Scores that are greater than or equal to 1.5 standard deviations below the mean for the child's age and gender for the APRS Total Score and Academic Success subscale are considered significant for screening purposes. The child's teacher should be queried about responses to specific APRS items to clarify the specific nature of possible academic difficulties.

In most cases, children with ADHD will be reported to be at or near grade level across all subject areas with no question of academic skills deficits. Ratings on the Academic Success subscale of the APRS would be expected to be within 1.5 standard deviations of the mean. These same children are typically reported to evidence problems with academic performance (e.g., poor completion and/or accuracy on independent seatwork) with below-average ratings for the APRS Total Score and Academic Productivity subscale. Further assessment of academic performance difficulties should be conducted, as discussed below.

If interview and rating scale data indicate potential academic skills deficits, further assessment of learning abilities will be necessary. Although typically a psychoeducational evaluation incorporating IQ and achievement measures is conducted, we prefer a behavioral assessment of academic skills deficits for a number of reasons (e.g., greater relevance to teaching strategies, stronger ecological validity). A behavioral assessment usually will include curriculum-based measurement probes (Shinn, 1989, 1998, 2010), direct observations of task-related behavior, review of written products, and problem-focused interviews with the teacher (for details, see Shapiro, 2011a; Shapiro & Kratochwill, 2000). The assessment of academic functioning should be conducted contemporaneously with further evaluation of ADHD in the context of an RTI framework, as discussed in Chapter 2.

Children referred for an evaluation of possible learning disabilities also should be screened for possible ADHD given that they are at higher risk for the latter disorder relative to their peers. This screening should be conducted even if the referral agent did not specify attention and/ or behavior problems as part of the reason for the evaluation request. Screening procedures for ADHD are discussed in detail in Chapter 2. These include questioning the teacher(s) about the presence of possible ADHD-related behaviors. This is most easily accomplished by having the teacher complete the ADHD Rating Scale–IV (DuPaul, Power, et al., 1998). Using DSM criteria, if six or more of the items in either the inattention or hyperactivity–impulsivity domains are rated as occurring "pretty much" or "very much" of the time, then further assessment of possible ADHD is warranted. If a lesser number of symptoms is reported, further assessment of ADHD would be pursued in cases where other assessment information warranted it.

Assessing Academic Performance Deficits

Even when children with ADHD do not demonstrate significant weaknesses in specific academic skills, they often have difficulty completing independent work in a timely fashion, obtaining accurate scores on classroom tests, studying for exams, taking notes on classroom lectures, and following through on homework assignments. In fact, behaviors related to academic performance are among the most important targets for change in any intervention program devised to address ADHD. Therefore, assessment of academic behaviors should be a standard component of an evaluation concerned with ADHD.

Some of the more important academic behaviors to assess include the completion and accuracy of independent seatwork, completion and accuracy of homework, and organizational skills (e.g., neatness of desk, accuracy of lecture notes). Methods for obtaining these data include direct observations of classroom behavior, teacher ratings, and collection of products (e.g., homework assignments, seatwork) completed by the student. These methods are discussed in greater detail in Chapter

2. It is expected that children with ADHD will complete significantly less work and/or complete tasks in a less accurate fashion than their classmates.

Differentiating between ADHD and Academic Skills Deficits

As reviewed previously, there is a great deal of overlap between ADHD and academic skills deficits or learning disabilities. Thus, many youngsters referred for an evaluation concerning ADHD will be found to exhibit symptoms of both ADHD and academic skills deficits. The vast majority of children with ADHD, however, do not have problems with academic skills per se. Rather, their problems with inattention and impulsivity lead to difficulties following directions; completing tasks in a consistent, accurate fashion; and obtaining test scores that accurately represent their knowledge. Thus, one of the goals of an evaluation where ADHD is evident, is to determine whether a student's academic problems are due to ADHD, learning disabilities, or both. What makes this discrimination particularly difficult is the ambiguity of the many definitions of learning disabilities, as well as the inconsistencies in learning disability definitions across school districts. Regardless of the definition of learning disability employed, the goals relative to an evaluation of ADHD are twofold. The first is to assess whether a child's apparent symptoms of ADHD meet criteria for this disorder. The second is to gather information to help judge the extent to which a student's academic problems are accounted for by difficulties with inattention, impulsivity, and overactivity.

Several factors should be considered in determining whether a child's problems with attention in school, impulse control, and activity level are due to ADHD or are secondary to academic skills deficits. These considerations are listed in the context of three possible scenarios:

1. If the data collected in the course of the evaluation, as described in Chapter 2, indicate clinically significant levels of ADHD symptoms evident across settings on a chronic basis, it is likely that the child's academic problems are secondary to ADHD. In this case, parent and teacher interview data, parent and teacher ratings, and the results of direct observations are consistent in placing the child's ADHD-related behavior in the extreme range for his or her gender and age. Further assessment of possible learning disabilities is warranted only if there is some question of below-average *ability* in one or more academic areas.

2. A second scenario is one in which the assessment data consistently indicate that few symptoms of ADHD are present and those

that are observed are exhibited primarily in academic situations (e.g., classroom instruction, independent seatwork). In such cases, parent and teacher interview data, parent and teacher ratings, and direct observation data will be in the normal range for ADHD symptoms. If academic problems are present, then hypotheses other than ADHD must be explored, including the possibility of academic skills deficits.

3. Conclusions based on the above two scenarios are relatively straightforward. More difficult professional judgments must be made in cases where assessment data are inconsistent relative to the frequency, severity, and cross-situational pervasiveness of possible ADHD symptomatology. For instance, a child's teachers may report significant ADHD symptoms, while his or her parents report few, if any, attention and behavior control problems. Although the general problem of interpreting inconsistent assessment data is discussed in Chapter 2, the specific discrimination between ADHD and academic skills deficits will be aided by considering the following:

a. Children with ADHD typically obtain clinically significant ratings on parent and teacher ratings of disruptive behavior problems in addition to ADHD (e.g., Aggression subscale on the CBCL). Children with learning disabilities in the absence of ADHD usually do not obtain high scores in these dimensions (Barkley, DuPaul, & McMurray, 1990). Furthermore, children with learning disabilities rarely are impulsive, disinhibited, and aggressive, whereas children with ADHD are more likely to display such difficulties (Barkley, in press).

b. Children with learning disabilities obtain average-range scores on measures that tap the situational pervasiveness of behavior (e.g., Home Situations Questionnaire [HSQ], Barkley, 1990; School Situations Questionnaire [SSQ], Barkley, 1990) and attention (e.g., HSQ-R, DuPaul & Barkley, 1992; SSQ-R, DuPaul & Barkley, 1992) problems, while those with ADHD usually receive high scores for the number of problem situations and the mean severity of behavior problems on these measures (Barkley, DuPaul, & McMurray, 1990).

c. Children with learning disabilities who do not have ADHD usually are observed to exhibit rates of on-task behavior and work completion that are no different from their normal counterparts when observations of independent seatwork are conducted (Barkley, DuPaul, & McMurray, 1990).

d. Students with learning disabilities also differ from those with ADHD with respect to the onset and pervasiveness of apparent ADHD symptoms. Usually, children who are exhibiting problems with attention and behavior control due to academic skills deficits lack an early childhood history of hyperactivity and problem behavior. The latter is a hallmark of ADHD as it is typically a disorder with an early onset. In contrast, the attention problems of students with learning disabilities usually arise in middle childhood (i.e., third or fourth grade) and are exhibited only in specific situations. Usually, attention problems are reported to occur only when they are receiving academic instruction and/or completing work in their most problematic subject areas. Alternatively, children with ADHD are likely to exhibit ADHD symptoms across most, if not all, school and home situations.

   e. Children with ADHD alone are likely to obtain scores on individual academic achievement tests that are similar to their peers, in contrast to the below-average scores usually obtained by students with learning disabilities.

Overall, children with academic skills deficits can be differentiated from those with ADHD on the basis of the onset, severity, and situational pervasiveness of observed ADHD symptoms. In particular, the more specific the attention and behavior problems are to academic situations and tasks, the more likely it is that these difficulties are secondary to academic skills deficits rather than to ADHD.

CASE EXAMPLE

David was an 8-year-old boy referred by his second-grade teacher. Concerns were raised regarding problems with inattention and difficulties of an academic nature. David was reported to exhibit significant difficulties completing assigned work within a reasonable time period and to daydream frequently during classroom instruction. He displayed these problems on an inconsistent basis across school days. The teacher was particularly concerned that David was making very slow progress with reading skills and had difficulties comprehending material he had just finished reading.

   An interview with David's mother indicated his birth, early development, and medical histories were unremarkable. His activity level as a toddler and preschooler was described as "normal for a boy." His father was reported to have evidenced learning problems and possible ADHD as a child, but no other significant problems were reported for family members. His mother reported no significant problems handling David's behavior at home and described his peer relationships as "excellent." David was not involved in special services or professional therapy at the time of the evaluation, although his mother did report recently placing him on a modified "sugar-free and food-additive-free" diet with resultant mild changes in behavior control. No formal behavior management strategies were being used in either home or school settings.

Initially the school team suggested several instructional modifications for implementation in the general education classroom. Although some improvement was noted, David's response to intervention was below goals set by the team. A subsequent psychoeducational evaluation was conducted by the school psychologist, which included intelligence testing and several individual achievement tests. Results suggested David was of average intelligence with a relative weakness in verbal abilities. Achievement testing indicated a number of deficits in language and reading functioning. Based on these results, the school team suggested that David receive academic support in reading and language arts skills several times per week with a resource room teacher.

Several measures were employed to evaluate whether David might have ADHD. A diagnostic interview with David's mother was conducted wherein only six of the 18 DSM-5 (American Psychiatric Association, 2013) symptoms of ADHD were reported as present on a frequent basis. These included distractibility and often shifting from one uncompleted activity to another. Notably, David was reported to evidence inattention only on tasks that were school related (e.g., reading), but was able to complete assigned household chores in a reliable fashion. No problems with impulsivity or overactivity were reported. Further reports indicated that David did not exhibit behaviors related to any other behavior disorder including oppositional defiant disorder, conduct disorder, depression, or anxiety disorder.

David's mother completed several rating scales to document the severity of his behavior control problems relative to other boys his age. Her responses on the CBCL resulted in a normal range profile (i.e., T-scores < 65) across all clinical scales including those related to ADHD. On the ADHD Rating Scale–IV, only five of the 18 symptoms of ADHD were reported to occur on a frequent basis. Ratings on the HSQ-R indicated mild attention problems were present only in selected home settings (e.g., when asked to complete homework). Scores on the Social Skills Improvement System (SSIS; Gresham & Elliott, 2008) were in the normal range. Thus, parent ratings did not indicate ADHD symptoms to be problematic, nor were these seen as pervasive across settings.

David's second-grade teacher completed similar questionnaires. Her responses on the Teacher Report Form of the CBCL resulted in borderline significant ratings (i.e., T-score = 66, or greater than the 93rd percentile) on the Attention Problems subscale. Remaining scales, including those related to other disruptive behavior disorders, were in the normal range. Scores on the SSIS did not indicate clinically significant levels of peer relationship difficulties. On the ADHD Rating Scale–IV, five of the 18 symptoms of ADHD were reported to occur on a frequent basis. On the SSQ-R, mild attention problems were reported to occur across most structured classroom settings. The most significant problems related to ADHD that were reported were with respect to concentration and completion of tasks, not with impulse control or hyperactivity. Thus, the symptoms reported by David's teacher were more consistent with ADHD, predominantly inattentive presentation.

David was observed in his regular classroom on several occasions using the Behavioral Observation of Students in Schools (BOSS; Shapiro, 2011b). Each observation took place during a time when David was assigned independent seatwork related to reading and language arts. Averaged over three 20-minute observations, David was observed to be actively or passively engaged approximately 80% of the time, although these percentages ranged from a low of 53% to a high of 90%. Thus, his task-related attention was quite variable across days. David exhibited off-task motor (e.g., fidgety restless) behavior during an average of only 28% of the observation intervals. David completed an average of 80% of the work assigned to him at a relatively low accuracy level (i.e., 74%). Although he did evidence some behaviors related to ADHD, his main problems were related to his understanding and accurate completion of assigned tasks.

In summary, most of the data collected in the course of this evaluation were not consistent with the conclusion that David met the criteria for a diagnosis of ADHD. In fact, only one piece of information, teacher ratings on the CBCL, was in the clinically significant range for this disorder. The remaining measures were in the normal range, including parent interview data, parent and teacher ratings on the ADHD Rating Scale–IV, parent ratings on the CBCL, and behavioral observation data. Behaviors related to ADHD were strictly in the realm of inattention and, more specifically, attention during academic tasks only. According to his parents, David was quite attentive to household chores and other nonacademic tasks assigned to him. Thus, David's problems with inattention were seen to be a reflection of his frustration in attempting tasks that were quite difficult for him rather than representing ADHD. Recommendations included further behavioral assessment of possible academic skills deficits to determine appropriate goals and procedures to increase his scholastic competencies. Although it was assumed that improving his academic skills would enhance his task-related behavior, the latter was directly targeted for change using a classroom-based contingency management program combined with a daily report card system (see Chapter 5).

Clearly, problems of learning and achievement will be high priorities for school-based personnel tasked with supporting students with ADHD. In addition, school-based professionals in these roles must also remain cognizant of co-occurring externalizing problems such as conduct disorder and oppositional defiant disorder.

ADHD AND OTHER EXTERNALIZING DISORDERS

As noted earlier in this chapter, oppositional defiant disorder and conduct disorder co-occur in approximately 30 to 50% of children and adolescents diagnosed with ADHD (Spencer et al., 2007). Conduct disorder involves serious misbehavior, that being usually aggressive or destructive, and is oriented toward people, animals, or property that may be characterized as belligerent, destructive, threatening, physically cruel, deceitful, disobedient, or dishonest (American Psychiatric Association, 2013). Often, behavior associated with conduct disorder also is illegal (e.g., stealing). In contrast, oppositional defiant disorder may be diagnosed when children or adolescents display consistent patterns of tantrums, arguing, and angry or disruptive behavior toward parents and/or other authority figures (American Psychiatric Association, 2013).

Connor and Doerfler (2008) studied 200 clinic-referred children and adolescents who were diagnosed with ADHD, with the intent of examining the extent to which clinical and/or functional impairment differences might be found between three groups: children with ADHD, children with ADHD and comorbid oppositional defiant disorder, and children with ADHD and comorbid conduct disorder. Their findings indicated, based on obtained parent ratings, that the combined ADHD + conduct disorder group was rated the highest of the three groups on levels of aggression and delinquency, followed by the ADHD/ODD group in the middle of these ratings, and the ADHD alone group having the lowest rated levels of aggression and delinquency. The combined ADHD/CD group also was found to have significantly higher scores, relative to the other two groups, on a measure of functional impairment. Connor and Doerfler suggested their findings indicate the need to consider child psychiatric diagnoses separately, and that the three groups reported on should receive differential treatment considerations, such as more aggressive treatments, higher doses of intervention, and more careful monitoring with the ADHD comorbid groups.

Similarly, Booster and colleagues (2012), in a study of 416 children with ADHD, found significantly more functional impairment among those with a comorbid disorder relative to ADHD alone. Specifically, these researchers found that children for whom ADHD was accompanied by a comorbid externalizing disorder (with or without a concomitant internalizing comorbidity) displayed poorer social skills than those with ADHD alone. They also found that children experiencing concomitant problems with ADHD and both an externalizing and internalizing comorbidity exhibited greater homework problems than their ADHD peers with fewer than two types of comorbidity. Finally, they reported that older children displayed significantly poorer social skills and greater homework problems as compared with younger children. These results formed the basis for concluding that practitioners need to pay careful attention to addressing both social skills and homework problems among children with ADHD and comorbid behavior disorders.

ADHD AND INTERNALIZING DISORDERS

Internalizing disorders of childhood include both depression and anxiety disorders. As noted previously, Spencer and colleagues (2007) reported that depression is likely to occur in every one out of two or three children with ADHD (e.g., 29–45%). Similarly, anxiety disorders occur in about 25% of cases of ADHD (Jarrett & Ollendick, 2008).

In an effort to elucidate comorbid ADHD and depression, Blackman, Ostrander, and Herman (2005) conducted a study to compare the clinical, social, and academic functioning children with co-occurring depression with ADHD (ADHD + depression), relative to children with ADHD alone, and children without ADHD. Their participants consisted of 130 children who were not experiencing problems, another 130 children were identified as experiencing ADHD related problems alone, and an additional 26 children were diagnosed with ADHD + depression. Consistent with many prior studies, children in both ADHD groups were significantly more impaired than typically developing controls. Furthermore, children in the ADHD + depression group were more impaired with respect to social competence than were children in the ADHD alone group; however, both ADHD groups were equally impaired regarding academic performance. These findings imply the need for caregivers to be cognizant of the potential need for greater supports in the area of social functioning for children and adolescents presenting with ADHD and depression.

Understanding the intersections of ADHD and depression may also require a further look at parenting, as clarified by Ostrander and Herman (2006). Here, these researchers examined the roles of parent behavior management and child locus of control in mediating the relationship between ADHD and depression. Their study involved a sample of 232 children with ADHD and 130 community controls. Results indicated that for older subjects (10 years and older), cognitive locus of control partially mediated the relationships between ADHD and parent management and depression. Findings also indicated that parent management partially mediated the relationships of ADHD with locus of control and depression. For children under 8 years of age, however, locus of control did not mediate the effects of parent management and ADHD on depression. Rather, for the younger group, only parent management—an environmental variable—explained the relationship between ADHD and depression. Finally, the results indicated that for children 8–9 years old, both locus of control and parent management partially were responsible for the ADHD–depression relationship; however, similar to the younger children, locus of control did not mediate the parent management–depression relationships.

On the basis of these findings, Ostrander and Herman (2006) suggest that effective interventions to treat and prevent depression in children with ADHD may vary depending on the child's age. For example, interventions to treat comorbid depression in younger children should target altering problematic parenting style, because they found that parenting marked by inconsistent expectations and unpredictable consequences was associated with symptoms of depression in children with ADHD. The researchers went on to say that "Parent management training to promote consistency, structure, and monitoring—either alone or in combination with cognitive interventions for the child—may help alleviate some of the internalizing symptoms in younger children with ADHD. For older children with ADHD who are also depressed, interventions need to expand beyond a focus on parenting practices and include altering negative cognitions around lack of perceived control" (Ostrander & Herman, 2006, p. 96).

ADHD WITH COMORBID ANXIETY

Anxiety disorders in children and adolescents can take several forms. The most common is generalized anxiety disorder in which children worry excessively about things such as family issues, school performance, and peer acceptance/relationship, for example. Separation anxiety disorder is a condition involving significant difficulties separating from or being away from parents. Children may also experience obsessive–compulsive disorder, which is characterized by thoughts (obsessions) that are unwanted and intrusive, as well as by feeling obligated to repeatedly perform rituals and routines (compulsions) in efforts to ease anxiety.

Two recent reviews can help further our understanding of both conceptual and practical issues in working with children presenting with comorbid ADHD and anxiety disorders. Schatz and Rostain (2006) reviewed available research from 1998 to 2005 on this particular comorbidity, with an eye toward explicating various cognitive and neurological explanatory models. The more practical findings of their review are summarized briefly here. First, their review suggested that anxiety in ADHD may partially ameliorate response inhibition deficits as well as impulsivity (i.e., anxiety symptoms may serve a protective role). Alternatively, there is evidence that anxiety in children with ADHD may further impair working memory deficits. Schatz and Rostain speculate that anxiety may help regulate impulsive behaviors associated with ADHD because of deficits in typical inhibitory mechanisms. Clearly, more research is needed to examine the degree to which anxiety symptoms diminish impulsivity associated with ADHD.

Jarrett and Ollendick (2008) also reviewed the literature on comorbid ADHD and anxiety, with the intent of both improving our understanding of this specific comorbidity, and informing future research and practice. Their efforts first framed available research around a set of contexts for informing explanations of the ADHD–anxiety relationship. These related contexts included genetics, temperament, neurological functioning, family influences, and temporal relationships (e.g., relative onset) between the two. Several conclusions follow from their review. First, ADHD and anxiety appear to have independent genetic transmission. Next, potential mechanisms for ADHD–anxiety comorbidity are postulated indicating a role for both neurological factors (e.g., interaction of both cortical and subcortical brain malfunction) and family influences (e.g., high levels of parent anxiety and overprotective approaches to parenting). Third, evidence supports that there are multiple pathways relating the two areas of functioning (e.g., evidence for both anxiety occurring first during development, and for ADHD occurring first). Finally, the primary and abundantly clear conclusion Jarrett and Ollendick draw from their review is that ADHD–anxiety comorbidity is not clearly understood as a function of extant literature; likely, the safest conclusion is that there are multiple viable explanations for the relationship.

From a practical point of view, Jarrett and Ollendick (2008) discussed the potential value of cognitive-behavioral therapy in treating comorbid ADHD–anxiety. Here the authors noted the work of Nigg, Goldsmith, and Sachek (2004) who discussed two potential pathways for the ADHD–anxiety relationship including early regulatory difficulties leading to problems managing anxiety, and another pathway wherein higher anxiety produces cognitive or regulatory dysfunction. The latter pathway involves intact executive functioning that is compromised by high levels of anxiety (Jarrett & Ollendick, 2008). They further suggest that future work on behavioral and cognitive-behavioral interventions might best focus on distinguishing (e.g., subtyping) based on these two pathways, and would likely be more successful with the latter pathway.

These same researchers have begun to explore intervention strategies for comorbid ADHD + anxiety. Jarrett and Ollendick (2012) designed and evaluated what they term an integrative treatment protocol for ADHD, comorbid with anxiety. The intervention consisted of a 10-week program combining parent training in behavior management and family based cognitive-behavioral therapy—targeting ADHD and anxiety, respectively. Working with eight children between the ages of 8 and 12, diagnosed with ADHD–anxiety disorders, the researchers found significant treatment effects on both ADHD and anxiety-related symptoms between pretreatment and posttreatment measures. This work is interesting in documenting concurrently delivered intervention strategies, for two different problems, to be effective simultaneously.

While Jarrett and Ollendick (2012) focused concurrently on both ADHD and anxiety-related symptoms, another recent treatment study has focused solely on the anxiety portion of comorbid ADHD–anxiety. Here, Houghton, Alsalmi, Tan, Taylor, and Durkin (in press) used a cognitive-behavioral approach to treating anxiety in nine 13- to 16-year-old adolescents with ADHD–anxiety. The weekly treatment protocol had each of the adolescent participants focus on four individualized anxiety-inducing events/times in their daily lives, and learn to use strategies intended to reduce their anxiousness. Outcome measures consisted of both self-recorded anxiety and self-report ratings of anxiety symptoms. Results indicated the cognitive-behavioral treatment approach produced significant decreases in anxiety across participants.

ADHD AND ADJUSTMENT PROBLEMS

In addition to experiencing comorbid learning and psychiatric disorders, children and adolescents with ADHD evince a wide range of adjustment problems and problems of daily living. As the following studies document, these problems vary by age and gender, and range from problems of adjustment and mood to educational problems, substance use, and risk for eating disorders.

Barkley, Fischer, Smallish, and Fletcher (2006) reported on a follow-up study of 19- to 25-year-old participants, originally seen a minimum of 13 years previously. Participants included those in a "hyperactive" group and a control group. The authors noted that 32% of the hyperactive group failed to complete high school. They were rated lower in job performance by employers relative to control group members, as well as had been fired from more jobs. In addition, by comparison with the controls, they had fewer close friends and more social problems. Also of note, more participants in the hyperactive group become parents (38% vs. 4%) as young adults, and had been treated for sexually transmitted disease (16% vs. 4%). These findings raise concerns about adaptive functioning in early adulthood that are similar to those of previously reported research, and add to the list of concerns, those of precocious sexual activity and early parenthood.

Another descriptive study focused on the experiences of adolescents with low, medium, and high levels of ADHD characteristics (Whalen et al., 2002). These researchers used unique methods of inquiry they refer to as "experience sampling." More than 150 participants kept a log of their behaviors, moods, and social contexts, two times per hour across two separate 4-day time periods. Adolescents with high levels of ADHD characteristics reported more negative affect/moods including anger, anxiety, stress, and sadness, as well as lower amounts of happiness and well-being. Additionally, participants with moderate levels of ADHD symptoms reported similar patterns of mood/affect relative to the low-level-ADHD characteristics group. Furthermore, male participants in the middle- and high-ADHD groups demonstrated higher levels of anxiety relative to low-ADHD males, but the low-ADHD females reported higher rates of anxiety relative to the other groups. Finally, the researchers reported elevated rates of nonacademic pursuits, and alcohol and tobacco use among the adolescents with ADHD characteristics, as well as more exposure to peers and less exposure to family members. These findings provide further evidence of the need to be concerned with the developmental trajectories, adjustment, and health/outcome risks of teens with ADHD, while also suggesting there may be gender differences in these risks.

Other researchers have also begun to explicate gender-related issues in the development of children and adolescents with ADHD. For example, Hinshaw, Owens, Sami, and Fargeon (2006) reported the results of a 5-year prospective study of girls with ADHD, ages 11–18, who had been diagnosed in childhood with ADHD. The study included a matched comparison group without ADHD. Girls with ADHD were found to be at risk for developing and/or displaying higher rates of both internalizing and externalizing symptoms. In addition, girls with ADHD scored significantly higher with respect to symptoms of eating disorders, and significantly lower with respect to social skills and academic performance. These results suggest the need to monitor adolescent girls with ADHD for a range of adjustment problems, including both academic and social skills problems, as well as eating problems/disorders.

It is clear that children and adolescents with ADHD are at risk for, and will present with, a wide range of behavior and adjustment problems across social, academic, employment, and daily living domains. The intervention and support needs indicated by these problems are the focus of the final sections of this chapter.

IMPLICATIONS OF COMORBIDITY FOR ASSESSMENT, MONITORING, AND INTERVENTION

High rates of comorbid academic, adjustment, and social problems in children and adolescents with ADHD create the need for a heightened level of attention and consideration of such co-occurring problems in school and mental health settings. For example, as already detailed in the assessment chapter of this book, diagnostic evaluations should always include broadband rating scales and broad-ranging informant interviews that can help screen for co-occurring problems. In addition, children and adolescents diagnosed with ADHD should be periodically screened and monitored for adjustment problems, especially throughout their adolescent years. The focus of such screening might include overall functioning in the areas of adjustment and mood, substance use, sexual activity, eating and body image (especially for females), and academics. With familial ADHD comorbidity in mind, initial evaluations and treatment planning should also include brief interview-based screening for ADHD and adjustment problems with parents.

IMPLICATIONS OF COMORBIDITY FOR TREATMENT

In keeping with the zeitgeist of contemporary treatment for ADHD and related problems, the first implication of comorbidity for treatment is that of relying on evidence-based treatments. As Pelham and Fabiano (2008) and Evans, Owens, and Bunford (in press) have concluded in their reviews of the ADHD treatment literature, behavioral intervention is the main evidence-based psychological treatment available, and it should be delivered with a focus on functional outcomes/impairments. As discussed in Chapter 2, functional analyses should be used to design interventions in the selection of target behaviors and identification of environmental factors (e.g., antecedents and consequences) maintaining these behaviors.

Using a functional impairment framework then, implies that supports for children and adolescents with ADHD will need to variously assess, monitor, and target for treatment the following areas of functioning: behaviors related to ADHD such as impulsive behavior and decision making; academic achievement and behaviors that enable it, such as work completion and accuracy, and academic organization; intrapersonal adjustment, including affect, mood, and emotion regulation; interpersonal relationships including those with peers and adults; and family adjustment relative to parenting and living with a child with ADHD. Further considerations of the severity, chronicity, and prioritization of current presenting problems can also be useful to creating a treatment/support plan. Attention to these factors will help the practitioner to avoid the problems inherent in a one-size-fits-all approach to the treatment of ADHD.

The determination of whether a student's academic, behavioral, and adjustment difficulties are due to ADHD, an academic skills problem, another disorder or adjustment problem, or some combination of all of these issues has direct implications for classroom intervention (Cantwell & Baker, 1991). The behaviors targeted for change, the treatment settings, and the specific interventions employed will vary as a function of assessment decisions. As discussed in Chapter 5, the usual treatment targets for a student with ADHD are behaviors related to classroom deportment, such as paying attention to instruction, staying seated, and following classroom rules. To the extent that academic performance difficulties are present, then certain scholastic behaviors will be targeted as well, including timely completion of seatwork and/or accuracy of written work. For those children with academic skills deficits, achievement-related behaviors and academic skill development are the primary targets for intervention. These would include not only behaviors related to independent seatwork but other academic survival skills as well, such as correct responding during reading group, accurate note taking during lectures, and providing correct answers to written test items. When a child is found to have both ADHD and an academic skills deficit, scholastic behaviors typically serve as the primary targets for intervention. This is due to the frequent finding that when academic performance is enhanced, classroom deportment often improves as well (DuPaul & Eckert, 1997; Hinshaw, 1992; McGee & Share, 1988). It is not unusual, however, to find circumstances where both academic and deportment behaviors must be targeted for change to obtain consistent and durable effects. Furthermore, for those youngsters who have ADHD and learning deficits, extrinsic motivational programming must be combined with academic interventions regardless of the specific behaviors targeted for change (Hinshaw, 1992).

Intervention programs designed to treat children with ADHD commonly are applied across a variety of settings given the cross-situational pervasiveness of symptoms of this disorder (Barkley, in press). For instance, token reinforcement systems may be applied across a variety of situations (e.g., playground, classroom, cafeteria) in both school and home settings in an attempt to enhance compliance with rules and attention to assigned tasks. In contrast, the primary intervention setting for children with academic skills deficits is the classroom. Although a number of classroom settings may be involved, treatment of academic difficulties rarely takes place outside of the classroom, yet strong arguments for adjunctive, home–school interventions have been made (Kelley, 1990). Those children with both ADHD and academic skills deficits will require treatment in multiple settings implemented by a number of professionals. In such cases, the need for effective communication and collaboration among the individuals involved in the child's treatment is obvious (see Chapters 5 and 9).

As discussed in subsequent chapters, the two most effective interventions for ADHD are stimulant medication (e.g., MPH) and contingency management procedures. Although the latter can involve changes to both antecedent conditions (e.g., more frequent prompts to pay attention) and consequences (e.g., positive reinforcement for task completion), motivational programming has received most of the emphasis in the ADHD treatment literature (DuPaul, Eckert, & Vilardo, 2012; Evans et al., in press; Pfiffner & DuPaul, in press). Thus, behaviorally based classroom interventions for ADHD usually include token reinforcement systems combined with response cost, wherein contingencies are available at school, at home, or in both settings in order to motivate the child to attend to assigned tasks and classroom rules (see Chapter 5 for details). In contrast, academic skills deficits are not directly enhanced by pharmacotherapy and are usually treated with psychoeducational programming designed to ameliorate presumed processing deficits that underlie the child's learning problems (Semrud-Clikeman et al., 1992; see also Crenshaw, Kavale, Forness, & Reeve, 1999, for a meta-analytic review of psychostimulant effects on behavioral and academic outcomes). The psychoeducational programming approach remains quite prevalent in this country despite a lack of evidence for its efficacy (e.g., Kavale & Mattson, 1983). Behaviorally and instructionally based interventions for academic skills deficits that have received empirical support include modifications to both antecedent and consequent conditions (see Shinn & Walker, 2010). Although motivational programming similar to that employed for ADHD has been found helpful in addressing academic skills deficits, there is an equivalent emphasis in the literature on changing antecedent stimulus conditions (e.g., rate of presentation of academic material). Thus, even though both ADHD and academic skills deficits can be treated behaviorally, the specific parameters of the intervention program will vary as a function of diagnostic status.

When children and adolescents present with comorbid ADHD and internalizing disorders, it appears that combinations of either behavioral and cognitive-behavioral treatment strategies are warranted, as seen with the Jarrett and Ollendick (2012) study discussed in an earlier section. Their combined treatment strategy was based on concurrently delivering two evidence-based treatments originally designed to target only one of the presenting problems (e.g., ADHD or anxiety problems). Programs and strategies that may be useful to consider in the presence of comorbid conditions could include, for example, the Coping Cat program for the treatment of child/adolescent anxiety (Kendall & Hedtke, 2006), the Adolescents Coping with Depression and Coping with Stress courses for the treatment and prevention of depression, respectively (free download available from the Kaiser Permanente Center for Health Research, 2013). For problems of comorbid ADHD and other externalizing behavior problems, parent- and teacher-delivered behavior management programs, such as those associated with the Incredible Years programs (see Webster-Stratton & Reid, 2014) and the Defiant Children/Defiant Teens programs (Barkley, 2013a; Barkley, Edwards, & Robin, 1999), will likely be helpful.

The intervention programs noted may be delivered in school-based settings by appropriately trained professionals or be delivered in community-based treatment settings. Furthermore, these programs could also be supplemented with appropriate individualized school-based counseling to help support the individual development and adjustment of students with ADHD (see Plotts & Lasser, 2013, for a thorough treatment of school-based counseling applications relevant to this discussion).

ADHD AND SPECIAL EDUCATION

Prior to 1991, students with ADHD were not eligible to receive special education services unless they qualified for such services on the basis of existing classification categories (e.g., specific learning disability, seriously emotionally disturbed). Thus, the vast majority of children with ADHD were placed in general education classrooms and minimal alterations were made to their instruction. Due to the intense lobbying efforts of a variety of professional and parent groups, a change in the interpretation of federal guidelines was issued by the U.S. Department of Education in 1991 (see Hakola, 1992). In this section, we provide suggestions to school psychologists on how to determine whether a specific child with ADHD requires special education services.

Presently, students classified as having ADHD may qualify for special education services in one of three ways. First, a child with both ADHD and another disability (e.g., learning disability) could qualify for special education services under one of the existing disability categories defined in the 2004 Individuals with Disabilities Education Act (IDEA).

A second possibility for special education eligibility is under the other health impaired (OHI) category. OHI includes chronic or acute health problems that result in limited alertness, which adversely affects educational performance. Thus, students with ADHD should be classified as eligible for services under the OHI category in instances where the ADHD is a chronic or acute health problem that results in limited alertness that adversely affects educational performance to the extent that special education services are needed.

The inclusion of ADHD as an OHI has been reaffirmed with the 2004 reauthorization of IDEIA (hereafter referred to as "IDEIA 2004"; Public Law 108-446). Furthermore, the OHI provision has been the most commonly applied criterion to judge a student's eligibility for special education services on the basis of having ADHD; the OHI category has been the fastest growing category over that past two decades. This provision clearly states that if the child's alertness is limited by chronic ADHD to the extent that his or her educational performance suffers, then the child may require special education services. The previous sentence describes most, if not all, children diagnosed with ADHD, as, by definition, it is a chronic disorder wherein they exhibit limited alertness and their academic performance is deleteriously affected. The difficult decision, therefore, is whether the child actually *needs* special education programming (i.e., the second criterion for determining special education eligibility, the first being the presence of a disability) to address these difficulties and/or academic competencies or whether interventions in the general education classroom will be sufficient.

A final criterion that could be used to determine a child's eligibility for instructional modifications on the basis of having ADHD is contained in Section 504 of the Federal Rehabilitation Act of 1973. Such modifications may or may not require the provision of special education services. This is a civil rights law that states that schools must address the needs of children with disabilities as competently as the needs of typically developing students are met. In order to qualify for Section 504 consideration, a student must have a mental or physical impairment that substantially limits a major life activity (e.g., learning, concentration, social interaction). Substantial limitations are evaluated with respect to the average student in the general population without the effects of mitigating measures (e.g., medication). Thus, even children with ADHD who are not eligible for special services under IDEIA 2004 (Public Law 108-446) could be considered in need of individualized intervention on the basis of Section 504.

If the above regulations are interpreted loosely, one could make a case that most children with ADHD are eligible to receive some degree of special education services. Given the high percentage of children already receiving such services and the limited database supporting the overall efficacy of special education, however, this may not be a prudent course of action. Rather, as is the case for children with other behavior disorders, one of the main criteria for receipt of special education services should be the child's response to interventions in the general education classroom (Gresham, 1991). Thus, the diagnosis of ADHD does not necessarily warrant the receipt of special education services, unless the child's behavior has not changed as a function of regular classroom interventions (Jimerson, Burns, & VanDerHeyden, 2007; National Association of School Psychologists, 2011).

From the standpoint of practice, a child diagnosed with ADHD who also is experiencing learning and/or achievement problems would likely be evaluated for special education eligibility purposes following a lack of responsiveness to interventions delivered within general education settings (see Telzrow & Tankersley, 2000). If that child is found eligible for special education services, a team of professionals would then design, implement, and evaluate an individualized educational program. If that child is found not eligible for special education services, school personnel would remain responsible for removing barriers to learning in the general education classroom/instruction. This removal of barriers has been referred to commonly as creating a 504 accommodation plan (see Zirkel & Aleman, 2000, for a thorough treatment of Section 504 and students with disabilities).

In designing accommodations, educators should consider both the potential accommodation itself and the barrier to learning that is being removed. For example, in providing a student with task modifications (TMs) in the form of allowing a choice of assignments, the barrier to learning of having one and only one assignment to work on is being removed. Similarly, allowing a student with ADHD to complete fewer items on an independent seatwork task (at the same level of accuracy expected of peers) is removing aspects of the assigned tasks known to exacerbate ADHD-related problems in the classroom—namely, repetitive work items. It should be noted, however, that there is scant empirical evidence supporting the use of educational accommodations (for a review, see Harrison, Bunford, Evans, & Owens, 2013). Thus, although typically recommended accommodations may have face validity, practitioners should be aware that these are not evidence based, for the most part.

Zirkel (2013) has designed a checklist for determining the legal eligibility for special education services in accordance with the regulations enumerated previously (see Appendix 3.1). Using this checklist as a guide, the following steps should be followed in determining whether a specific child will require special education services for ADHD:

1. Conduct an evaluation of ADHD and related difficulties, as discussed in Chapter 2. If the child is found to meet the criteria for ADHD, then, by definition, he or she has a chronic condition that significantly limits alertness, thus satisfying two components of the eligibility criteria for special education services under the OHI category.

2. If the child is found to exhibit behaviors related to one of the existing classification categories of IDEIA 2004 (e.g., learning disability; Public Law 108-446), then special education services may be warranted.

3. If the child does not qualify for special education services under one of the existing categories, then two more determinations must be made. First, does the child's ADHD-related behavior in the classroom significantly limit his or her educational performance? This can be determined using academic performance data, as discussed in Chapter 2. Usually, some aspect of a child's academic achievement is deleteriously affected by his or her ADHD symptomatology. Thus, some form of intervention will be necessary as Section 504 stipulates such action given that the disability substantially impairs a major life activity (i.e., learning). The typical initial step is to design and implement an intervention program in the general education classroom (see Chapter 5). Such programs will include modifications to the child's instructional program based on behavioral principles. Second, the child also may be referred to his or her physician for consideration of a trial of psychotropic medication, as discussed in Chapter 7.

4. The last, and most critical, criterion for special education eligibility is whether the child *needs* such services because of his or her ADHD. This criterion could be interpreted in a variety of ambiguous ways. Therefore, the most objective way to reach a decision regarding this criterion is through evaluating the efficacy of general education classroom interventions (Gresham, 1991; Jimerson et al., 2007). Baseline data should be collected on a number of target behaviors prior to implementing a specific intervention (including medication). After implementing the recommended treatment(s), data are collected again on the same variables to assess behavioral change. If the child does not exhibit significant improvement following a trial of general education classroom

intervention(s), one of three possible courses of action is followed. First, changes could be made to the intervention program in the general education classroom. Second, the child could receive some form of special education programming. Third, changes could be made in general education interventions and special education programming could be provided.

5. Whether special education services are provided or not, interventions addressing the child's ADHD will be necessary. The efficacy of both general and special education interventions should be evaluated on a continuous basis to determine when changes in programming and/or placement are necessary.

SUMMARY

Most children with ADHD will exhibit significant problems with academic performance, such as slow or insufficient work completion, inconsistent accuracy on seatwork and homework, and poor study skills. Furthermore, about 25 to 40% of these children will display academic skills that are significantly below average, and therefore will be characterized as having a learning disability. The fact that academic problems are consistently associated with ADHD has direct implications for the assessment and treatment of these students. The evaluation of ADHD must not only be directed toward behavior control difficulties but should include measures of academic performance as well. Furthermore, such children should routinely be screened for academic skills deficits, with additional assessment of academic functioning conducted as necessary. In similar fashion, intervention programs designed to treat ADHD must include target behaviors related to academic performance. In the case of children who have both ADHD and academic skills deficits, treatment must be directed toward ameliorating both conditions simultaneously.

Many students with ADHD will present with comorbid problems of adjustment, including learning deficits, anxiety, depression, other conduct problems, and difficulties of interpersonal adjustment. Such comorbidity may occur either simultaneously or developmentally. Typically, functional impairment will increase with comorbidity (Crawford et al., 2006), and may become more intense over the course of development from childhood to adolescence (Harrison, Vannest, & Reynolds, 2011). It is incumbent upon school-based professionals to be aware of these issues and problems, and to work together with families and community-based professionals to provide appropriate information, screening, monitoring, and supports, as necessary to maximize the likelihood of school success for students with ADHD.

Finally, federal guidelines allow for the provision of special education services to children with ADHD when they meet the criteria for learning disabilities, emotional disturbance, or OHI limiting their educational performance. Special education eligibility decisions should be made on the basis of a reliable assessment of ADHD, the degree to which the child's ADHD impacts academic and social functioning, and the success of general education classroom interventions in ameliorating academic and behavioral difficulties related to ADHD.

APPENDIX 3.1. Zirkel Checklist for Performing Eligibility for Special Education Services

Yes   No

Under the IDEA

A. CHILD FIND
  1. Reason to suspect both C1 and C2 below?
  2. If YES for A1, initiating evaluation within reasonable period?

B. EVALUATION
  1. Appropriate?
     • For example, various sources (including standardized tests, grades, behavioral data, parental information, and any independent educational evaluations [IEEs])
     • For example, all areas of suspected disability

C. ELIGIBILITY
  1. Preponderant evidence of meeting the criteria of an IDEA classification.

     a. Other health impairment (OHI)
        • A chronic or acute health problem resulting in limited alertness (i.e., credible diagnosis of ADHD)?
        • If state law or district policy/practice requires a physician to make this diagnosis, the obligation is on the district, not the parent.
        • In any event, the district may not condition the evaluation (or services) on medication of the child.

        —OR—

     b. Specific learning disability (SLD)
        • Basic psychological processing disorder (i.e., credible diagnosis of ADHD)?
        • Severe discrepancy or response-to-intervention (RTI) criteria?

        —OR—

     c. Another IDEA classification (e.g., emotional disturbance [ED])

  2. If YES for C1a, C1b, or C1c, does this classification adversely affect the child's educational performance to the extent of necessitating special education?

Adapted with permission from Zirkel, P. A. (2013). ADHD checklist for identification under the IDEA and Section 504/ADA. *West's Education Law Reporter, 293* 13–27. See original article for notes.

Under Section 504

A. CHILD FIND

   1. Reason to suspect C1 through C3 below?

B. EVALUATION

C. ELIGIBILITY

   1. Preponderant evidence of meeting these three criteria

      a. Mental or physical impairment (i.e., credible diagnosis of ADHD)?

        —AND—

      b. Limiting a major life activity—expanded under the Americans with Disabilities Act Ammendments Act of 2008 (ADAAA) (effective 1/1/09)
- For example, learning
- For example, concentration
- Other: social interaction, behavioral control?

        —AND—

      c. Substantially—similarly liberalized under the ADAAA
- Still, compared to the average student in the general population
- But, without the effects of mitigating measures (e.g., medication)

CHAPTER 4

Early Screening, Identification, and Intervention

By definition, ADHD is a disorder of childhood onset with behavioral symptoms exhibited prior to 12 years old (American Psychiatric Association, 2013). Children typically are not diagnosed with ADHD until the onset of formal schooling (i.e., kindergarten and first grade). Although preschool educational programs are typically play oriented and offer more free-choice activities than later schooling, the preacademic tasks, social activities, and art projects comprising schooling during these years require sustained attention and compliance with rules for short periods of time. Thus, children with ADHD-related behaviors could significantly disrupt structured activities, transitions from one activity to another, and group interactions (e.g., circle times). Furthermore, preschoolers who are physically overactive and more impulsive than their peers may have difficulties sharing, waiting turns, and controlling frustration even during less-structured activities such as free play. Thus, given the potential for early onset of ADHD symptoms, it is important for school personnel, particularly those working with young children, to be aware of (1) how this disorder manifests in early childhood, (2) how to identify young children at risk for ADHD, and (3) how to design programs for reducing symptoms and enhancing academic, social, and family functioning.

ADHD IN YOUNG CHILDREN

Despite the myriad difficulties associated with ADHD symptoms in young children, the vast majority of research studies on this disorder have been conducted with elementary school-age children (see Barkley,

2006). Although issues such as rapid developmental changes between ages 2 and 6 make diagnosis of preschool-age children somewhat tenuous (Lahey et al., 1998), research provides evidence that symptoms of ADHD emerge at a very young age (Egger, Kondo, & Angold, 2006; Spira & Fischel, 2005; Sterba, Egger, & Angold, 2007; Strickland et al., 2011; Wolraich, 2006) and are associated with significant deviations in brain structure (Mahone et al., 2011). Furthermore, ADHD-related characteristics seen in young children mirror those of older children with respect to prevalence, subtypes, and gender differences, offering support for an accurate nosology.

Estimates of ADHD prevalence in young children vary greatly. Lavigne, LeBailly, Hopkins, Gouze, and Binns (2009) found a prevalence rate of approximately 8.8%, while Keenan, Shaw, Walsh, Deliquadri, and Giovanelli (1997) found that 5.7% of 5-year-olds in a low-income sample met diagnostic criteria for ADHD. In an epidemiological study of disorders in a large community-based sample of 4-year-olds, Lavigne and colleagues found ADHD in 6.8 to 15.1%, depending on the severity of impairment. Regardless of differences in prevalence rates across studies, ADHD is among the most common childhood disorders, affecting a large percentage of the population of preschool age children.

ADHD in young children is associated with significant impairment in behavioral, social, and preacademic functioning with affected children approximately 2 standard deviations below their non-ADHD counterparts in all three areas (DuPaul et al., 2001). Furthermore, children (N = 303) from the Preschool ADHD Treatment Study (PATS; Greenhill et al., 2006) were found to have significant impairment that was correlated with ADHD severity, with younger children exhibiting the greatest levels of symptom severity. Overall, the majority of the PATS sample (69.6%) had one or more comorbid disorders with oppositional defiant disorder, communication disorders, and anxiety disorders being the most common. Finally, in a longitudinal study Lahey and colleagues (1998) found that preschool children diagnosed with ADHD continued to show functional impairment 3 years later and that symptom severity was the most significant marker of persistence into middle childhood. Together, this research strongly supports the early emergence of a constellation of symptoms characteristic of ADHD that is both atypical of preschool-age children and associated with significant and chronic impairment across settings.

Given that ADHD tends to be chronic, at least 70 to 80% of preschool-age children with this disorder will continue to exhibit significant ADHD symptoms during elementary school (Lahey et al., 2004; Riddle et al., 2013). Children exhibiting high levels of hyperactive and impulsive behaviors (i.e., combined or predominantly hyperactive–impulsive types of ADHD) are at higher than average risk for developing other disruptive behavior disorders (i.e., oppositional defiant disorder and conduct disorder) along with academic and social deficits (Campbell & Ewing, 1990). In addition, 59 to 67% of children with ADHD, whose difficulties are persistent at school entry, will continue to show significant symptoms of disruptive behavior disorder during middle childhood and early adolescence (Pierce, Ewing, & Campbell, 1999) and nearly 90% will fall short of being considered well adjusted as adolescents (Lee, Lahey, Owens, & Hinshaw, 2008). Young children with ADHD who also exhibit significant symptoms of oppositional defiant disorder and/or conduct disorder have the greatest risk for continued ADHD in middle childhood and this risk is not diminished by early treatment with stimulant medication (Riddle et al., 2013).

Aberrant mother–child interactions, as well as disruptive and aggressive social behaviors, are related to ADHD at a young age. Mothers of young children with ADHD issue significantly more commands, criticism, and punishment than mothers of nondiagnosed children (Barkley, 1988). In addition, mothers of preschool-age children with ADHD report greater levels of parenting stress than do mothers of similar-age normal children or even parents of older children with ADHD (DuPaul et al., 2001; Fischer, 1990). As a result, parents of young children with this disorder cope with behavior difficulties in a less adaptive fashion than do parents of young children without ADHD (DuPaul et al., 2001; Keown & Woodward, 2002). In preschool/daycare settings, children with ADHD exhibit high levels of disruptive, noncompliant, and possibly physically aggressive behaviors (Campbell, Endman, & Bernfield, 1977; DuPaul et al., 2001). These behaviors not only affect interactions with adult caregivers but also could negatively impact peer relationships. In fact, peer rejection is strongly associated with aggression, as rated by peers and teachers, among preschool-age children (Milich, Landau, Kilby, & Whitten, 1982). This finding is not surprising given that children with ADHD who also are aggressive disrupt the play activities of other children and are excessively demanding and noisy during peer interactions (Campbell et al., 1977; Campbell, Schliefer, & Weiss, 1978). In some cases, ADHD-related behaviors are severe enough to warrant removal from preschool or daycare classrooms, thus reducing the opportunities for children to develop age-appropriate social interaction and preacademic skills (Blackman, Westervelt, Stevenson, & Welch, 1991).

Young children with ADHD may be more likely to utilize medical services relative to their normal counterparts for at least two reasons. First, the vast majority (57%) of children with ADHD are reported by their parents to be accident-prone and 15% of this population has experienced four or more serious accidental injuries (Barkley, 2001). Several studies have shown that young children with ADHD, particularly boys, may be at higher risk for bone fractures, lacerations, head injuries, and other physical injuries than are controls (e.g., Lee, Harrington, Chang, & Connors, 2008). Furthermore, young children with ADHD appear to be at greater than average risk for accidental poisonings, presumably due to high rates of impulsive and overactive behavior (e.g., Lahey et al., 1998). In fact, Lahey and colleagues (2004) found that young children with ADHD were seven times more likely to sustain an accidental injury than their non-ADHD peers when assessed over a 4-year period. Furthermore, the injuries of children with ADHD are more likely to be severe (including loss of consciousness) compared with the injuries of children without ADHD (e.g., Mangus, Bergman, Zieger, & Coleman, 2004). Finally, young children with ADHD are more likely than their typically developing peers to experience injuries throughout their lifetimes (Schwebel, Speltz, Jones, & Bardina, 2002). This increased and chronic injury risk remains high even when other possible contributing factors (e.g., age, gender, SES, IQ) are taken into account.

A second reason for the higher than average medical utilization rates for young children at risk for ADHD is that a growing number of preschool-age children receive psychotropic medication (e.g., MPH) to reduce symptoms of the disorder. In fact, approximately 1.2–2% of 2- to 4-year-olds are prescribed stimulant medication, presumably for treatment of ADHD (Zito et al., 2000). Furthermore, approximately 67% of daycare centers in one state reported giving medication to young children for ADHD (Sinkovits, Kelly, & Ernst, 2003). Finally, 17% of Lahey and colleagues' (2004) sample of 4- to 7-year-olds with ADHD was prescribed stimulants in their first assessment wave with the percentage growing to 48.4% 3 years later. Thus, it can be assumed that a significant percentage of young children with ADHD are prescribed stimulant medication requiring medical oversight.

Children's early experiences with literacy and numeracy have a significant influence on later academic skills. For example, research has demonstrated that children's experience with early literacy activities, such as those that increase phonemic awareness (Snow, Burns, & Griffin, 1998) and early numeracy activities (Gersten, Jordan, & Flojo, 2005), make a significant difference in their later language and literacy skills and mathematics achievement. Unfortunately, young children with or at risk for ADHD experience significant difficulties with early literacy and numeracy skills. For example, DuPaul and colleagues (2001) found that preschoolers meeting diagnostic criteria for ADHD obtained significantly lower scores on a test of cognitive, developmental, and academic functioning compared with a sample of typically developing peers. On average, children with ADHD received scores 1 standard deviation below the expected mean for their age and relative to mean scores obtained by typically developing controls. This academic achievement gap is similar to that found for older children and adolescents with ADHD (Frazier et al., 2007) and suggests that academic impairment precedes school entry for many young children with ADHD. Not surprisingly, 3- and 4-year-old children with ADHD are significantly more likely to receive special education services relative to non-ADHD peers (Marks et al., 2009). In fact, Marks and colleagues (2009) found approximately 25% of their sample of children with ADHD received special education services relative to about 5% of control sample children.

In sum, the behavioral, medical, social, and academic difficulties associated with ADHD typically begin at an early age and are usually unremitting (DuPaul & Kern, 2011). Thus, the best opportunity to prevent significant behavioral, academic, and social deficits; to reduce the need for medical intervention; and to boost academic functioning of children with ADHD during the early elementary grades (i.e., kindergarten and first grade) involves early identification and intensive intervention during the preschool years.

SCREENING AND DIAGNOSTIC PROCEDURES

In order to identify young children who are at risk for ADHD, one must use reliable and valid methods to (1) screen for those youngsters who require further assessment and (2) assess behaviors related to ADHD and other disruptive behavior disorders. Although psychometrically sound assessment methods are available, evaluating preschool-age children for ADHD is fraught with difficulties. Chief among these is the fact that typical children in this age range often engage in inattentive, impulsive, and highly active behaviors. In many cases, these behaviors may simply be a manifestation of being a young child. A related concern is the ephemeral nature of behavior difficulties exhibited by young children. Although about 50% of young children exhibiting ADHD symptoms will show chronic difficulties in this area, the corollary is that these symptoms will remit in about 50% of affected children (Campbell & Ewing, 1990). Furthermore, behavior in young children can be highly inconsistent across time and settings. Finally, differentiating behaviors that are a manifestation of ADHD versus other disorders (e.g., autism) is particularly challenging in young children given the natural variability in skill and ability development in this age group. Thus, screening and diagnosis of ADHD in young children must be conducted in a conservative manner while remaining cognizant of developmental considerations.

Screening

There are two approaches to screening for at-risk children: classroom-based and individual screening. Classroom-based screening is a proactive procedure designed to identify those children at risk for ADHD or related disruptive behavior disorders *before* a teacher or parent referral is made. Stated differently, given the prevalence of ADHD in the general population, it is assumed that one or two children in every classroom may have this disorder. Rather than waiting for concerns to be voiced regarding these children, methods can be used to identify them at the earliest point possible. For example, the Early Screening Project (Feil, Walker, & Severson, 1995) employs a multiple gating procedure to identify young children at risk for behavior disorders. Initially, the preschool teacher is asked to rank all children in terms of severity and frequency of externalizing behaviors. The top three children are then passed to the next "gate," wherein the teacher provides behavior ratings on a psychometrically sound questionnaire. Those children who receive teacher ratings that exceed normative criteria (e.g., 1.5 standard deviations above the mean) are then passed to the next gate where systematic behavioral observations and parent ratings are collected. If the latter measures result in scores that exceed normative criteria, then a classroom intervention is designed and implemented and/or the child is referred for a more comprehensive evaluation.

In contrast, individual screening is a reactive procedure wherein assessment takes place *after* a teacher or parent referral. This process is very similar to that described for Stage I of our assessment model (see Chapter 2). Thus, whenever a preschool teacher or parent states concerns about a young child's attention, impulse control, activity level, or behavior control, screening for possible ADHD is warranted. Furthermore, given the strong association between symptoms of this disorder and difficulties attaining early reading and math skills, screening for ADHD should take place when teachers or parents indicate concerns regarding a child's learning letters or numbers.

As is the case for older children, the primary assessment methods used here are teacher or parent ratings of ADHD behaviors and/or a brief parent or teacher interview. To aid in this process, McGoey, DuPaul, Haley, and Shelton (2007) devised a preschool version of the ADHD Rating Scale–IV. The latter contains the 18 DSM-IV-TR symptoms of ADHD that have been adapted for use with preschoolers. Specifically, behavioral items include examples of how symptoms might be manifested by young children (e.g., difficulties following instructions manifested by having problems making the transition from one activity to another).

Given that DSM-5 (American Psychiatric Association, 2013) retained these same symptoms as part of the diagnostic criteria for ADHD, this measure continues to have utility for screening purposes. Thus, if a significant number of symptoms are reported to occur often or very often, then further assessment of ADHD may be necessary. Another option for screening is the Conners Rating Scale (Conners, 2008), which contains an ADHD Index including the 18 DSM-IV-TR symptoms of ADHD. Normative data for this index are available by age and gender allowing one to determine the degree to which the frequency of ADHD-related behaviors deviates from other children of the same gender and age. For screening purposes, a relatively liberal threshold (90th percentile) is suggested for determining whether additional assessment of ADHD is warranted.

As part of the screening process, the following questions should be considered:

1. How much of the child's disruptive behavior is due to "immaturity"? Is the child immature in many areas of development in addition to attention span and distractibility? Have the child's behaviors improved over time and with careful attention to their amelioration? If not, a referral for an ADHD evaluation may be warranted.

2. Are the classroom expectations age appropriate? For example, are children expected to sit still for too long? The curriculum may be too focused on academics and/or may be requiring skills beyond the child's instructional levels. Are the disruptive behaviors a function of frustration?

3. Are the classroom rules clear? Have these rules been taught to the children? Is the teacher's discipline style clear and consistent? Is the child oppositional and defiant toward the classroom rules?

4. Parents and professionals often are reluctant to "label" a child at a young age. They and the child's teacher may be more comfortable waiting until kindergarten or first grade to see whether the child "grows out of it" (i.e., behavior becomes less difficult to manage). Alternatively, if a child exhibiting ADHD-related behaviors receives no intervention during the preschool years, the "wait-and-see" approach may result in increased frustration in school activities, the development of poor peer relationships, and diminished self-esteem relative to school success. Thus, one must ask whether the benefits of identification and intervention at this age outweigh the costs.

When screening data warrant further assessment, then a multimethod protocol should be used as described in Stage II of our assessment model (see Chapter 2). Although the questions guiding the process and the process itself are the same as with older children, there are several important differences. First, different assessment measures must be used with preschoolers than with older children. Specifically, one must use rating scales and other instruments that have been developed for use with preschoolers. At a minimum, assessment methods must include an adequate and representative normative sample of 3- to 5-year-olds. Some measures that meet this criterion are delineated below. Second, given the variable nature of preschoolers' behavior, observations and ratings need to sample behavior over a wider range of time and settings than with older children. For example, teachers should be asked about behavior over the entire school year and parents should rate behaviors over a 6-month period. Observations need to be conducted during both structured (e.g., circle time) and unstructured (e.g., free-play) activities. Finally, primary emphasis should be given to parent report of ADHD symptoms because parents typically spend the most time with young children. When additional adults (e.g., daycare personnel) spend considerable time with a child, then interview and/or rating scale data should be collected from these individuals.

A number of interviews and behavior rating scales have been developed for assessing the disruptive behavior of young children. Preschool versions of structured diagnostic interviews such as the Diagnostic Interview for Children and Adolescents (Reich, 2000) and the Diagnostic Interview Schedule for Children (DISC; Columbia University DISC Development Group, 2000) are available. Although these interviews are somewhat lengthy (30–60 minutes), they provide a comprehensive and reliable way to assess symptomatic behaviors of various disorders that might affect preschoolers. Rating scales that contain items specifically addressing the behavior of young children also are available for completion by parents (or other caretakers) as well as by preschool teachers. Broadband parent scales include the Preschool and Kindergarten Behavior Scale (PKBS-2; Merrell, 2003), the Early Childhood Inventory–4R (ECI-4R; Gadow & Sprafkin, 2010), a young child version of the Child Behavior Checklist (CBCL; Achenbach & Rescorla, 2001), as well as the Behavior Assessment System for Children-2 (BASC-2; Reynolds & Kamphaus, 2004). Similar rating scales are available for teachers including the PKBS-2, Conners Rating Scale, ECI-4R, Teacher Report Form of the CBCL, and the BASC-2. Narrowband scales that can be used to obtain parent and teacher report of ADHD symptoms include the Preschool ADHD Rating Scale–IV (McGoey et al., 2007), ADHD Symptoms Rating Scale (ADHD-SRS; Phillips, Greenson, Collett, & Gimpel, 2002), and the Conners Teacher Rating Scale–Revised for Preschoolers (Purpura & Lonigan, 2009).

Another critical component of the multimethod assessment of ADHD symptoms in young children is direct observation of child behavior in classroom and/or home settings. For example, DuPaul and colleagues (2001) used an adaptation of the Early Screening Project social behavior coding system (Feil et al., 1995) to obtain information regarding the behavior of young children at risk for ADHD in structured (e.g., listening to teacher reading) and unstructured (e.g., free-play) situations in their preschool classrooms. This system uses a combination partial interval (15-second) system for negative behaviors, a whole interval system for positive behaviors, and a momentary interval system to record activity changes. The category of negative social behavior includes negative social engagement, disobeying established rules, off-task behaviors, and tantrumming. Positive social behavior includes positive social engagement, parallel play, and following established rules. Activity change is measured independently of negative and positive social behavior and is defined as a child engaging in an activity other than the activity engaged in at the start of the previous observation interval. DuPaul and colleagues found that young children with ADHD exhibited significantly higher rates of negative social behavior in structured situations than did typically developing peers.

Observations of parent–child interactions across a variety of situations may be helpful not only in determining the developmental deviance of a young child's behavior but also to provide information that could be helpful in designing behavioral interventions for the home. DuPaul and colleagues (2001) observed parent–child interactions in a clinic playroom setting across four different controlled situations, each of which was 10 minutes in duration, in the following order: The first situation consisted of a parent allowing his or her child to play with toys in a free-play situation (FPS). The second situation consisted of a parent providing minimal attention to his or her child in a low adult attention situation (LAAS). The third situation involved a parent supervising his or her child's activity (e.g., puzzle making and drawing) in a parent-supervised situation (PSS). The final observation situation required each child to complete tasks (e.g., cleaning up playroom) in a parent-directed task situation (PDTS). Parent behaviors that were coded included alpha (i.e., direct) commands, beta (i.e., indirect and vague) commands, positive behavior, negative behavior, questions, and reinforcement of child compliance. Child behaviors included activity, compliance, noncompliance, inappropriate behavior, and on-task behavior. For all but the activity category, the percentage of observation intervals was calculated. The activity score represented the number of intervals when activity changes occurred.

This parent–child interaction coding system was found to discriminate between young children with ADHD and normal peers (DuPaul et al., 2001). Children with ADHD exhibited more than twice the level of noncompliance and greater than five times the level of inappropriate behavior displayed by controls when asked to complete activities and tasks by their parents. Furthermore, parents of children with ADHD exhibited negative behavior toward their children three times more frequently than parents of controls, particularly when asking their children to complete activities and tasks. Interestingly, minimal group differences in interactions were found during the LAAS, suggesting that for many young children with ADHD escape from parent-directed tasks is a prime motivation for noncompliant behavior (as opposed to displaying negative behavior to gain parental attention). Thus, this system can be helpful in suggesting directions for functional assessment.

Along these lines, it is imperative that functional assessment data be collected. The components of a functional behavioral assessment for young children are no different than those for older children (see Chapter 2) and include parent and teacher interviews as well as behavior observations. In most cases, assessment data will be descriptive such that antecedent and consequent events will be delineated as they naturally occur in home or school environments. When possible, experimental analysis procedures as described by Boyajian, DuPaul, Wartel Handler, Eckert, and McGoey (2001) can be used to more definitively identify the function(s) of a specific target behavior. More details regarding functional assessment with young children are provided later in this chapter (see "Multicomponent Early Intervention" section).

By definition, a diagnosis of ADHD requires children to show either academic or social impairment as a function of their symptomatic behaviors (American Psychiatric Association, 2013). Children must not only exhibit the requisite number of inattentive or hyperactive–impulsive symptoms but also must show some functional deficits in relation to these symptoms. There are at least three ways that impairment in functioning can be assessed (Healey, Miller, Castelli, Marks, & Halperin, 2008). First, parents and teachers can be asked about possible impairment as part of the diagnostic interview. For example, many structured interviews include an item asking parents whether the symptoms they have observed have caused problems with academic or social functioning. Of course, this is a very general indicator of functional impairment that does not provide precise data and may have rather limited reliability and validity.

A more precise method of documenting functional impairment is through parent and teacher ratings. Practitioners can ask respondents to complete a broad-based impairment rating like the Impairment Rating Scale (Fabiano et al., 2006) and the Children's Problem Checklist (CPC; Healey et al., 2008) or more specific ratings of key areas like the Social Skills Improvement Systems (SSIS) Rating Scales (Gresham & Elliott, 2008) and the Preschool Learning Behaviors Scale (McDermott, Leigh, & Perry, 2002). Information from these scales can delineate the degree to which children show impairment in these areas relative to a normative population.

The third and most precise method for assessing academic and social functioning is to use direct measures in each area. Norm-referenced tests of early language, math, and reading abilities like the Bracken Basic Concepts Scale–Revised (Bracken, 1998) will provide age-appropriate information about early academic skills. Criterion-referenced tests specific to early academic skills may be of even greater value given that obtained data may translate more directly to instructional strategies. For reading and language, Phonological Awareness Literacy Screening (Invernizzi, Sullivan, & Meier, 2001) and Dynamic Indicators of Basic Early Literacy Skills (DIBELS; Kaminski & Good, 1996) have good psychometric properties with the early childhood population. Fewer measures are available for early math skills but include the Early Numeracy Skills Assessment (ENSA; Sokol, 2002) and the Preschool Numeracy Indicators (Floyd, Hojnoski, & Key, 2006; Hojnoski, Silberglitt, & Floyd, 2009).

Fewer methods and measures are available to directly assess social skills and peer status. Behavioral observations of children's behavior in unstructured and/or playground settings can be conducted to document the frequency of positive and negative social behaviors relative to peers (see prior discussion of direct observations of behavior). Although seemingly objective, observations of social behavior are limited because data are only available for a small cross-section of time. This is especially problematic for assessment of low-rate behaviors like physical aggression. Assessment of peer social status typically involves collection of sociometric measures wherein children report on who they like and dislike. Such information may be helpful in documenting children's acceptance or rejection by peers; however, these are sensitive data to obtain because educators and parents may consider it inappropriate to ask children to judge their relationship with others (particularly to identify peers they do not prefer) and, thus, are rarely used outside of research investigations.

Once assessment data are collected, the results must be interpreted in a similar fashion to the interpretation process described in Stage III of our assessment model (see Chapter 2). Diagnostic decisions must be made in the context of the degree to which assessment data are consistent with DSM-5 (American Psychiatric Association, 2013) criteria for one of the three presentations of ADHD. Several caveats are important to consider here. First, a diagnosis of ADHD is made less confidently in young children because of the inherent variability of behavior in this age group, as well as possible diminishment of symptoms over time. In fact, in our work with preschoolers, we use the term *at risk for ADHD* to describe young children who meet DSM-5 (American Psychiatric Association, 2013) criteria for this disorder. This terminology acknowledges the severity of the symptoms while allowing for the possibility that these symptoms are merely precursors of the disorder and may remit with maturation. Also, we have found that qualifying the diagnosis with the term *at risk* is more acceptable to parents and teachers of young children who are concerned about the potential long-term stigma attached to a diagnostic label applied at an early age.

Another consideration at the interpretation stage is the degree to which apparent ADHD symptoms may have other causes. Although all of the alternative hypotheses enumerated in Chapter 2 for older children also are relevant for the evaluation of younger children, the need to differentiate ADHD from autism and other developmental disabilities is paramount in this age group. Autism and related pervasive developmental disorders are most likely to be identified in the preschool years (American Psychiatric Association, 2013). Furthermore, children with developmental disabilities may exhibit inattention, impulsivity, and high levels of gross motor activity. Particularly when parent and teacher concerns are voiced regarding a child's language and social skills, the practitioner should include measures to screen for symptoms of autism. For example, the Autism Diagnostic Interview–Revised (Lord, Rutter, & Le Couteur, 1994) can be used to put parent and/or teacher report of autism symptoms into the context of a structured diagnostic interview. In addition, observations of child behavior, such as the Childhood Autism Rating Scale (Schopler, Reichler, & Renner, 1988), may be helpful in screening for behaviors related to autism.

As is the case for older children with ADHD, intervention strategies should be designed, evaluated, and modified based on assessment data (see Stages IV and V of our assessment model in Chapter 2). As part of the treatment plan, it is prudent to recommend periodic reevaluation of a child's ADHD diagnostic status to accurately ascertain whether the disorder is chronic. For example, a subsample of measures could be read-ministered once per year through early elementary school. Given that symptoms of this disorder can remit over time in some young children, one should track the trajectory of ADHD-related behaviors to aid in short- and long-term treatment planning.

EARLY INTERVENTION
AND PREVENTION STRATEGIES

The most effective interventions for ADHD have been psychostimulant medication (e.g., MPH) and behavior modification applied across home and school settings (MTA Cooperative Group, 1999; Pelham & Fabiano, 2008). Although most efficacy studies have been conducted with elementary school-age children (i.e., 6- to 10-year-olds), empirical investigations with young children with ADHD also have provided support for these treatments (for a review, see Charach et al., 2010; Ghuman, Arnold, & Anthony, 2008). More specifically, stimulant medication and parent education applied in isolation have led to positive effects on behavior relative to control conditions. Behaviorally based parent education programs appear to be an effective strategy for young children with conduct problems because this treatment can disrupt the coercive parent–child interactions that often are the source of problematic behaviors (Wierson & Forehand, 1994). Of particular note is the parent education program developed by Webster-Stratton (1996) that incorporates a videotape-based discussion model versus the more traditional didactic model of parent training. This program has extensive empirical support for its effectiveness in the treatment of young children with conduct problems (e.g., Webster-Stratton, Reid, & Hammond, 2001) and has been identified as an empirically supported treatment for conduct disorder (Eyberg, Nelson, & Boggs, 2008).

Prior comprehensive reviews of treatment for young children with or at risk for ADHD have examined studies of psychotropic medication, parent education programs, and school-based behavior modification (Charach et al., 2011; Ghuman et al., 2008; McGoey et al., 2002). Very few studies of multicomponent treatment (e.g., parent education plus preschool-based intervention) were found in these reviews. The extant empirical literature supports the use of each of these treatments for ameliorating ADHD symptoms and related behaviors in young children. To illustrate what is known regarding the treatment of early childhood ADHD, examples of each treatment approach and supporting evidence are provided below.

Psychotropic Medication

The most widely studied treatment for ADHD in preschoolers has been psychotropic medication, specifically psychostimulant compounds. The vast majority of investigations have examined the effects of MPH, although dextroamphetamine and lithium carbonate also have been studied. Most studies have focused on the extent to which medication reduces ADHD symptoms and related problem behaviors. Ghuman and colleagues (2008) conducted a systematic review of the pharmacotherapy literature relevant to young children with ADHD and located 24 published studies during the period 1967–2007, the vast majority of which were investigations of stimulants. Although findings have differed across individual studies, most placebo-controlled investigations of stimulants have shown significant reductions in ratings and observations of ADHD-related behaviors with approximately 80% of treated children showing a positive response (Ghuman et al., 2008).

The most comprehensive study of stimulant medication (MPH) for young children with ADHD is the PATS (Kollins et al., 2006). A sample of 303 children (76% boys) between 3 and 5.5 years old who met DSM-IV-TR criteria for ADHD were initially enrolled in the study. Participating children went through several phases prior to the controlled medication trial phase including screening, parent education, and open-label safety lead-in. As a result, of the 261 children whose families completed the 10-week parent education phase (using the Community Parent Education [COPE] program; Cunningham, Bremner, & Secord, 1998), 37 (14%) exhibited sufficient improvement such that parents no longer sought medication treatment (Greenhill et al., 2006). An additional 45 (17%) children withdrew following parent education because parents did not want medication, children no longer met inclusion criteria, or families moved and were lost to follow-up. Sixteen children withdrew during or following the open-label safety lead-in phase, thus leaving 165 children who were enrolled in the placebo-controlled crossover medication trial (147 of whom completed the trial).

Children who participated in the 9-week controlled medication trial phase were assessed across 5 weeks of dosage titration (placebo, 1.25-mg, 2.5-mg, 5-mg, and 7.5-mg MPH) with each dosage used for 1 week. Statistically significant reductions in combined parent and teacher ratings of ADHD symptoms relative to placebo were found for the three highest dosages (i.e., all dosages except 1.25 mg; Greenhill et al., 2006). Symptom ratings did not differ among the three highest dosages; however, there was a significant linear dose–response effect indicating stepwise reductions in ADHD symptoms as dosage increased. Group-level findings for methylphenidate effects are qualified by substantial differences in medication response across individuals. Specifically, relatively equal percentages of children (ranging from between 15 to 22%) were found to show optimal responses to each of the four active methylphenidate dosages. Furthermore, 12% of the children were found to show either no response or optimal response to placebo rather than an active dose of methylphenidate. Approximately 30% of parents reported their children to exhibit a moderate to severe adverse side effect during one or more of the active medication phases (Wigal et al., 2006). As has been found for older children with ADHD (see Connor, 2006b), the three most commonly reported adverse side effects included decreased appetite, trouble sleeping, and weight loss. All three of these side-effects occurred significantly more often during methylphenidate than placebo conditions. Of additional concern, for the 95 children who remained on methylphenidate following the controlled medication phases of the study, annual growth rates were 20% below expectations for height and 55.2% less than expected for weight (Swanson et al., 2006). Thus, the use of stimulant medication in this age group must be considered by balancing possible benefits of symptom reduction against probable reductions in growth velocity, although long-term studies of growth reduction are rare.

There are several important limitations to medication studies with this population including (1) absence of measures assessing adherence with medication protocols, (2) minimal study of behavioral effects and impact on important areas of functioning (e.g., academic achievement) in real-world preschool classrooms, and (3) short-term (e.g., several weeks) study of effects (DuPaul & Kern, 2011; McGoey et al., 2002). Furthermore, several investigations (including the PATS study) have reported that parents took their children off medication following completion of the study. Therefore, it appears that at least some parents did not perceive medication to lead to clinically meaningful changes in their children's behavior and/or were concerned about adverse side effects. Thus, the most prudent conclusion is that MPH and other stimulants are effective in reducing ADHD symptoms and related problem behaviors in young children; however, the extent to which pharmacotherapy is necessary in this age group beyond alternative interventions remains to be determined. In fact, the American Academy of Pediatrics ADHD treatment guidelines (2011) specifically recommend that behavioral intervention should precede pharmacotherapy in treating young children.

Preschool-Based Behavioral Intervention

In contrast to pharmacotherapy, relatively few studies have investigated the effects of behavioral and/or educational interventions in preschool classrooms. This is both surprising and sobering given the short- and long-term implications of disruptive behavior in preschool and elementary school settings. Furthermore, many of the "classroom" interventions studied thus far have been examined in laboratory rather than preschool settings, thus limiting the generalizability of obtained results. As an example of a classroom-based investigation, McGoey and DuPaul (2000) evaluated the effects of a behavioral intervention combining positive reinforcement and response cost on the disruptive behavior of four preschool-age children with ADHD. The children's teachers were asked to reinforce appropriate behaviors and to discourage inappropriate behaviors by the contingent awarding or removal of token reinforcers (i.e., buttons), respectively. Daily rewards were earned by children depending on the number of buttons they had earned during the school day. Direct observations of behavior indicated decreases in disruptive behavior during intervention relative to baseline conditions. The teachers and students reported this intervention to be acceptable and effective.

In general, it appears that as is the case for older children with ADHD, classroom interventions based on behavioral principles are effective in reducing disruptive behaviors in preschool settings. This conclusion is tempered by several limitations of the literature including small sample sizes and a lack of treatment integrity, long-term follow-up, and generalizability data (McGoey et al., 2002). In addition, interventions have been applied using a "one-size-fits-all" approach with the underlying assumption that all young children with ADHD will respond to a particular intervention. More work is necessary along the lines of Boyajian and colleagues (2001), who designed preschool interventions using functional assessment data. The latter allow for individualizing behavioral interventions in an attempt to optimize outcomes.

Parent Education in the Use of Behavioral Interventions

A number of investigations have provided evidence that parent-mediated behavioral interventions can enhance compliance and reduce inappropriate behavior in young children with ADHD and similar disruptive disorders. Positive effects on child behavior appear to result from changes in the way the parents issue commands and respond to their children when the latter are cooperative. For example, Strayhorn and Weidman (1989) conducted a controlled study of parent education with a sample of 98 parents of preschool-age children with ADHD. Parents were randomly assigned to a control or an experimental group; those in the latter group were taught to implement positive reinforcement for compliant behavior in the context of parent–child interaction training. The experimental group demonstrated statistically significant improvements on parent ratings of child behavior as well as in direct observations of parent–child interactions in the clinic setting. Parents also reported a high degree of satisfaction with training outcomes. These same investigators found that group differences were maintained a full year after treatment, attesting to the maintenance of treatment-induced behavioral change (Strayhorn & Weidman, 1991).

As is the case for preschool-based behavioral interventions, parent education in behavior management appears to be an efficacious treatment for young children with ADHD. However, this conclusion should be tempered by similar limitations including a lack of treatment integrity assessment, reliance on indirect outcome measures (e.g., parent behavior ratings), and lack of data regarding generalization across settings (McGoey et al., 2002). Furthermore, most parent education training studies taught parents to implement multiple behavioral interventions (e.g., positive reinforcement, response cost, and time-out from positive reinforcement). Thus, it is difficult to discern which specific intervention strategies are effective and whether a comprehensive treatment package is necessary to obtain behavior change. Finally, most studies have included primarily white, middle-class samples, thus limiting the degree to which results can be generalized to diverse populations. Given that the parent education literature consistently has documented the limited effects of this treatment approach for single mothers from low socioeconomic backgrounds (Nixon, 2002), further work with more diverse samples is critically important.

COMMUNITY-BASED PREVENTION AND INTERVENTION

Despite empirical evidence that psychosocial interventions may help reduce the family and school difficulties of preschoolers with ADHD, it appears that these interventions are not implemented frequently in community or nonresearch settings. In short, there is a gap between what is needed by these children, what is known to work to address these needs, and what is actually provided in the real world. Eckert, DuPaul, McGoey, and Volpe (2002) surveyed parents of young children at risk for ADHD (N = 101), community-based service providers (e.g., early childhood educators, pediatricians, and school psychologists; N = 137), and national experts and researchers in the field of ADHD (N = 25) regarding the needs of preschoolers with this disorder. There was general agreement among the three samples that parents and preschool teachers required information and ongoing support relevant to behavioral and educational interventions. Although parents perceived that they were getting helpful information from their child's physician and teacher, they reported less satisfaction with parent support groups and other community sources. Service providers reported ongoing needs for early intervention services, parent education, and educational consultation. Experts reported a gap between research and practice, as well as a general need for more research on effective interventions with this age group.

The gap between research and practice does not appear to be due to a lack of acceptance or comfort with possible interventions on the part of parents and preschool teachers. Quite the contrary: Parents not only perceive the need for education in structured parenting strategies, surveys indicate that they find effective behavioral interventions, especially those incorporating positive reinforcement, to be highly acceptable and preferable to medication treatment (Wilson & Jennings, 1996). In similar fashion, Stormont and Stebbins (2001) found that preschool teachers rated various behavioral and educational interventions to be important in the management of young children with ADHD, and importance ratings were highly correlated with their comfort level with these strategies. Teacher ratings of importance and comfort level were not correlated with years of experience, education level, or other demographic factors. Thus, parents and preschool teachers are in critical need of information and support in understanding and treating young children with ADHD. Although the empirical literature supports a number of treatments, there is a clear gap between research and community-based practice. In the following section, we advocate for greater involvement of school psychologists in early intervention with this population and articulate a prevention/intervention model that can be implemented by mental health, educational, and health professionals.

Prevention of Difficulties Associated with ADHD

As stated earlier in this chapter, early-onset ADHD symptoms are associated with a number of chronic difficulties that compromise children's success in a number of critical arenas (see top of Figure 4.1). By far, the two most problematic outcomes are the subsequent development of oppositional defiant disorder and for conduct disorder symptoms and academic underachievement. Over 50% of children, especially boys, with ADHD will be diagnosable with oppositional defiant disorder or conduct disorder at some point in their childhood (Barkley, 2006). Social development is dependent, at least in part, on the interaction between behavioral dispositions of children (e.g., ADHD) and parents' behavior management skills (Tremblay et al., 1992). The greatest number of reinforcers are delivered by the people who have the most contact with children (i.e., parents); therefore, positive exchanges with primary caregivers make a significant contribution to children's social development (Patterson, Reid, & Dishion, 1992). A key tenet of Patterson's theory (Patterson et al., 1992) of the development of antisocial behavior is that the latter begins in the home during the toddler/preschool years. More specifically, children learn that their own aversive behavior (e.g., crying, defiance) turns off the aversive behavior of parents (e.g.,

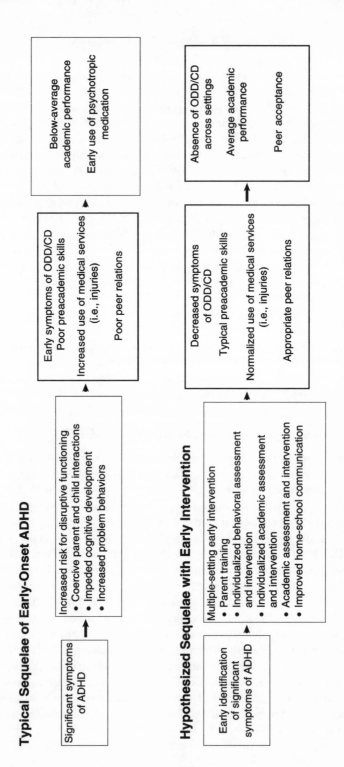

FIGURE 4.1. Typical and hypothesized sequelae of early-onset ADHD.

commands). Over time and with repeated trials, coercive interactions train children to use aversive behaviors as a method to control unpleasant and chaotic situations (Dishion, Patterson, & Kavanagh, 1992). As children develop, these coercive exchanges intensify in frequency and severity, leading to aversive behavior that generalizes across settings, is persistent over time, and results in rejection by parents and peers (Reid & Eddy, 1997).

The major variable underlying this coercive process is parents' skill and effectiveness in setting limits and in monitoring children's behavior (Dishion et al., 1992). Symptoms of ADHD are significantly associated with disrupted family management practices and can increase the probability of coercive parent–child exchanges (Dishion & Patterson, 1997). The key to change is to alter parental disciplinary practices, including reducing the frequency of coercive exchanges (while concomitantly increasing positive exchanges) between parents and children. Furthermore, parents must be encouraged to consistently monitor their children to prevent antisocial behavior (e.g., physical aggression) and to prevent accidental injuries associated with impulsive behavior. Intervention is much more likely to be successful if conducted during what Patterson refers to as the "basic training" stage (i.e., preschool) rather than later in life when the coercive interaction style is well entrenched, antisocial behaviors are firmly established, and parent behavior is more distally related to child behavior (Patterson et al., 1992; Reid & Eddy, 1997). Given that preschoolers with ADHD are more likely than their nondisabled peers to show aggressive/defiant behavior in school settings, there is a pressing need to alter teacher–student interaction style as well.

The second common outcome associated with ADHD in early childhood is academic underachievement. As we stated earlier in this chapter, academic deficits often are evident from the very beginning of a child's schooling and persist throughout his or her school years. Numerous research studies have demonstrated that children's early experiences with literacy and numeracy have a significant influence on later academic skills. For example, research has demonstrated that children's experience with early literacy activities (i.e., phonemic awareness) makes a significant difference in their later language and literacy skills (e.g., Hart & Risley, 1995). Some research also suggests that early instruction in number activities may significantly reduce failure in early mathematics (e.g., Griffin, Case, & Siegler, 1994).

Other than the investigation of individual treatment components (e.g., parent training and stimulant medication), there have been very few attempts to research the effects of comprehensive prevention/early intervention with this population. McGoey and colleagues (2002) conducted a pilot investigation of a community-based intervention program for young children with ADHD. A total of 57 children (3 and 4 years old) identified as having ADHD were referred by community service providers (e.g., pediatricians), preschool teachers, and parents. Children were randomly assigned to a combined intervention group or to a community treatment control group (wherein families obtained psychological, pediatric, educational, and/or psychiatric services available in the community). Complete results were available for 23 early intervention participants and 22 community control participants.

The combined intervention program included (1) weekly parent training sessions (using the program developed by Webster-Stratton, 1996) for 3 months followed by monthly parent training sessions for 9 months, (2) preschool-based behavioral interventions for 3 months followed by teacher consultation for the first 6 months of the following school year, and (3) open medication trials (MPH or dextroamphetamine) for those children who did not respond to the psychosocial interventions.

Dependent measures were collected periodically over a 15-month period and included parent and teacher behavior ratings, observations of parent–child interactions and preschool behavior, documentation of injury rates and medical utilization, parent ratings of stress and family functioning, and a brief test of children's cognitive development. Furthermore, at two points in time, parents and teachers of children in the combined intervention group were asked to complete several consumer satisfaction ratings.

Results of this pilot investigation indicated that relative to community treatment controls, children who received the combined intervention showed statistically significant improvements in behavior control (at home and at school), their parents had reduced stress, and the family experienced more adaptive coping. The primary effect of the combined intervention was to alter the trajectory of child behavior over time relative to the community control participants. For example, the negative linear trend in teacher-rated antisocial/aggressive behavior (on the PKBS; Merrell, 1994) was significantly steeper for the combined intervention group (slope = −1.06) than for the community control group (slope = −0.2). In particular, the continued provision of teacher consultation seemed to help the combined intervention children to maintain a downward trend in antisocial behavior. Parents and teachers uniformly reported the combined intervention procedures to be highly acceptable and moderately effective. Although very few children who received early intervention were placed on psychotropic medication, statistically significant changes in medical utilization and cognitive development were not obtained in this pilot investigation.

At the individual level of analysis, the specific effects of preschool interventions based on functional assessment data were examined using single-subject designs employing more continuous data collection (Boyajian et al., 2001). Results indicated that determining the function of aggressive behavior (e.g., escape motivated vs. attention motivated) helped to develop classroom-based interventions that markedly reduced the frequency of aggressive behavior for three boys with ADHD relative to baseline conditions (see Figure 4.2).

Shelton, Woods, Williford, Dobbins, and Neale (2002) reported similar results with a comprehensive early intervention protocol for 184 young children at risk for ADHD. These preschoolers attended Head Start programs and were from diverse ethnic backgrounds. Behavioral interventions were implemented in home and preschool settings and were individualized using consultation procedures. After 1 year of intervention, children receiving early intervention showed reduced ADHD symptoms and aggression relative to an assessment-only control group.

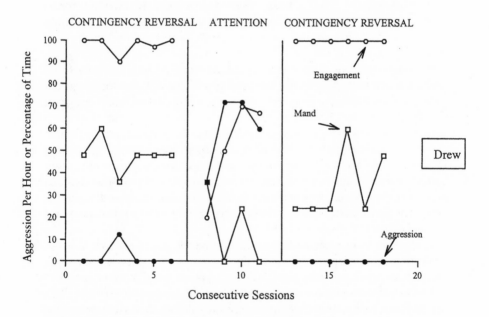

FIGURE 4.2. Level of aggression, requests (mands), and percentage of engagement in the contingency reversal (i.e., intervention) and baseline (attention) phases for Drew. From Boyajian, DuPaul, Wartel, Handler, Eckert, and McGoey (2001). Copyright 2001 by the National Association of School Psychologists. Reprinted by permission.

Although significant differences were not obtained regarding parenting competence, parenting stress, or family support, parents and teachers reported high satisfaction with the services they received.

Barkley and colleagues (2000) investigated the effect of a multicomponent prevention program for young children with disruptive behavior disorders. Although this program did not specifically target preschoolers with ADHD, their results are instructive regarding the promise and limitations of an early intervention approach with this population. A total of 158 children attending public school kindergarten who exhibited significant behaviors associated with ADHD and oppositional defiant disorder were randomly assigned to four experimental groups: parent education only, full-day treatment classroom only, combination of parent education and treatment classroom, and a no-treatment control. The parent education program developed by Barkley (1997b) was used on a weekly basis for 10 sessions followed by an additional five monthly booster sessions. Behavioral interventions were implemented in kindergarten classrooms using the model developed at the University of California–Irvine (see Pfiffner et al., 2006). Classroom strategies included token reinforcement, response cost, group cognitive-behavioral self-control training, group social skills and anger control training, and a daily report card system.

Comprehensive data regarding child, family, and classroom functioning were collected at the beginning and end of the kindergarten year. The two groups that received the classroom treatment program showed significant improvements in adaptive behavior, social skills, and symptoms of ADHD and oppositional defiant disorder according to parent and teacher report, as well as direct observations in the classroom. Unfortunately, no significant effects were found for the parent education component, perhaps because many parents did not attend these sessions on a consistent basis. Neither treatment component improved academic achievement or performance on clinic-based measures of attention and cognitive skills.

The results of these three promising investigations are consistent in indicating that psychosocial interventions primarily composed of behavioral strategies can reduce ADHD and oppositional defiant disorder symptoms over the short term, particularly in classroom settings. Peer interactions and social skills also may be enhanced by early intervention efforts. None of these multicomponent programs were associated with improvements in academic achievement, which is a critical limitation. Furthermore, it is unknown whether short-term gains in behavioral functioning will maintain over time. In fact, Shelton and colleagues (2000) found that the initial gains in classroom functioning realized by Barkley and colleagues (2000) were not sustained after 2 years.

Multicomponent Early Intervention Model

In light of the promise and limitations of prior efforts at prevention and early intervention with young children at risk for ADHD, researchers at Lehigh University and Lehigh Valley Health Network in eastern Pennsylvania have developed a comprehensive, community-based early intervention program that comprises multiple components. This intervention model is specifically designed to reduce and/or prevent the most problematic outcomes associated with ADHD symptoms in early childhood (see bottom of Figure 4.1). Systematic data were collected over several years to ascertain short- and long-term outcomes associated with implementation of intensive school and home programming relative to a parent education only condition. We believe that school psychologists and other educational personnel should be key participants in the design and implementation of early intervention programs such as this multicomponent protocol in their local settings.

The components of this intervention focus on three domains (behavior problems, academic readiness/skills, and child safety) across two settings (home and school). Specific intervention components include parent education, assessment-based behavioral intervention at home and at school, preacademic readiness instruction at home and at school, and home–school communication.

Parent Education

Parent education focuses on the domains of behavior problems, academic readiness/skills, and child safety. Training typically is delivered to parents in groups of 10 who participate in 20 sessions over a 1-year period led by a school psychologist or special educator. Of the 20 sessions, 12 consist of the original procedures outlined by Cunningham and colleagues (1998) using the COPE program. This program has been found effective in reducing noncompliance and aggression among at-risk children (for a review, see Cunningham, 2006). The remaining eight sessions include two introductory sessions (e.g., providing basic information about ADHD and related disorders), five sessions addressing functional assessment and promotion of academic readiness skills (described below), and one session devoted to injury prevention and home safety. Each parent education session lasts approximately 90–120 minutes.

The 12-session COPE program entails educating parents regarding effective behavioral procedures, such as positive reinforcement for compliance and use of problem solving and mild punishment techniques to address problem behavior. Key behavioral concepts are delineated through videotaped vignettes of parent–child interactions followed by group discussion. In addition to the COPE program, parents are provided information and support regarding several related concepts and procedures. Philosophical components of the functional behavioral approach are a focus throughout parent training. Parents are introduced to the fundamental concepts concerning functions of behavior. For example, situations in which particular interventions are not likely to be effective (e.g., time-out in the context of escape-maintained problem behavior) are discussed. Using a consultative problem-solving process (Sheridan & Kratochwill, 2008), parents are taught strategies for determining the function of challenging behaviors at home and then introduced to interventions that are matched to behavioral function. Instruction is provided in developing antecedent interventions (i.e., making changes in the environment to reduce the likelihood of problem behavior), skill building (teaching children alternative means to get their needs met), and providing consequences in a manner that is least likely to reinforce behavior.

Because a primary focus of the multicomponent early intervention model is to enhance academic and school readiness, two parent education sessions focus on this area of development. Four major topics are included in these sessions. The first is developing early literacy skills using the Ladders to Literacy curriculum (Notari-Syverson, O'Connor, & Vadasy, 1998). The second topic is "understanding your child's curriculum," wherein parents are helped to understand vocabulary they are likely to encounter as their child enters elementary school (e.g., phonics, readiness). The third topic that is covered is "reading to your child." Videotaped vignettes are used to illustrate reading at various developmental levels including appropriate questions and expectations. The fourth major topic is "understanding your child's interests and attention span." This topic includes helping parents to select materials and learning opportunities that are likely to be motivational for their children.

Promotion of child safety is targeted in one session and is addressed in additional sessions throughout parent training. The primary method for accomplishing this is the use of The Injury Prevention Program (TIPP; American Academy of Pediatrics, 1999). Specifically, parents are provided with TIPP handout materials and group discussion of safety issues and strategies ensues. The implementation of safety promotion strategies also is imbedded into behavioral interventions designed as part of the parent training. Specifically, safety-related behaviors will serve as targets for intervention.

Assessment-Based Intervention: Home

Functional behavioral assessment and intervention is facilitated through a collaborative consultative model (e.g., Sheridan & Kratochwill, 2008).

Parents participate in a behavioral consultation procedure with a school psychologist or special educator once every month, as necessary, to facilitate the development and implementation of individualized intervention plans for each child. As part of this process, a functional behavioral assessment is conducted collaboratively wherein parents and the psychologist collect descriptive assessment data regarding possible antecedents and consequences surrounding challenging behavior. Hypotheses regarding the functions of behaviors are tested in the home using a brief functional analysis procedure (Northup et al., 1991). This assessment procedure requires approximately 90 minutes. Once hypotheses are developed regarding potential functions of problem behaviors, conditions are devised to confirm these functions. For example, if a parent request to complete a task is hypothesized to be associated with problem behavior, parents will be asked to provide multiple requests during a 5- to 10-minute observation period. To establish experimental control, this request session is alternated with a no-request session. If high rates of problem behavior are observed during the request session and low rates are observed during the no-request session, the function (escape) of problem behavior is experimentally supported. If differential rates of the problem behavior are not observed, alternative hypotheses are developed.

After the functional behavioral assessment has been completed and a behavioral function is identified, an individualized intervention is developed for each child/family. Interventions typically consist of three components including antecedent strategies, skill building, and consequent approaches. Parents are trained to implement specific interventions through didactic instruction, modeling, practice, and feedback. Finally, a goal is established for the target behavior.

In subsequent months, parents are contacted periodically to discuss whether treatment goals are being met. Existing interventions are reviewed and problems with interventions assessed and remedied. Intervention decisions are made collaboratively by the parent(s) and psychologist based on data collected by the parents and parental report. Once a goal for a target behavior has been reached, maintenance is programmed and, if necessary, a new target behavior is selected, thus restarting the consultation process.

Assessment-Based Intervention: School

As in the home, functional behavioral assessment and intervention is facilitated through a collaborative consultative model in the preschool setting (see Table 4.1). Teachers receive behavioral consultation from the same psychologist or special educator who is working with the children's

TABLE 4.1. Steps to Functional Analysis and Intervention Evaluation

1. Consultant conducts Problem Identification Interview with teacher to determine problem behavior and possible environmental events (e.g., attention from teacher) maintaining behavior.

2. Consultant conducts Brief Functional Analysis with child in preschool classroom. This step involves:

   a. Analogue assessment to get initial data on what environmental events might be following problem behavior.
   b. Replication of conditions that produced the highest and lowest rates of problem behavior to check on reliability of analogue assessment.
   c. Contingency reversal to see if problem behavior will decrease and appropriate replacement behavior (e.g., verbal request) will increase if the latter is followed by the same environmental event (e.g., attention) that was found to follow problem behavior in the analogue assessment.

3. Consultant implements intervention based on results of contingency reversal. Each child's teacher gradually takes over implementation of the intervention after observing the consultant. Intervention effects are evaluated by looking at changes in problem behavior and appropriate, replacement behavior across baseline and intervention conditions.

Note. From Boyajian, DuPaul, Wartel, Handler, Eckert, and McGoey (2001). Copyright 2001 by the National Association of School Psychologists. Reprinted by permission.

parents. Initially, a functional behavioral assessment is conducted in each child's preschool classroom consistent with guidelines developed by the Pennsylvania Department of Education (Bambara & Knoster, 1995). This functional behavioral assessment process includes the following five steps: (1) conduct a functional assessment, (2) develop hypothesis statements, (3) design an effective behavioral support plan, (4) evaluate effectiveness, and (5) modify support plan as needed. Preschool teachers are asked to collect data across 2 weeks regarding the antecedent and consequent events for a single problem behavior. Based on information from this assessment, hypotheses are collaboratively formulated by the teacher and the psychologist. These hypotheses are tested by the psychologist using brief reversals (e.g., Kern, Childs, Dunlap, Clarke, & Falk, 1994). For example, if assessments identify escape from difficult work to be the function of behavior problems, work difficulty will be systematically manipulated across brief (e.g., 5–15 minutes) periods of time. If problem behavior systematically varies with work difficulty, hypotheses will be confirmed. Interventions then are individually developed based on the assessment information. These interventions typically consist of antecedent modifications, skill development, and consequent strategies. As was the case for parents, teachers are trained to implement specific interventions through didactic instruction, modeling, practice, and feedback. A treatment goal is selected collaboratively between the teachers and the psychologist, and teachers are asked to collect data on a target behavior to monitor progress toward achieving that goal.

In subsequent months, teachers are contacted to review progress toward intervention goals. Existing interventions are reviewed and problems with interventions are assessed and remedied. Once a goal for a target behavior has been reached, maintenance is programmed and, if necessary, a new target behavior is selected.

Children with ADHD typically do not fully benefit from the preschool experience because they miss preacademic information due to inattention and may be excluded from playtime as punishment for disruptive behavior. Furthermore, the classroom ecology is changed by the presence of a child with ADHD because the classwide level of disruption may increase. Thus, the preschool teacher must evaluate the physical space, the daily schedule of activities, and his or her teaching techniques to help the child with ADHD to succeed, and to manage the class as a whole. Classroom interventions for ADHD in preschool settings have not been studied in any detail to date. Thus, as part of the consultation process, preschool teachers are asked to consider possible accommodations, as delineated below.

1. *Redesign the physical space.* Tables where more formal activities, such as those designed to teach early academic skills, should be positioned away from indoor climbers, block areas, water tables, or other distractions (e.g., bright, three-dimensional bulletin boards). Use shelves or furniture as boundaries to play areas (e.g., book corner, dramatic play area) so that there are physical cues as to the type of play that is appropriate in a given area. These types of environmental arrangements may help the child to focus on one activity at a time while minimizing the probability of becoming distracted by other classroom activities.

2. *Adopt a step-by-step approach to activity setup.* For example, rather than setting up an art activity by placing paper, crayons, scissors, and glue on a table all at once, the teacher would provide materials necessary for only the first step in the process (e.g., paper and crayons for coloring). As children complete each step of the activity, materials successively are added and then removed from the table when no longer needed. This reduces distractions and minimizes potential disruptions. During the presentation of activity directions, the child with ADHD should be seated as close as possible to the teacher with an uninterrupted view of the teacher's demonstrations. Finally, chairs should be spaced so that children are not seated too close together.

3. *Evaluate and modify the daily schedule and activity transitions.* The teacher should be encouraged to critically examine the content and timing of scheduled activities. Specific modifications will vary as a function of the classroom. Several questions could be considered. Is it preferable to schedule two short circle times versus one longer one? The former may be more adaptable to children with a short attention span. What time of the day does the child sit better for activities? Perhaps the schedule could be adjusted based on observations of the child's behavior. Must everyone actually form a line to go outside? Can transitions be shortened so that there is less waiting (e.g., to get everyone dressed to go outside, to serve snack to everyone)? Finally, it may be beneficial to "talk through" transition times. For example, impending transitions can be announced, as can the requirements for completing the present activity.

4. *Vary the curriculum.* To maximize interest level, the teacher should be encouraged to be creative in planning innovative and engaging activities (e.g., flannelboard stories, puppet shows) for the entire class and should include those of special appeal to the child with attention and behavior problems.

5. *Give individual directions clearly.* The teacher should not assume that the child will follow directions presented to the group on a consistent basis. While giving directions, the teacher should make eye contact and gently touch the child to encourage attention. Commands should be made in a straightforward, direct manner (e.g., "Johnny, please pick up these toys") rather than posed as a question or favor (e.g., "Johnny, could you do me a favor and pick up these toys?"). Multistep directions should be broken down into individual steps. Finally, the child should be asked to repeat directions to ensure attention and understanding.

6. *Increase the ratio of adults to children.* Recruit and use volunteers (e.g., grandparents, college students) to provide the child with ADHD more individualized attention during structured activities, circle times, and transitions. Also, having extra help can ensure greater consistency and follow-through on any interventions that might be implemented.

Assessment and Training of Preacademic Skills: Home

Ladders to Literacy: A Preschool Activity Book (Notari-Syverson et al., 1998) is used as a curriculum guide to create early literacy experiences. The program is readily individualized, offering choices, self-direction, and multiple opportunities for practice, thus making it appropriate for children at a variety of developmental levels. Activities and experiences contained in *Ladders to Literacy* fall into three broad areas that have been identified to influence children's literacy development. These are print/book awareness, meta-linguistic awareness, and oral language.

Ladders to Literacy contains activities designed for "busy parents" that are simple and can be completed in the context of other activities (e.g., while washing the dishes, while driving the car). For example, one activity suggests that parents ask their child to predict what will happen next when reading a familiar story. Parents are provided activities on index cards for easy access. They are instructed to complete at least one activity daily, lasting approximately 15–20 minutes.

Parents also are exposed to several activities to assist their child with early numeracy skills. These activities are designed to reinforce number identification and linearity. For example, children are exposed to number lines and thermometers, which provide visual representations of the early numeracy concepts of bigger/smaller and going up/going down.

Assessment and Training of Preacademic Skills: School

Assessments based on children's preschool curricula occur on a monthly basis. In addition, phonemic segmentation fluency, letter-naming fluency, and picture-naming fluency are assessed using the DIBELS (Kaminski & Good, 1996). A modified version of the DIBELS focusing on numeracy skills is used to allow for dynamic assessment of premath abilities. Specific skills assessed include numeric character naming, counting, character–set matching, set–set matching, and pattern matching. These data will help teachers to individualize instruction on an ongoing basis.

The *Ladders to Literacy* program is used as the instructional intervention because it contains an extensive curriculum for early childhood teachers. Each activity is used to teach or reinforce a specific skill (e.g., awareness of sounds). Activities are categorized into three levels of task demand including "high demand/low support," "medium demand/ medium support," and "low demand/high support." These correspond to the demand of the task on the child and the level of adult assistance needed to complete the activity. This system of categorization facilitates selection and scheduling of tasks depending on child characteristics and ongoing demands on the teacher. In addition, tasks contain multiple skills or goals along with adaptations for children with disabilities (e.g., hearing, motor, or visual impairments). Thus, they are suitable for children with diverse needs.

Home–School Communication

Preschool teachers are asked to send brief notes home to parents so that the latter can review the day's academic and behavior issues. In these notes, teachers provide parents with a brief description of the lesson plan for the day (e.g., "We reviewed words that begin with C today"). If a child is having difficulty, teachers are asked to provide parents with a simple exercise to improve the skill. Teachers also are asked to report any behavior problems that were exhibited by children that day, as well as examples of positive behaviors or areas of improvement in that regard. Parents are guided by the psychologist or special educator in providing positive consequences (e.g., praise and rewards) for appropriate school behavior and performance.

Another possible strategy to support home–school communication and consistency is conjoint behavioral consultation (CBC; Sheridan & Kratochwill, 2008). CBC involves the collaborative partnership of parents and teachers, assisted by a consultant, to identify and address child academic, behavioral, and/or social needs. A four-stage process is followed including conjoint needs identification, conjoint needs analysis, plan implementation, and conjoint plan evaluation. During the conjoint needs identification phase, parents and teachers identify target behaviors and decide how to collect data on those behaviors. For conjoint needs analysis, the group reviews the collected data, hypothesizes what is maintaining the behavior, and creates a plan to address the target behavior. The parent and teacher implement the plan and the group has a plan evaluation meeting after a specified period of time (e.g., 4 weeks) to discuss the need for continuation, modification, or discontinuation of the original plan. CBC has been demonstrated as an effective service delivery model for improving the behavioral functioning of older students with ADHD (for a review, see Sheridan & Kratochwill, 2008).

In sum, the purpose of the multicomponent early intervention protocol is to address the areas of greatest risk for young children exhibiting behaviors symptomatic of ADHD. Specifically, the objective is to prevent more serious antisocial behaviors from developing as well as to promote early literacy and numeracy skills. Data from our ongoing research program provides support for continued use of the early intervention protocol along with suggested areas for modification.

MULTICOMPONENT EARLY INTERVENTION: FINDINGS AND FUTURE DIRECTIONS

The multicomponent early intervention model described in this chapter was evaluated in the context of a randomized clinical trial (i.e., the Early Intervention for ADHD [EIA] project; DuPaul et al., 2013; Kern et al., 2007). The purpose of the trial was to evaluate the multicomponent early intervention protocol relative to parent education alone in reducing

ADHD-related problem behaviors and, hence, the negative sequelae that typically follow. The participant inclusion criteria for the EIA project were highly similar to entry criteria for the PATS (Greenhill et al., 2006), discussed previously in this chapter. A multiphase screening process was conducted wherein children were identified as meeting DSM-IV-TR criteria for one of three subtypes of ADHD based on parent diagnostic interviews as well as parent and teacher ratings of ADHD symptoms. Children with autism, low cognitive ability, or conduct disorder were excluded. Most (76%) of the sample met criteria for oppositional defiant disorder.

After screening, 137 children met inclusion criteria. Using a randomized design, children were assigned to either a multicomponent intervention (MCI) group (N = 73) or a parent education (PE) group (N = 64). Groups did not differ at baseline with respect to child age, gender, parent occupation, parent education, ADHD subtype, presence of oppositional defiant disorder, or receipt of psychotropic medication. The MCI group received intervention, as described in this chapter, over 2 years delivered in both home and preschool/daycare settings.

The PE group received only parent education over the course of 2 years. The Early Childhood Systematic Training for Effective Parenting (STEP; Dinkmeyer, McKay, Dinkmeyer, Dinkmeyer, & McKay, 1997) curriculum was used, with sessions pertaining to general child rearing (understanding child behavior, discipline, social–emotional development). This was supplemented with sessions pertaining to ADHD information (e.g., characteristics, prevalence), child health and nutrition, cognitive and language development, safety, parent self-care, and preparation for school.

Treatment outcomes were evaluated using standardized assessments in the form of questionnaires completed by parents and preschool/daycare teachers, preacademic skills assessments administered to children, and direct observations. Analyses of 1- and 2-year outcomes were conducted using hierarchical linear modeling. Results indicated there were no significant group differences between the two treatment groups *at 1 year* after the onset of intervention (Kern et al., 2007). Importantly, statistically significant growth ($p < .01$) occurred for almost all of the dependent measures (16 of 18) examined at that time point. That is, negative trajectories were found for aggressive behavior, delinquent behavior, and symptoms of ADHD, oppositional defiant disorder, and conduct disorder. In addition, statistically significant positive slopes were obtained for teacher and parent-rated social skills as well as early literacy skills.

Similar results were obtained for an expanded set of 46 dependent measures assessed every 6 months *over 2 years*. Specifically, statistically significant ($p < .05$) linear slope was found for 30 measures, all of which were in the expected direction (i.e., negative slope for parent and teacher behavior problem ratings, as well as observations of noncompliant and off-task child behavior, with positive slopes for parent and teacher ratings of social skills and direct assessment of academic skills). Significant quadratic slope (indicating a change in direction of slope) was found for 14 of the measures. Typically, these showed initial steep changes with slopes gradually tapering off over time (e.g., see Figure 4.3).

Significant differences between MCI and PE groups in linear and/or quadratic slope were found for nine measures, including ratings of parent stress and family coping, teacher ratings of oppositional behavior, and direct observations of off-task, noncompliance, and positive social engagement in preschool and home settings. Most of these differences in 2-year outcome favored the MCI group, including family coping, ratings of parent distress and problematic parent–child interactions, direct observations of classroom off-task behavior and positive behavior in parent–child interactions, and teacher ratings of oppositional behavior. Two years after the onset of treatment, the percentage of children meeting DSM-IV-TR criteria for ADHD and oppositional defiant disorder was reduced from 100% at baseline to 61.5% (ADHD) and from 76 to 46.2% (oppositional defiant disorder). Furthermore, following 2 years of treatment, only 8.3% of the sample would have met the initial inclusion criteria (i.e., DSM-IV-TR criteria plus extreme parent and teacher behavior ratings) for entry into the study. None of the participants met criteria for conduct disorder after 2 years and only 29.1% were receiving

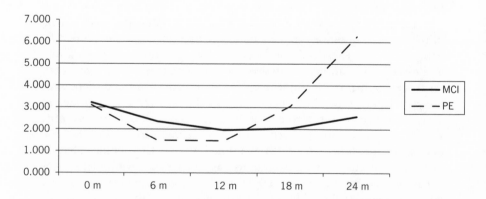

FIGURE 4.3. Mean percentage of observation intervals when off-task behavior was observed during structured classroom activities as a function of treatment group (MCI, multicomponent intervention; PE, parent education) and time (baseline [0 months] through 24 months of treatment).

psychotropic medication. Although there were no statistically significant differences between groups with respect to diagnostic and medication outcomes, the direction of differences in most cases favored the MCI group. Also, the rates of diagnosis and impairment (see Figure 4.4), as well as percentage of children receiving psychotropic medication (see Figure 4.5), were less than that obtained by Lahey and colleagues (2004) with their untreated sample of young children with ADHD followed over a 2-year period.

These findings indicate that early intervention had a significant impact on home and preschool behavioral functioning and possibly on preacademic and home safety skills. In general, children in both groups improved significantly, in contrast to the more typical flatline or worsening of behavioral outcomes found in this population (e.g., see Lahey et al., 2004). Although there were few differences between the two early intervention groups, the MCI approach may be stronger for certain outcomes (e.g., noncompliance, off-task, and reduction of medication use) in the second year of treatment, particularly in the preschool or elementary school setting. These outcomes suggest that certain subgroups experienced differential benefits from this more intensive intervention. Furthermore, parents in the MCI group rated treatment strategies as significantly more acceptable than parents in the PE group at the 6- and 12-month assessment phases. No significant group differences in treatment acceptability were found at 18 and 24 months. Overall treatment

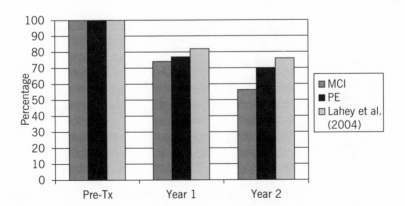

FIGURE 4.4. Percentage of young children with ADHD meeting diagnostic and impairment criteria for ADHD as a function of early intervention. Comparison data are provided for participants in the Lahey et al. (2004) study, as these were young children with ADHD not receiving systematic intervention. Pre-Tx, pretreatment.

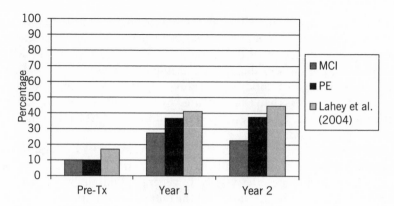

FIGURE 4.5. Percentage of young children with ADHD receiving psychotropic medication across phases of an early intervention study. Comparison data are provided for participants in the Lahey et al. (2004) study, as these were young children with ADHD not receiving systematic intervention. Pre-Tx = pretreatment.

acceptability for both groups was in the moderate range. Teachers also reported MCI intervention strategies to be moderately acceptable and effective.

Individual response to treatment varied considerably within both groups. We calculated individual effect sizes for 6-month outcomes for each participant using parent and teacher ratings of oppositional behaviors (Conners' T-scores). Ratings of oppositional behavior were used because behaviors targeted for intervention were primarily noncompliance and aggression. Effect sizes were calculated using the formula (pretreatment rating – 6-month treatment rating)/group SD. A positive treatment response was identified for those participants who obtained an effect size of 0.5 SD units or greater. In the PE group, 27% of the sample showed a positive response based on parent ratings, 42% based on teacher ratings, and 9.1% responded positively in both settings. Results were similar for the MCI group with 27.5% showing a positive response based on parent ratings, 33.9% on teacher ratings, and 7.1% in both settings.

Findings from the EIA study were promising for several reasons and also raise important questions for future research (DuPaul & Kern, 2011). First, significant improvements were seen for some children who received an intervention of relatively mild intensity, in the form of parent education. Alternatively, a significant minority of children did not respond to intervention, including some in the MCI group who received individualized assessment-based interventions in both home and school.

Thus, it is imperative to further evaluate responsiveness to varying intensities of intervention. A second important question is whether a less intensive parent education program would be equally effective in light of variable education session attendance among parents. Specifically, some children responded to a relatively low-intensity intervention and thus may not require twenty 2-hour sessions over many months. In fact, a three-tier early intervention model may be viable wherein children who exhibit a sufficient response to only parent and teacher education remain in that protocol, while children who are not responsive to parent and teacher education alone move to more intensive intervention strategies (for greater detail on a tiered approach to early intervention, see DuPaul & Kern, 2011). This tiered approach has the additional potential advantage of greater cost-effectiveness and feasibility given limited resources for early intervention in the community.

SUMMARY

ADHD is a disorder that typically begins early in life, with most symptoms becoming evident prior to elementary school. Yet, until recently, minimal research has been conducted to aid practitioners in identifying and supporting young children at risk for this disorder. In this chapter, we have described methods for (1) screening preschool children to identify those youngsters requiring further assessment and intervention; (2) adapting our multimethod assessment model for the evaluation of ADHD in young children; and (3) intervening early to reduce the frequency and severity of ADHD-related behaviors, as well as to prevent the emergence of common outcomes (e.g., academic deficits and conduct problems) associated with this disorder. Given the chronicity of ADHD and associated impairments in many children, it is hoped that early identification and intervention may enhance the school, social, and family functioning of these children such that more expensive and intensive services are not necessary later in life. Although this assumption requires empirical verification, in keeping with repeated calls for school psychologists to be preventionists (Power, 2002), we strongly believe that school practitioners should be engaged with these children and their families and teachers as early as possible.

CHAPTER 5

Interventions and Supports in Elementary School

Children spend 6–8 hours per day, 5 days per week in classroom and other school settings throughout each school year. These educational environments require children to follow rules, interact appropriately with other children and adults, participate in adult-directed instructional activities, learn what is being taught, and refrain from disrupting or disturbing the learning and activities of others. For teachers, imparting the knowledge and skills comprising the curriculum and teaching children to behave in a manner consistent with organizational, social, and cultural expectations are demanding tasks. The work of teachers is even more demanding when it involves children diagnosed with ADHD, as the behaviors characteristic of these children can interfere with students' classroom learning (i.e., both children with ADHD and their classmates). In addition, the behaviors characteristic of children with ADHD also can impede positive social interactions with peers and teachers in educational settings.

The purpose of this chapter is to present and discuss school-based intervention and support strategies for promoting the learning and prosocial behavior of elementary school-age children diagnosed with ADHD, and for facilitating the smooth conduct of classroom teaching where these children are involved (see Chapter 6 for interventions for secondary school students with ADHD). We begin with a discussion of contextual considerations and conceptual foundations for these interventions. Next we discuss interventions based on contingency management and academic skill instruction, as well as cognitive-behavioral approaches. We complete the chapter with a discussion of considerations for supporting teachers responsible for students with ADHD.

CONCEPTUAL FOUNDATIONS OF INTERVENTIONS FOR CHILDREN WITH ADHD IN CONTEMPORARY SCHOOL CONTEXTS

By definition, the behavioral difficulties experienced by children with ADHD are both chronic and impairing, thus rendering school success an elusive goal. As previously noted, these children are at risk for experiencing a host of school-related problems including skill acquisition difficulties, work completion difficulties, and grade retention (Lahey et al., 2004). And, the nature and extent of presenting problems for these children often (but not always) leads to eligibility for special education and placement in a specialized behavior and/or academic support program. In secondary school, students with ADHD are at risk for earning poor grades and dropping out of school. These risks indicate the importance of identifying and delivering effective educational and behavioral supports for these children.

Given the challenging and chronic nature of ADHD, we recommend that involved professionals take a systematic and ongoing approach to designing, implementing, and evaluating classroom-based supports that combines both preventive and remedial approaches to dealing with presenting problems, and that involves multiple intervention agents or approaches. To facilitate such an approach, the strategies presented are reviewed based on empirical support for them in the research literature of education, psychology, and behavior support, as well as the National Association of School Psychologists (2011) position statement on *Students with Attention Deficit Hyperactivity Disorder*. In addition, we review promising and recently investigated approaches to behavioral and instructional management pertinent to children with ADHD.

To begin, we examine our assumptions. The first is that a diagnosis of *ADHD should be considered a serious concern with concomitant problems that will be enduring over time* and will be associated with difficult-to-manage behavior in classroom settings (Barkley, 2006). Children diagnosed with ADHD likely will experience academic and social learning difficulties across many, but not all, classroom situations and throughout their school-age years (Mannuzza & Klein, 2000). To date, the vast majority of research in the area of interventions for children with ADHD has focused on issues and strategies pertaining to managing social behavior and deportment in the classroom, primarily via medication and contingency management. However, this focus on optimizing children's social behavior, behavioral maladjustment, and prevention of antisocial behavior represents only "one side of the coin" regarding ADHD. The other side is focused on optimizing the academic achievement and performance of identified children.

Social and academic problems can be seen as related. Viewing them as such leads to our second assumption. Specifically, we assume that *both social and achievement problems of childhood can be understood as instructional problems* (Bambara & Kern, 2005; Skiba & Peterson, 2003). That is, we as educators and psychologists have a critical role to play in providing instruction to promote both academic and social skill development such as to prevent and solve problems in these areas.

In a related fashion, then, our third assumption is that *professionals involved with children with ADHD should take an educative approach to behavior problems* (Sugai et al., 2000). From this perspective, interventions for behavior problems have as their explicit goals to teach identified children the skills and knowledge necessary to replace problem behaviors with acceptable ones. An educative approach represents an alternative to interventions that are solely child focused and primarily concerned with the elimination or reduction of problem behaviors.

Taking an educative approach to behavior problems leads us to our fourth assumption: *Dealing effectively and in an educative manner with behavior problems will require the development and implementation of programmatic behavior and teacher support plans* (Bambara & Kern, 2005). Contemporary approaches to prevention of school-based problems, often referred to as "positive behavior support" programs, employ school- and classwide approaches to facilitate the learning and behavior of all students (see Sugai et al., 2000, for a thorough treatment of this topic). In doing so, such programs have the ability to "jump-start" individually focused intervention/support strategies.

Finally, it is assumed that *persons responsible for supporting behavior of children with ADHD will have completed appropriate professional training* (see Power, Mautone, & Ginsburg-Block, 2010, for a discussion of professional training needs in the area of school-based interventions). Such training should include conceptual and practical preparation with regard to intervention design, delivery, and outcome evaluation.

Given these assumptions, classroom-based intervention strategies for ADHD should be grounded in the guidelines for interventions presented in Table 5.1. First and foremost, the development and evaluation of interventions for ADHD are empirically based. Treatment strategies are chosen based, in part, on their demonstrated efficacy in the research literature. For example, there is clear evidence that manipulating environmental events in the classroom leads to significant changes in behavior among students with even the most severe symptoms of this disorder (see meta-analysis by DuPaul, Eckert, & Vilardo, 2012). Furthermore, the actual success of an intervention program for an individual student is assessed by using appropriate outcome evaluation measures. For example, curriculum-based measurement data regarding a child's academic

TABLE 5.1. Guidelines for the Design, Implementation, and Evaluation of Interventions for Learning and Behavior Problems

1. Intervention development, evaluation, and revision are *data-based* activities.
2. Intervention development, evaluation, and revision are driven by *child advocacy* and focused on attainment of clearly identified, socially valid *child outcomes*.
3. Intervention procedures must be thoroughly identified and defined, as well as implemented with integrity by persons with clearly delineated responsibilities.
4. Effective interventions produce or lead to increased rates of appropriate behavior and/or improved rates of learning, not solely decreases in undesirable or disturbing behavior.
5. Prior to its implementation, an intervention's effects on the behaviors of the identified child, the teacher, and on the classroom are unknown.

skills development can be used to set appropriate targets for and assess the benefit of academic interventions (Shinn, 2010).

Second, the child's needs are paramount in the selection of intervention strategies. Treatment goals are delineated relative to socially valid outcomes for the child with ADHD, as judged by consumers such as parents, teachers, and students themselves. Third, given that a team of professionals typically is involved in the treatment of students with ADHD, the responsibilities of each team member must be delineated clearly to ensure that intervention strategies are implemented with integrity. Fourth, the focus of treatment is primarily on *increasing* the frequency and/or duration of appropriate behaviors (e.g., academic productivity and accuracy) rather than primarily on *decreasing* disruptive classroom behavior. Finally, each child's response to intervention is presumed to be unique, and therefore the salutary effects and aversive side effects of a particular treatment are unknown prior to its implementation. This perspective implies the need for ongoing and comprehensive evaluation of all intervention strategies.

In addition to our assumptions about students with ADHD, and the noted intervention guidelines, we rely on several other conceptual and practical foundations in designing interventions for students with ADHD-related difficulties. First, school professionals often rely on reactive and punitive procedures in attempting to change the behaviors of impulsive and inattentive students. Such procedures are likely to be successful only when they are used sparingly, with minimal affect, and in the context of a positively reinforcing environment. Alternatively, an approach more likely to be successful is a balanced approach wherein both *proactive and reactive* strategies are employed. Specifically, antecedent events that typically precede inattentive and disruptive behaviors should be manipulated to prevent problematic interactions from arising. In addition, reactive strategies should not be confined to punitive approaches but rather, should emphasize delivery of positive reinforcement when attentive and appropriate behaviors occur.

Another conceptual principle useful in designing effective interventions for students with attention problems is to intervene at the point of performance (Goldstein & Goldstein, 1998). This principle maintains that to be optimally effective, strategies must be implemented in close proximity (i.e., in time and place) to the occurrence of the target behavior. For example, if the behavior of concern is attention to and completion of math work, then the most effective intervention strategies will be those used in math class at the time when students are expected to complete math work. Interventions further removed in time and place from the behavior of interest are likely to be less effective. This guiding principle is based on evidence that impulsivity is a primary deficit underlying the attention difficulties and other symptoms of ADHD (Barkley, 2006). Changing or preventing impulsive behavior typically requires that interventions be implemented when and where the problem behaviors, or their replacement behaviors, occur.

In addition to intervening at the point of performance, intervention design for students with attention problems needs to be individualized. That is, we need to avoid a "one-size-fits-all" approach, based on the notion that all children sharing the ADHD diagnosis or behavior profile have the same support needs (DuPaul, Eckert, & McGoey, 1997). This process of individualizing intervention plans should take into account (1) the child's current level of academic skills; (2) the topography and possible functions of a child's inattentive/problem behavior; (3) the target behaviors and/or outcomes of greatest concern to the teacher, parents, and/or student; and (4) elements of a teacher's approaches to classroom management and instruction that might limit the effectiveness of some interventions. Individualized interventions should be developed through a consultative problem-solving process using assessment data and collaborative interactions among teachers, parents, and other school professionals (DuPaul et al., 2006; Sheridan, Kratochwill, & Bergan, 1996).

Finally, recognition that interventions for students with ADHD can and should be mediated by a number of individuals is another important contemporary intervention design issue. Specifically, effective support strategies can be implemented by teachers, parents, peers, and the identified students themselves (Jitendra, DuPaul, Someki, & Tresco, 2008). When available, computers also can be used to improve task engagement and/or work completion, especially with drill-and-practice types of activities. The guiding principle here is that the classroom teacher should not be expected to be solely responsible for addressing all difficulties related to a student with ADHD. Other important resources (e.g.,

TABLE 5.2. Possible Mediators for School-Based Interventions

Intervention type	Elementary	Secondary
Teacher-mediated	Instructional strategies Token reinforcement systems	Study skills instruction Contingency contracting
Parent-mediated	Goal setting Contingency contracting Home-based reinforcement Parent tutoring	Negotiating Contingency contracting Home-based reinforcement
Peer-mediated	Peer tutoring	Peer coaching Peer mediation

Computer-assisted	Reading and math
	    instruction
	Fluency-building practice
	    exercises
		Learning and instructional
		    supports
		Homework supports
		Word processing

Self-directed	Self-monitoring	Self-monitoring Self-evaluation

Note. Adapted from DuPaul and Power (2000). Copyright 2000 by the American Psychiatric Association. Adapted by permission.

peers) in the classroom and home environments (e.g., parents) can be used to support and deliver interventions, thus creating a more comprehensive and perhaps cost-effective intervention strategy. Table 5.2 contains a matrix of some of the most effective intervention strategies in the context of both academic settings (i.e., elementary vs. secondary level) and mediating agent. These specific strategies are described later in this chapter, after the following sections addressing more general considerations in treatment design for students with ADHD.

BASIC COMPONENTS
OF CLASSROOM-BASED INTERVENTIONS

As already noted, there is a tendency to focus on the manipulation of consequences when designing classroom interventions for children identified with ADHD (for a review, see DuPaul, Eckert, & Vilardo, 2012). Here, intervention research has emphasized the use of positive reinforcement and positive reinforcement coupled with mild forms of punishment (e.g., response cost and time-out from positive reinforcement). In the field of applied behavior analysis in general, research over the past two decades has emphasized the prevention and management of behavior and achievement problems through antecedent manipulations and environmental arrangements (Mayer, Sulzer-Azaroff, & Wallace, 2014; Sugai et al., 2000). Similar emphases are warranted in the area of classroom-based management of children with ADHD.

Intervention procedures based on principles of human behavior have a long and well-documented history of effectiveness in ameliorating children's learning and behavior problems in school settings, including children with ADHD (Mayer et al., 2014). For example, these behavior change strategies have been successful in reducing the disruptive, off-task behavior of children identified with ADHD and increasing their academic productivity (Evans et al., in press; Pelham & Fabiano, 2008). Given the difficulties hypothesized to underlie the problems exhibited by children with ADHD (e.g., problems with impulsivity, self-control, and delayed responding), this finding is not surprising. It may be that behavioral interventions increase the overall level of appropriate classroom behavior through provision of external cues and prompts (e.g., rules, directions, contingencies) that supplement those "privately" operating (i.e., self-directing thoughts) for the target student. In designing behaviorally based interventions for classroom problems related to ADHD, the following issues warrant consideration:

1. A thorough assessment of the specific presenting problems, including a functional assessment, should be conducted to guide the design and selection of intervention components (e.g., target behaviors and their function[s], instructional strategy, motivational program).

2. Children diagnosed with ADHD typically require more frequent and specific feedback than their classmates to optimize their performance. As such, initial phases of interventions aimed at ADHD-related problems should incorporate contingencies that can be delivered in a relatively continuous manner. Leaner schedules of reinforcement should be introduced gradually. Related to the issue of timing of reinforcement, in one study (Rapport, Tucker, DuPaul, Merlo, & Stoner, 1986) children with ADHD tended to choose smaller, more immediate rewards over larger, delayed rewards contingent upon completion of academic work. These results serve to emphasize the need to attend to the general notion that to be effective, contingencies need to be in place at the "point of performance."

3. Contingent positive reinforcement should be the primary component of a behaviorally based intervention program for problems related to ADHD. But some evidence exists to suggest that exclusive reliance on reinforcement may distract the child from the task at hand. Alternatively, this concern may be ameliorated by the use of positive reinforcement coupled with the use of mild negative consequences (e.g., prudent

reprimands; Abramowitz, O'Leary, & Rosen, 1987; Rosen, O'Leary, Joyce, Conway, & Pfiffner, 1984) and redirection of the child toward appropriate task behavior. The effectiveness of verbal reprimands and redirections can be enhanced through *specificity* of communication regarding the teacher's concerns and through *consistent delivery immediately* following the occurrence of problem behavior (Pfiffner & O'Leary, 1993). Furthermore, treating children with dignity and respect requires that reprimands and redirection statements be made in a *brief, calm, and quiet* manner. As much as possible, reprimands should be delivered *privately* while making eye contact with the child.

4. When student behavior during independent work periods is targeted for change, initial task instructions should involve no more than a few steps. The child then should be asked to repeat directions back to the teacher to demonstrate understanding. Similarly, student homework and related tasks/projects should be assigned one at a time, with more complex tasks broken into smaller units. In some cases, the overall amount of assigned work would be reduced for the child with ADHD. The length and complexity of the workload would be increased gradually as the child demonstrates successful independent completion of increasingly larger units. Repetitive material (e.g., reassigning erroneously completed worksheets) should be avoided. Alternatively, an assignment focused on the same skill or concept area could be substituted to avoid boredom and potential exacerbation of attention problems.

5. Academic products and performance (e.g., work completion and accuracy) are preferred as targets of intervention as compared with specific task-related behaviors (e.g., attention to task or staying in one's seat) for several reasons. First, this preference promotes teacher monitoring of important student outcomes. Second, this preference promotes attention to the organizational and academic skills (e.g., working with the appropriate materials for an assignment, soliciting formative feedback on initial task performance) necessary for independent learning and for completing academic assignments. Third, a focus on active academic responding does not violate the "dead man test for behavior" (i.e., desired behavior) articulated by Lindsley (1991). Albeit morbid, it is nonetheless instructive to consider this "rule" that stated "If a dead boy could do it, it wasn't behavior" (Lindsley, 1991, p. 457). In practice, then, employing treatment targets such as "sitting still" and "remaining quiet" violate the dead man test. Finally, this preference for active and engaged academic responding as a treatment target promotes a focus on behavior that is incompatible with inattentive and disruptive behavior, and as such may lead to multiple desired outcomes, including a reduction in disruptive behavior (Pfiffner & O'Leary, 1993).

6. Preferred activities (e.g., free-choice activity time, access to a classroom computer) should be used as reinforcers whenever feasible, rather than tangible rewards (e.g., stickers and consumable items). Such contingencies may include making access to a preferred classroom activity contingent upon completion of an assignment in a less preferred subject area (e.g., completion of a math worksheet leads to access to reading activities; see Shimabukuro, Prater, Jenkins, & Edelin-Smith 1999). Also in this vein, the specific rewards or reinforcers employed should be varied or rotated as needed to prevent disinterest with them, and thus with the program (i.e., reinforcer satiation). Finally, rather than assuming that specific activities will be motivating for the child, reward menus should be developed through direct questioning of the child as to what he or she wants to earn or by observing his or her preferred activities.

7. To enhance the positive incentive value of classroom privileges, employ a priming procedure with the child prior to academic assignment periods. Priming involves teachers and students reviewing a list of possible classroom privileges *prior* to beginning an academic work period wherein students choose which activity they would like to participate in following the work period.

8. The integrity or fidelity with which an intervention program is implemented must be monitored and evaluated (Gresham, 1989, 2009). Such monitoring can serve as the basis for making changes in program components, justifying additional resource needs, and/or developing and providing additional training materials or coaching with those carrying out the procedures. An intervention integrity checklist such as the one developed by Gresham is an example of one method for monitoring program integrity. Gresham (1989) employed this checklist to assess the accuracy of implementation of a classroom response–cost lottery system. An independent observer evaluated the degree to which the classroom teacher completed the 11 main steps of this intervention on a daily basis. Thus, intervention integrity could be evaluated for each component across implementation days. Such information is invaluable in determining the need for additional teacher training and support in implementing classroom interventions. This type of checklist, of course, would be altered to reflect the specific components of a particular intervention procedure.

CONTINGENCY MANAGEMENT PROCEDURES

Contingency management involving reinforcement of appropriate academic and social behavior should be viewed as the cornerstone of classroom-based behavior management strategies for all students, including those with ADHD. By definition, a *positive reinforcer* is an event, condition, or stimulus that increases the future likelihood of an action or behavior that it immediately follows (Mayer et al., 2014). For children with ADHD, the research literature indicates that several different behavior management strategies based on positive reinforcement can favorably enhance classroom behavior. In fact, the meta-analysis conducted by DuPaul, Eckert, and Vilardo (2012) indicated that manipulation of antecedent and consequent events in the classroom was associated, on average, with a moderate to large effect size with respect to behavior change. Contingency management interventions have had less pronounced effects on academic achievement in this population.

A representative range of such strategies includes the use of positive reinforcement (often in the form of token reinforcement) coupled with penalties or redirection contingent on problematic behavior, time-out from positive reinforcement, and DBRCs to influence in-school behavior.

Token Reinforcement Programs

Contingent social praise and attention can be effective in producing positive behavioral change with many children. Typically, however, praise alone is insufficient to bring about consistent improvement in the classroom behavior and academic performance of children with ADHD (Pfiffner & DuPaul, in press). Behavioral strategies that incorporate secondary generalized reinforcers (e.g., token economies) can provide the reward immediacy, specificity, and potency that often are required for children diagnosed with ADHD. Behavior management systems incorporating these components have been shown to be highly successful in enhancing the academic productivity and appropriate behavior of inattentive children (e.g., DuPaul, Guevremont, & Barkley, 1992).

Designing a school-based token reinforcement system involves the following steps:

1. One or more problematic classroom situations are targeted for intervention. These situations may be determined through a teacher interview and/or use of an objective rating scale such as the School Situations Questionnaire–Revised (SSQ-R; DuPaul & Barkley, 1992). Direct observations in the classroom should be used to validate the selection of these problematic situations and behaviors (see Chapter 2). Typically, classroom work periods requiring independent completion of tasks present the greatest difficulty in terms of behavior control for children with ADHD.

2. Target behaviors are selected. They typically include academic products (e.g., number of math problems completed in a given amount of

time) or specific actions (e.g., appropriate interactions with peers during recess). In general, products are preferred due to the relative ease of their collection and monitoring. In addition, academic productivity typically involves behaviors that are incompatible with inattentive and disruptive behavior.

3. Types of secondary reinforcers (i.e., tokens) to be used are identified; these may include multicolored poker chips, check marks or stickers on a card, or points on a card stand. Younger children (e.g., up to 9 years old) generally prefer tangible rewards (e.g., poker chips), whereas older children and adolescents respond more positively to points or check marks. Token economy systems typically are considered too complicated for children under 5 years of age. With preschool-age children, the use of primary reinforcers (e.g., parental or teacher praise, hugs, or other social attention) contingent upon the occurrence of appropriate behavior is recommended.

4. The values of target or goal behaviors must be determined. That is, the number of tokens earned by completing each target behavior or its subcomponents should be determined by task difficulty, with completion of more difficult or time-consuming tasks worth more tokens than less involved assignments. More complex behaviors are broken down into their component parts (e.g., "successful work completion" can be defined as completing a certain number of items within a specified time period, attaining a certain level of accuracy, and reviewing the work before requesting the teacher's feedback) to allow children to earn tokens for partial completion of a task or reaching a certain performance criterion. In these instances, a task analysis may be necessary to explicitly delineate the components of expected behaviors.

5. The teacher and the student should jointly develop a list of privileges or activities within the classroom and/or school for which tokens may be exchanged. The list should include low-, medium-, and high- "cost" items. It can be beneficial to ask parents to collaborate on the development of this list and, in addition, to make privileges available at home in exchange for tokens. The amount of tokens or points necessary to "purchase" each privilege can be determined collaboratively among those individuals involved in the program. As a rough guide, estimate the maximum number of tokens that could be earned on a daily basis and divide this sum evenly among available reinforcers, then add or delete tokens to the cost of each item in accordance with the "value" of the privilege or activity to the child.

6. The value of the tokens should be taught or demonstrated to involved children (i.e., via token-backup reinforcer exchanges

accompanied by discussion), and initial criteria for earning tokens should be set to ensure early success. Take, for example, a child for whom the percentage of assigned math problems completed is chosen as a target behavior. The child typically completes somewhere between 50 and 60% of math problems. An initial completion rate of 50% might be the criterion selected for the first few days of the program.

7. Tokens are exchanged for classroom privileges on at least a daily basis. However, as a rule, shorter delays between receiving tokens and exchanging them for backup reinforcers will result in a more effective program. Although tokens can serve as immediate rewards of an interim nature, they may lose their value as reinforcers if they cannot be "cashed in" until after a long period of time has elapsed.

8. The effectiveness of the intervention program should be evaluated in an ongoing fashion, using multiple outcome measures. Based on the results of this ongoing evaluation, new behavioral targets may be added, old ones deleted or modified, and privileges rotated or varied. Also, the delivery of tokens and the timing of token exchanges may be altered. Response cost procedures (as discussed later) also may be incorporated into the system when some improvement in appropriate behavior has been achieved, yet disruptive or inattentive behaviors remain problematic.

9. Following initial implementation and behavioral improvement, several additional procedures may be necessary to ensure the generalization of obtained effects across time and settings. First, any additional problematic situations must be identified and targeted for change by implementing the above strategies (i.e., Steps 2–8). It is erroneous to assume that one need only obtain performance in one situation for such behavior to spontaneously generalize to other settings (see Abikoff, 2009, for a discussion of treatment generalization and ADHD). Second, the use of tokens and backup reinforcers should be faded in a gradual fashion. For example, rather than continuing to provide tokens following successful completion of each step in an academic task, reinforcement would be provided contingent upon completion of several steps first, and then following completion of the entire assignment. Eventually, the system would evolve into a contingency contract as discussed below in an effort to promote generalization of treatment gains, as well as to promote sustainability of student support.

Response Cost

Contingency management strategies consisting solely of positive reinforcement procedures are rarely effective in maintaining appropriate levels of academic and social behavior among children with ADHD (Pfiffner & O'Leary, 1993). In fact, several studies have documented the effectiveness of levying mild penalties following inappropriate (i.e., off-task) behavior in promoting consistent behavioral change (Pfiffner & O'Leary, 1987; Pfiffner, O'Leary, Rosen, & Sanderson, 1985; Rosen et al., 1984). For example, in addition to prudent reprimands and verbal redirection, penalties involving the loss or removal of privileges, points, or tokens (i.e., response cost) contingent upon inattentive, disruptive behavior has proven beneficial when used in combination with reinforcement-based procedures.

The concurrent use of token reinforcement and response cost has been demonstrated to increase the levels of on-task behavior, seatwork productivity, and academic accuracy of children with ADHD (Coles et al., 2005; DuPaul, Guevremont, & Barkley, 1992; Rapport, Murphy, & Bailey, 1980, 1982). In several cases, obtained classroom improvement was equivalent to that obtained with stimulant medication (Rapport et al., 1982). For example, Rapport (1987a, 1987b) describes a token delivery system that incorporates response cost. The student and teacher are each supplied with a card stand or electronic apparatus (e.g., the Attention Training System; Gordon, 1983) serving to display point totals earned by the child. Points are earned for in-seat, academically engaged behavior on a fixed-interval schedule and are deducted following incidents of off-task behavior. Points are awarded or deducted by the teacher changing the card displayed on his or her card stand (or by pressing a button on a remote control device). With this system, students change their own cards to match the teacher's or receive/lose points on the electronic apparatus via the remote mechanism controlled by the teacher. Thus, "token" delivery and deduction are accomplished on a remote basis by the teacher, allowing for simultaneously teaching and/or involvement in activities with other students. As with other token systems, at the conclusion of an academic work period a child's accumulated points are traded for various backup reinforcers (e.g., a choice activity).

Several issues should be considered in the use of response–cost procedures. For example, response–cost is a form of punishment, and its use could result in the child taking a negative view of the entire token system. Thus, in introducing the program and its components to the student and the teacher, emphasis should be placed on the program's positive aspects (e.g., emphasize that the student will have a chance to earn points and rewards for completing work accurately). In addition, initial and ongoing efforts should be made to adjust and arrange contingencies such that the child is earning more points than he or she is losing. For example, students may initially test the system by deliberately engaging in off-task behavior to see whether they will lose points. To prevent teachers from being caught up in a "point reduction game" of this sort, it is recommended that point reductions not occur more than once per minute regardless of the frequency of off-task behavior. Also, the teacher should be instructed to look away from the child immediately following point reductions (Rapport, 1987b). Finally, a child's point total should never fall below 0; when a point total is 0, all disruptive, off-task behavior should be ignored. If 0 point totals are a common occurrence, the contingencies may need to be revised so that point reductions do not occur for minor infractions. Once the child begins to experience success and is invested in the system, the criteria for point reductions can become more stringent in efforts to further improve classroom behavior and performance.

Contingency Contracting

Contingency contracting is a behavior management technique that involves the negotiation of a contractual agreement between a student and a teacher (DeRisi & Butz, 1975). Typically, the contract stipulates the desired classroom behaviors and consequences available contingent upon their performance. As with a token economy program, specific academic and behavioral goals are identified for the child to meet in order to gain access to preferred activities or other rewards. Contracting typically involves a direct connection between target behaviors and primary contingencies rather than the use of secondary reinforcers such as tokens. As such, there may be a longer time delay between behavior completion and reinforcement than with a token economy program. A sample contract appears in Figure 5.1.

Although contingency contracting is a relatively straightforward procedure, several factors may directly influence its efficacy with the ADHD population. First, the age of the child is an important consideration. Contracting procedures typically are unsuccessful with children under the age of 6, perhaps due to a lack of sufficiently developed rule-following skills and an inability to delay reinforcement for longer time periods on the part of young children. A second consideration is the length of the time delay between the required behavior and reinforcement. For example, a procedure requiring an 8-year-old child with ADHD to accurately complete math problems at a rate of 80% of assigned problems each day for a 1-week time period before earning a reward is doomed to failure. Timing of reinforcement is a crucial issue in implementing behavior management programs with children, especially

I, (Insert student's name here) _____ , agree to do the following:

1. Complete all my written math and language arts assignments, with at least 80% accuracy, before lunch time.
2. Give my teacher my full attention when he or she is speaking to the class or go to my reading group.
3. Remain quiet, and follow directions when lining up for recess, lunch, or music class.
4. Follow all playground rules (e.g., take turns, no fighting) during recess.

Each day that I do these things I will be allowed to choose **one** of the following:

1. 15 minutes time at the end of the school day to play a game with a classmate.
2. Use a classroom computer for work or play for 15 minutes.
3. Assist my teacher by completing some errands (e.g., take attendance forms to the main office) or in class jobs (e.g., collect student math assignments).

If I have a successful week, I will have earned one of the special weekend activities with my parents, such as a trip to the park, a bicycle ride, or having a friend visit at my house. If I do not complete these classroom responsibilities, then I will lose the opportunity to participate in daily free-time activities.

I agree to fulfill this contract to the best of my abilities.
Signed:

_____   _____
(Student's signature)   (Teacher's signature)

_____
(Date)

FIGURE 5.1. A sample classroom behavior contract for a student with ADHD.

those with ADHD. To increase the probability of improved outcomes in the example given, access to preferred activities should be provided at the conclusion of the successful work period or school day.

The choice of target behaviors and the manner of incorporating them into an intervention program are important determinants of a behavioral contract's success. For example, during the *initial* stages of a contracting procedure care should be exercised to avoid large numbers of goals, extremely high standards of quality, and completion of complex (e.g., multistep) tasks. For the child with ADHD, these types of initial requirements likely will lead to failure. A preferable approach would be to target a few simple behaviors or products so that the child can achieve success right from the start. More difficult or complex goals could be incorporated gradually into later iterations of the contract such that terminal objectives are reached with minimal failure along the way.

A final consideration of importance in designing a behavioral contract is the identification of appropriate reinforcers. All too often identified reinforcers take the form of activities or items that are assumed by school personnel to be motivating for children. Assumptions about the reinforcer preferences of the children we work with are a good starting point for designing contracts and contingency management procedures. However, reinforcer preferences can be very idiosyncratic, and as such it is suggested that individual reward menus be derived. Two alternatives for doing so are suggested. First, it is advisable, especially with older children, to negotiate directly with the student regarding possible privileges. Direct negotiation not only ensures identification of potent reinforcers, but also enlists the student's cooperation and investment in the contractual process. Second, naturalistic observations can be conducted to identify a child's preferred activities for use as reinforcers. Such observations might include identifying those off-task behaviors (e.g., drawing, playing with objects at seat) that the child frequently engages in while assigned to do independent work. This strategy would be helpful especially when a child is unable to provide suggestions for rewards.

Time-Out from Positive Reinforcement

Another type of mild punishment strategy that may be appropriate for classroom use consists of various forms of time-out from positive reinforcement. Time-out from positive reinforcement, as its name implies, involves restricting the child's access to positive reinforcement (e.g., teacher and peer attention). An adaptation of Barkley's (2013a) procedures designed for use within the home may be most applicable. To be effective, time-out procedures should be (1) implemented only when there is a reinforcing environment to be removed from, (2) implemented when the function of the child's disruptive behavior is to gain teacher or peer attention, (3) implemented swiftly following a rule infraction, (4) applied with consistency, and (5) employed for the smallest amount of time (e.g., 1–5 minutes) that proves effective. Lack of available reinforcement is the most salient feature determining the effectiveness of this procedure, *not* the amount of time spent in actual time-out. If the child is to be moved to a time-out area, this area should be located in a relatively dull location within the classroom (*not* a separate room, closet, cloakroom, or hallway) to allow for monitoring of the child's activities. Criteria for terminating the time-out period should include (1) a time-out period sufficiently long enough to be effective (i.e., 1 minute for every 2 years of age of the child); (2) a short period of calm, nondisruptive behavior required prior to its termination; and (3) the child's expressed willingness to correct, amend, or compensate for the misbehavior that led to the time-out contingency. Finally, children who leave the time-out area without permission should have their time interval lengthened by a fixed amount for each violation, or lose points or tokens if a token economy system is also being used.

An illustrative example of the use of time-out is provided by Fabiano and colleagues (2004) who compared three variations of time-out from positive reinforcement. These researchers examined the effects of time-out procedures of longer duration (15 minutes), shorter duration (5 minutes) and an escalating/de-escalating time-out, relative to no time-out on the problematic behavior of 71 children with ADHD participating in a summer treatment program. The time-out intervention was implemented in conjunction with an overall treatment program in all cases, and the effects were uniformly positive. That is, each form of time-out was effective in reducing intentional aggression, noncompliance, and property destruction as compared with no time-out, with no differences in effectiveness detected between the time-out conditions tested.

To summarize, restrictive procedures such as time-out should be employed only in the context of ongoing positive reinforcement programming. Furthermore, time-out contingencies should be an intervention of last resort following implementation of a hierarchy of both positive and less restrictive behavior management procedures. For example, inappropriate behavior would lead initially to brief, prudent reprimands, followed by response cost, followed by time-out with head down at desk, followed by time-out in a corner of the room. More severe disruptive behaviors (e.g., physical aggression) should lead to immediate application of the more restrictive time-out procedures or to other procedures consistent with classroom or school rules. When used, time-out procedures need to be monitored very carefully, as they are not considered viable ongoing management strategies, but rather are best viewed as short-term behavior reduction techniques.

DBRCs and Home-Based Contingencies

Home-based contingency management procedures, based on the child's behavior and/or academic performance at school, can be used as an effective supplement to classroom-based contingency management. These procedures have several beneficial features. First, on a daily basis the child receives direct feedback from his or her teachers as to performance in several areas of classroom functioning. Second, parents receive daily information about the child's classroom performance, thus providing an ongoing forum for teacher–parent communication. For children experiencing classroom difficulties, this schedule of communication is preferable to waiting for a parent–teacher conference or an end-of-the-term report card. Third, in many, but not all, cases, when a daily report card program leads to symptom reduction, students also show improvement in academic functioning (Owens, Johannes, & Karpenko, 2009). Fourth, more than 70% of students with ADHD can be expected to show behavioral improvement within the first month of a daily report card program with additional gradual improvement over the course of several months of treatment (Owens et al., 2012). Finally, the system circumvents some of the practical limitations (e.g., restricted range of possible reinforcing activities) of classroom-based contingency management systems because it involves the parents in providing reinforcement for in-school behavior.

An example of a home-based reinforcement program for a student with ADHD has been proposed (DuPaul, Guevremont, & Barkley, 1991) that employs a daily report card similar to the one displayed in Figure 5.2. For each child, several behavioral goals are identified, such as paying attention to class activities, completion of assigned work, accuracy of work, and following rules. The specific goals should vary with respect to the presenting problems of the individual student (e.g., interactions with classmates may be targeted if the child is prone to arguing and fighting with peers). The columns of the card can be used to convey information across different subject areas or periods of the school day. Thus, if the child has more than one teacher, they all may participate. The teacher enters ratings (on a 5-point scale from "excellent" to "extremely poor") of the child's performance in the appropriate area of the card, initials the card, and provides comments where necessary. Ratings and comments are made in ink to prevent their alteration by the child. The student is responsible for giving the card to each teacher and bringing it home on a daily basis.

Given the use of quantitative ratings, school–home notes can be used within a token economy system based at home. For example, the teacher provides quantitative ratings of performance in each goal area, as discussed above. When the card is brought home, the parent(s) briefly discusses the positive and negative ratings with the child. Then, specified point values are assigned to the numbers on the card and summed to yield the net total points earned for the day. For example, each teacher rating of "1" could be converted to 25 points, each "2" to 15 points, each "3" to 5 points. Ratings of "4" or "5" would result in the deduction of 15 and 25 points, respectively. To produce positive behavior change, a home token reinforcement program must be arranged such that these points can lead to the "purchase" of backup reinforcers (e.g., household privileges, television time, spending a night at a friend's home). As with

---

DAILY STUDENT REPORT CARD

Student name: _____   Date: _____

Please rate the student in each of the areas listed, as to how well he or she
performed in school today. Please use ratings of 1 to 5, based on the following
scale: 1 = excellent, 2 = good, 3 = fair, 4 = poor, 5 = extremely poor or did not
work.

	Class periods or subject:					
Behaviors:	1	2	3	4	5	6
Participation						
Classwork						
Turned in homework						
Interactions with other students						
Teacher's initials						

Add comments here and on back if needed: _____

FIGURE 5.2. Daily report card for use in a home-based reinforcement program
for ADHD. From Barkley (1990). Copyright 1990 by The Guilford Press.
Adapted by permission.

other token programs, this system's effectiveness is dependent upon its
motivational value and the availability of a variety of backup reinforcers.

Kelley (1990) and Volpe and Fabiano (2013) have written texts
that provide thorough coverage of this topic, focused on developing and
using daily report cards as a means of communication among parents,
teachers, and children. A variety of daily report cards are presented in
their texts, all of which could be adapted for use with students who
are exhibiting ADHD-related behaviors. For example, a school–home
note that could be used with a secondary school-level student might
emphasize, for example, behaviors such as homework completion and
test grades. Daily reports such as these allow the teacher to alert parents
about upcoming homework assignments on a regular basis, as well. At
the secondary level, teachers typically prefer to complete school–home
notes on a weekly rather than a daily basis.

Several factors may limit the effectiveness of home-based reinforcement programs (Rapport, 1987a). One primary drawback of such
a system is that, by definition, it involves a delay in the provision of
reinforcement. Given that children with ADHD have difficulty delaying

reinforcement (Barkley, 2006), home-based reinforcers may be less powerful relative to classroom-based contingencies that are more immediately linked to the behaviors of interest. This issue is particularly important in working with children younger than age 6. Second, school personnel have limited means for assessing parental implementation of the procedures. Finally, when home-based reinforcers are used, parents should be discouraged from relying solely on material rewards, which can lose some of their potency over long periods of time. Instead, parents should be provided with assistance in developing an array of potential reinforcers of an activity, social, or material nature. These reinforcers should be salient to the child, readily available in the home or community, inexpensive if they involve a monetary cost, and rotated on a regular basis to prevent boredom with the "same old rewards." It is particularly important to use reinforcers that are viewed as "necessities" by the child (e.g., watching television, playing video games, riding bicycle) rather than an exclusive reliance on "luxury" items that the child could live without (e.g., going to a favorite restaurant, a trip to the amusement park).

In view of the limitations to home–school communication systems enumerated above, it is worthwhile to delineate the factors that will enhance the efficacy of home-based contingencies. These factors are listed in Table 5.3. First, daily and weekly goals are specified in a positive manner. As noted earlier, to pass the "dead man test," target behaviors involve the active performance of classroom responsibilities (e.g., work completion) rather than an absence of inappropriate behavior. Second, both academic and behavioral goals are included. In an effort to increase

TABLE 5.3. Components of Effective Home–School Communication and Contingency Programs

1. Parental cooperation and involvement are solicited prior to implementation.
2. Student input into goals and contingencies is solicited, particularly with older children and adolescents.
3. Daily and/or weekly goals are stated in a positive manner.
4. Both academic and behavioral goals are included.
5. A small number of goals are targeted at a time.
6. The teacher provides quantitative feedback about student performance.
7. Feedback is provided by subject or class periods.
8. Student performance is communicated on a regular basis (either daily or weekly).
9. Home-based contingencies are tied to school performance. Both short- and long-term consequences are employed.
10. Goals and procedures are modified, as necessary.

the chances of initial success, one or two goals should be readily attainable by the child. This will serve to "hook" the child into cooperating with the system before increasing standards or expectations for performance. Third, it is important to employ only a few goals at a time so that the student and teacher are not overwhelmed by the system. Fourth, teacher feedback about the child's performance should be quantitative. Although qualitative statements can be informative, they are often vague and nonspecific (e.g., "Johnny had a good day today"). Fifth, feedback is provided by subject or class period. This provides the student with specific information about performance, allows for more frequent feedback, and circumvents a loss of motivation if the child experiences difficulties in the early part of the day. In the latter situation, if ratings on the daily report card were based on the entire day's performance, it is likely that the child would still obtain low ratings even if his or her behavior improved over the course of the day. Sixth, home–school communication occurs on a daily or weekly basis to facilitate the provision of frequent reinforcement. Seventh, a hierarchy of short- and long-term privileges at home are tied directly to teacher ratings on the daily report card. It is unlikely that a child with ADHD will exhibit improvement in the absence of external reinforcement. Eighth, parents should be involved in planning the home–school communication program from the onset to ensure their understanding of and cooperation with the procedures. Older children and adolescents should be included in planning the program for the same reasons. Ninth, goals and procedures are modified on an ongoing basis in accordance with student progress or lack thereof.

Another possible parent-mediated intervention involves having parents provide home-based academic support to their children. For example, Hook and DuPaul (1999) evaluated the effects of a *parent tutoring* intervention for four second- and third-grade students with ADHD who exhibited reading difficulties. Parents were trained to monitor their children's reading using passages provided by the children's teachers. Tutoring was implemented over a 4- to 8-week period using a multiple-baseline, across-participants experimental design. Reading achievement was assessed at home and at school using brief curriculum-based reading probes that were administered two times per week across experimental phases. All four children showed gains in reading on home-based probes, with more variable improvements evident on school-based reading probes. The results indicated that parent tutoring may be a promising intervention for enhancing reading achievement for some children with ADHD, particularly those whose parents are invested in their child's education.

In summary, parent-mediated strategies, particularly home-based contingency systems, can be effective in enhancing school performance, especially when used to supplement classroom-based behavior change procedures (e.g., cover periods of the school day when the latter procedures are not in effect). Students who display ADHD-related behaviors that are considered milder in severity should be particularly responsive to home–school programming. As with other contingency management strategies, attention to the details of identifying target behaviors and reinforcers, linking the two, and monitoring and managing the system to ensure its integrity will be critical to successful outcomes.

Functional Behavioral Assessment

The contingency management strategies discussed previously focus on altering target behaviors primarily through the manipulation of consequences following the occurrence of targeted problem and appropriate behaviors. From a technical standpoint, these procedures focus on what behavior looks like, or its topography, rather than what function a behavior serves for an individual student. Technical advances in classroom-based behavior management, however, make prominent the notion of linking intervention to an assessment of behavioral function.

Functional assessment strategies include interviews, observations, and environmental manipulations (e.g., changing a seating arrangement) intended to identify environmental variables that reliably precede or reliably follow problem behaviors of concern. Such variables are then hypothesized, in a behavior analytic formulation, to prompt or promote the occurrence of problem behavior, in the case of preceding variables. And in the case of variables reliably following problem behavior, these are hypothesized to reinforce or maintain problem behavior (see Bambara & Kern, 2005).

Understanding the factors that maintain the problem behaviors, along with the situations that appear to set the stage for those behaviors, is an essential first step in planning successful interventions. For example, consider a target student's out-of-seat behavior that is reliably occasioned by the teacher's presentation of a classwide, in-seat math work assignment. In this instance one potential intervention could involve provision of teacher assistance at the beginning of that assignment to ensure that directions are understood, the student has all necessary materials, and the student is able to independently complete the work assigned. This would be a preventive or proactive strategy.

Alternatively, consider the same student and behavior but a different identified function of the problem behavior. In this instance, suppose the student's out-of-seat behavior reliably results in teacher attention (e.g., "Ryan, do you need help with your assignment? Let me look at your work and see if I can help."). Here it would be hypothesized that Ryan's out-of-seat behavior is reinforced via teacher-delivered attention. At least one component of a *functional* approach to intervention would include behavior management strategies intended to strengthen a socially acceptable alternative behavior that would produce the same type of reinforcement—in this case teacher attention. For example, the teacher might use a strategy that included providing attention contingent upon Ryan being in his seat and/or working on independent in-seat assignments, and withholding attention when out-of-seat behavior occurs. Alternatively, he or she might work with Ryan to develop an unobtrusive signal that he can use to readily obtain teacher attention and assistance with challenging academic work.

In a representative study, Stahr, Cushing, Lane, and Fox (2006) used functional assessment strategies to guide the development of classroom-based interventions for a fourth-grade student diagnosed with ADHD. The interventions used were linked to problems hypothesized to serve the functions of escape from difficult tasks and access to teacher attention for another student. Results of this work suggested that interventions based on functional assessment strategies, in conjunction with self-management strategies, resulted in significant improvements in on-task and appropriate attention-seeking behaviors.

Understanding the factors that maintain problem behaviors, along with the situations that appear to cue or prompt those behaviors, is an essential first step in individualizing interventions (DuPaul et al., 1997). For example, consider the disruptive classroom behavior (e.g., verbal disruptions, speaking out of turn) of an identified student. Assume that we know the behavior is reliably occasioned by the teacher's instructional presentation of new math material. It is highly probable in such circumstances that the child's disruptive behavior is motivated by the desire to avoid and/or escape from math instruction. Here, then, one potential intervention could involve provision of teacher assistance at the beginning of that activity to ensure that rules and expectations are understood, that the student has all materials needed to participate in the instruction, and that the student is able to clearly see and hear the teacher's presentation. This would constitute a preventive or proactive strategy. Flood and Wilder (2002) used this type of strategy to identify the conditions under which a student with ADHD exhibits high rates of off-task behavior. Based on the hypothesis that difficult academic assignments elicited the behavior of concern, these researchers taught the student to communicate his need for instructional assistance at such times, resulting in significant improvement in desired classroom behavior.

Alternatively, consider the same student and behavior but a different formulation of the problem. Suppose, for example, the student's disruptive behavior reliably results in teacher attention (e.g., "James, please stop disrupting the lesson. Don't you remember the class rules?"). These circumstances might lead to a hypothesis that James's disruptive behavior is being reinforced through teacher-delivered social attention. At least one component of a functional approach to intervention would include behavior management strategies intended to strengthen an alternative behavior that would produce the same type of reinforcement—in this case, teacher attention. For example, the teacher might use a strategy that included providing attention contingent upon James responding appropriately to a question posed by the teacher and/or otherwise maintaining appropriate attention to the lesson, and withholding attention when disruptive behavior occurs.

Once the function of a child's behavior is determined, then an intervention is designed that leads to functionally equivalent behavior. Functionally equivalent interventions provide access to desired consequences contingent upon appropriate behavior rather than the problematic behavior. Connections between behavioral functions and possible functionally equivalent interventions are displayed in Figure 5.3. For example, if a child is engaging in disruptive behavior in a classroom to gain teacher attention, then the intervention should arrange for teacher attention to be contingent only upon the display of appropriate behavior, while disruptive behavior is ignored (i.e., differential reinforcement of incompatible behavior). It is assumed that function-based interventions will be more effective than strategies implemented based on broader diagnostic data and/or a trial-and-error approach. Furthermore, because function-based interventions provide access to desired consequences, it is presumed that these strategies will result in outcomes that are maintained over time.

Based on a formulation of this type, Ervin, DuPaul, Kern, and Friman (1998) used functional assessment strategies to guide the development of classroom-based interventions for four adolescents diagnosed with ADHD. For two of these students, the interventions used were linked to problems hypothesized to serve the functions of escape from written tasks and access to peer attention, respectively. The former student was allowed to complete written assignments using a computer rather than writing by hand—the problem behavior was hypothesized to be escape motivated. The latter student was provided with peer attention contingent on the display of on-task behavior—it was hypothesized that the problem behavior was maintained by peer attention. Results of this work suggested that the classroom interventions based on functional assessment strategies resulted in significant improvements in the task-related behavior of both students.

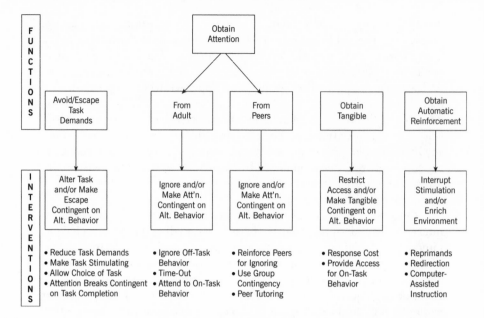

FIGURE 5.3. Possible functions for child behavior and associated interventions. From DuPaul and Ervin (1996). Copyright 1996 by the Association for Advancement of Behavior Therapy. Reprinted by permission.

COGNITIVE-BEHAVIORAL MANAGEMENT STRATEGIES

A primary goal of treatment for ADHD is to enable a student to develop adequate levels of self-control. The latter term implies that a child will exhibit age-appropriate social and academic behaviors on an independent basis (i.e., with a minimum of accommodation on the part of the environment). Although this is a desirable treatment goal, it is quite difficult to obtain in practice given the chronic and multifaceted nature of ADHD. Self-regulation interventions for ADHD are composed of strategies incorporating self-monitoring, self-reinforcement, and/or self-instruction (Barkley, 1989). These strategies, especially those incorporating self-instruction, sometimes have been referred to as *cognitive-behavioral interventions* given their emphasis on changing children's thinking, behavior, and their interaction. Self-regulation interventions have become increasingly popular as treatments for a variety of classroom difficulties, including ADHD (see Shapiro & Cole, 1994). In general, despite their apparent potential in ameliorating ADHD symptoms, these interventions, particularly self-instruction training, have not been uniformly successful (Abikoff, 1985). Nevertheless, we will review findings relevant to self-monitoring and self-reinforcement approaches enumerated above while highlighting procedures that are of relevance for practitioners (see also Chapter 6 for description of self-regulation interventions for adolescents with ADHD).

Self-Monitoring

Children can be taught to observe and record the occurrence of their own behaviors. For instance, a child with ADHD might be taught to recognize and record instances of on-task behavior during academic work. Typically, an auditory or visual stimulus (e.g., beep from a tape recorder, hand signal from the teacher) is used periodically throughout a specific time period to signal the child to observe his or her current behavior. The child then records whether he or she was on-task on a grid or chart taped to his or her desk. This type of self-monitoring can be used alone or, more typically, in combination with other self-management procedures. Although this intervention has not been studied extensively with children diagnosed with ADHD, attention-related behaviors have been found to increase as a function of self-monitoring, especially when combined with self-reinforcement or external reinforcement (e.g., Barkley, Copeland, & Sivage, 1980). Also, some research indicates that it may be more effective to have the child monitor task completion and/or accuracy than to simply monitor attentive behavior (e.g., Lam, Cole, Shapiro, & Bambara, 1994).

Self-monitoring may be a particularly viable intervention for adolescents with ADHD, especially when organizational skills are a concern. For example, Gureasko-Moore, DuPaul, and White (2007) evaluated the use of a self-monitoring strategy for three seventh-grade students with ADHD. All of these participants were reported by their teachers to have significant problems being prepared and organized for class (e.g., coming to class with correct textbook, pencils, and notebook). A checklist of preparatory behaviors was constructed for each student by his or her teacher. This checklist was used to determine the percentage of preparatory steps completed across experimental phases in the context of a multiple-baseline, across-participants design. Following a baseline phase, a school psychologist provided brief training in self-monitoring to each participant. All three students showed substantial gains in the percentage of steps completed as a function of self-monitoring. In fact, several weeks later, students were observed to complete nearly 100% of required preparatory behaviors on a consistent basis, even without external prompting and reinforcement.

Self-Reinforcement

The most promising self-regulation intervention for ADHD requires students not only to monitor their behavior but also to evaluate and reinforce their own performance (Barkley, 1989). In fact, the combination of self-monitoring and self-reinforcement has been found effective in improving on-task behavior, academic accuracy, and peer interactions for students with ADHD (Barkley et al., 1980; Hinshaw, Henker, & Whalen, 1984). These effects are enhanced further when stimulant medication is used in combination with these procedures (Barkley, 1989).

Self-reinforcement strategies may be particularly helpful for addressing ADHD-related problems in two situations. First, a student can be taught to monitor and reinforce his or her own behavior while fading the use of an externally based, contingency management program (Barkley, 1989). The premise is that positive behavioral change will be maintained despite the reduction in teacher feedback or other forms of reinforcement. Of course, backup reinforcers (e.g., classroom or home privileges) *must* be used as teacher monitoring and feedback are faded. The fading of backup reinforcement must take place over an extended time period. A second situation where self-reinforcement is an appropriate treatment for ADHD is at the secondary level where teachers and students are reluctant to employ contingency management procedures. Thus, self-management may be a more acceptable intervention at the secondary level, and therefore presumably more likely to be implemented on a consistent basis.

An example of self-monitoring and self-reinforcement procedures useful for ameliorating ADHD symptoms is based on the work of Rhode, Morgan, and Young (1983). They used these strategies to facilitate the mainstreaming of six elementary students with "behavioral handicaps." The initial stages of the program involve the use of a token reinforcement program and verbal feedback from the teacher based on teacher ratings of student behavior during specific intervals in the classroom. Ratings are provided using a 6-point criterion hierarchy: 5 = excellent—followed all classroom rules for entire interval, work 100% correct; 4 = very good—minor infraction of rules (e.g., a talk-out or out-of-seat) but followed rules rest of interval, work at least 90% correct; 3 = average—did not follow all rules for entire time, but no serious offenses, work at least 80% correct; 2 = below average—broke one or more rules to the extent that behavior was not acceptable (e.g., aggressive, noisy, talking) but followed rules part of the time, work approximately 60–80% correct; 1 = poor—broke one or more rules almost entire period or engaged in higher degree of inappropriate behavior most of the time, work between 0 and 60% correct; and 0 = unacceptable—broke one or more rules entire interval, did not work at all or work all incorrect. Separate evaluations of behavioral and academic performance can be made using this system. Teacher-provided points are exchanged for backup reinforcers in school or at home as in a standard token economy.

Once students demonstrate behavioral and/or academic gains, they are trained in evaluating their own behavior using the criteria listed above. At this stage, the teacher's ratings continue to be used to determine how many points students have earned. In addition, students can earn 1 bonus point for matching teacher ratings exactly. If student ratings deviate by more than 1 point from teacher ratings, students do not earn any points for that interval. Thus, contingencies are associated with both behavioral improvement *and* rating one's performance in a manner similar to the teacher.

Over the course of time, the teacher ratings are gradually faded such that the student ratings are the primary arbiter for earning backup reinforcement. This is facilitated by (1) the use of random "matching challenges" that occur on a periodic basis, and (2) the gradual reduction in frequency of these matching challenges. For example, the initial cutback in teacher ratings may involve a matching challenge that occurs every other day, on the average. Then the teacher matches are faded to every third day, once weekly, and once biweekly, on the average. If, at any point in time, the student's performance deteriorates and/or the teacher suspects inflation of student ratings, then matching challenges are conducted more frequently.

In the program described by Rhode and colleagues (1983), the students eventually employed self-ratings only, with no backup reinforcers. This led to maintenance of significant behavioral improvements across resource and regular classroom settings. This self-reinforcement system has been extended to children with ADHD and related disruptive disorders in elementary (Hoff & DuPaul, 1998), middle (Shapiro, DuPaul, & Bradley, 1998), and high school (Smith, Young, Nelson, & West, 1992) settings. Thus, the use of variations of this program could have applicability for the treatment of ADHD-related behaviors across a wide age span. Nevertheless, it is important to note that a key variable influencing the success of these procedures is the continued use of external reinforcers contingent on student ratings. It is unlikely that the effectiveness of this intervention would be maintained if backup reinforcement was reduced or eliminated earlier in the sequence of program steps.

Designers of self-regulation interventions need to keep in mind that children with ADHD often lack the skill to be accurate judges of their own behavior. Because they may have a tendency toward recalling their positive behaviors and not recognizing the problem behaviors that affect their ratings, a brief discussion or reminder of the behaviors that led to a lower rating may be useful (Hinshaw & Melnick, 1992).

Several recent examples provide good models for developing and implementing self-regulation interventions. For example, as noted previously, Gureaske-Moore and colleagues (2007) worked with six middle school students identified with ADHD, to improve classroom preparation and homework completion rates using self-management strategies. The students were taught to use checklists and logs to monitor their own behaviors. In addition, students were guided to evaluate the data relative to identified goals, in collaboration with a school psychologist. The self-regulation strategies resulted in significant improvements in classroom preparation and homework completion across all student participants.

In another example, Evans and colleagues (2009) engaged 28 middle school students with ADHD in a project aimed at improving school-related organization behaviors. The project specifically focused on student academic binders, and used a monitoring tool called the organization assessment sheet (OAS), which contained items referring to assignment notebooks, separate class folders, homework folders, and specific organizational strategies using particular sections of the binder. Students were taught to monitor and evaluate their behavior relative to identified expectations for being well organized, and reinforcers were delivered contingent upon high rates of demonstrated binder organization. Nearly all (26 of 28 students) demonstrated significant improvements in organization, and the researchers also found significant correlations between specific items on the OAS and student math grades.

In one other example of self-regulation interventions, Plumer and Stoner (2005) demonstrated improvements in peer-related social behaviors for three, third- and fourth-grade students with ADHD. This project is notable in that the self-monitoring and evaluation that formed the heart of the intervention was guided by a process of peer coaching delivered by students from the same classroom as the target students. The primary components of the intervention involved individual students and a peer in daily goal setting, behavior monitoring at recess and lunchtime, behavior evaluation relative to the daily goals, and assignment of points based on performance. The points could be exchanged for items on a menu of reinforcers. Significant improvements in positive social behaviors were obtained across participants, as a result of the intervention.

Designing a self-regulation system in a classroom for children with ADHD would involve teaching children to use the system, providing clear descriptions of the expected behaviors, and drawing up a list of privileges students would like to earn. The goal of such a system is to eventually train children to monitor their own behavior in the classroom, without constant feedback from the teacher.

EFFECTIVE INSTRUCTIONAL STRATEGIES

In addition to the documented benefits of contingency management strategies, students identified with ADHD are likely to benefit from prevention-oriented behavior- and classroom management strategies. Furthermore, children with this disorder may require remedial or supplemental instruction aimed at improving basic academic skills, learning, and study. In general, ameliorating the classroom difficulties experienced by target students should involve multiple prevention and intervention approaches including (1) active and ongoing teaching of classroom rules, routines, and expectations for appropriate classroom behavior; (2) grading practices and contingencies to support the rules, routines, and expectations; (3) changes in instructional routines and curricula to improve rates of learning; (4) ongoing monitoring of progress in basic skill areas (i.e., reading, writing, math, and spelling); and (5) teaching students to be competent at organizing and studying academic materials.

In considering the classroom learning and performance of children with ADHD, several variables will need to be analyzed, ranging from the child's basic academic skills to the observable classroom behaviors that are potentially interfering with the child's classroom performance. A nonexhaustive list of such variables is provided in Table 5.4. For many children experiencing achievement and/or behavior problems in the classroom, a first step in pursuing problem resolution is to determine whether the problem is a skills or a conditions problem so that an appropriate intervention might be designed. One of the difficulties facing professionals serving children with ADHD, however, is that classroom difficulties

TABLE 5.4. Skills and Conditions to Consider in Evaluating and Treating Classroom-Based Problems Associated with ADHD

Skills	Conditions
Reading skills	Severity of ADHD symptomatology
Writing skills	Classroom management and motivational strategies
Spelling skills	
	Instructional routines
Math skills	
	Curricula
Study skills, organizational skills, and self-management skills	Home–school communication
Social and interpersonal skills	Community-based interventions (e.g., medication)

are likely to be a combination of *both* skills and conditions problems. Because of this likely interaction, multiple interventions typically will be implemented across settings and intervention agents.

The strategies discussed in this section are those with empirical support for their effectiveness in ameliorating some of the difficulties listed in Table 5.4. However, it must be noted that these routines, strategies, and approaches to teaching have only recently begun to be researched specifically with respect to their effects on the learning and behavior of children with ADHD. Researchers at Lehigh University, including the first author of this book, have developed and tested a consultation model (Promoting Academic Success for Students [PASS]) for designing academic interventions for students with ADHD. This data-based decision-making model includes elements of consultative problem solving (Bergan & Kratochwill, 1990), curriculum-based measurement (Shinn, 1998), and functional assessment of academic behavior (Witt, Daly, & Noell, 2000). The academic outcome data collected (reported later in this chapter) has shown the cost-effectiveness of instructional interventions based on this model relative to more typical "trial-and-error" approaches to intervention design. For now, we begin our discussion with a focus on proactive teacher behaviors (i.e., proactive strategies occurring prior to the display of problem behaviors).

Instructional Management and Remediation in Basic Skill Areas

Classroom-based research efforts involving children with ADHD have tended to focus on the issues of behavior management as discussed in the previous sections of this chapter. In contrast, relatively little research has been conducted regarding instructional, curricular, or classroom environment manipulations aimed at enhancing the learning and academic performance of these children. Our speculation is that this phenomenon is a result of a combination of two variables. First, disruptive behaviors frequently are paramount concerns to teachers, and lead them to refer children to specialists. Second, historically, research knowledge and practices regarding ADHD and related problems have emerged from within the domains of medical and clinical professionals rather than from the educational arena. However, this set of circumstances has begun to change as educational researchers have now investigated intervention approaches including peer tutoring, computer-assisted instruction, task and instructional modifications, and strategy training on the learning and achievement of students with ADHD. These strategies are described below following a brief discussion of some basic issues in instruction, as well as strategies for remediation in basic skill areas such as reading, writing, and spelling.

A complete treatment of the topic of instructional strategies and interventions is well beyond our scope, and numerous books are available on the topic (e.g., see Shinn & Walker, 2010, for thorough coverage of interventions for academic and behavior problems; see Archer & Hughes, 2011, for coverage of effective teaching). However, it is our hope that this presentation will spark the further development of needed classroom-based research and practices linking instructional strategies to improved outcomes for students with ADHD.

Basic Instructional Processes

As reviewed and discussed by Archer and Hughes (2011), effective teaching involves the sequential arrangement of six primary instructional functions: review, presentation, guided practice, corrections and feedback, independent practice, and weekly/monthly reviews. For example, *review* involves checking for prerequisite skills and knowledge, and discussion of previously taught material and information relevant to the current lesson. Next, *new information or material* (i.e., facts, discriminations, basic concepts, and relations) is presented in manageable steps or units, using clear positive and negative examples. Once the new material and examples have been presented, students are provided with numerous opportunities for *guided practice* with high rates of success. Then, based on student performance during the practice exercises, teachers provide students with *feedback and corrections*, and reteaching of material as needed to strengthen the new learning. When students are able to respond correctly a high percentage of the time to questions and problems involving the new material, they are ready for independent practice. *Independent practice* is intended to build fluency and autonomy with newly learned material, so that students can apply the new learning to various problems and understand it within a variety of contexts. Finally, *weekly and monthly reviews* are provided, again in the interest of building fluency and independent application of the learned material.

These teaching functions promote student learning for two primary reasons. First, the strategies ensure that students are provided with the opportunities to learn what they are supposed to learn. Second, working through cycles of review, practice, feedback, corrections, and more practice, teachers ensure that students are performing accurately and becoming more fluent. Doing so helps to avoid situations in which students repeatedly practice or perform their schoolwork inaccurately, thereby strengthening "mis-rules" (e.g., add when I see a "–" sign and subtract when I see a "+" sign). Furthermore, these factors can be manipulated and individualized with respect to difficult-to-teach material or students. For example, more opportunities to practice and a greater frequency of feedback might be provided around material broken down into smaller units when teaching a student who is experiencing difficulty in a particular subject area.

The instructional support and remediation strategies discussed later incorporate factors that have been associated with improved performance among children with ADHD. These include opportunities to learn via active responses to teacher directions and instruction, coupled with opportunities for the provision of frequent feedback and corrections. These strategies are presented only briefly here, with the intent of providing the interested reader with direction for further reading or study.

Reading Skills

Research findings suggest that success in reading in the early school years is related to later school achievement and adjustment (National Reading Panel, 2000). As such, skill in reading is a critical building block for a child's successful school experience. Children with ADHD appear to be at greater risk for reading problems than their typically developing peers (DuPaul et al., 2001; O'Reilly, 2002). Reading instruction and remediation can be construed broadly as divisible into the two related areas of *decoding* and *comprehension.*

Gaining meaning from written information involves the decoding of text. The importance of children learning to decode text is such that the National Research Council (1998) and the National Reading Panel (2000) have discussed the importance of *all children* receiving instruction in phonics as part of early reading instruction. Similarly, other leading researchers in the field of reading instruction (Adams, 1990; Carnine, Kame'enui, & Silbert, 1990; Denton & Vaughn, 2010) suggest that systematic phonics-based training should be a part of a student's kindergarten through grade 3 years of reading instruction. Grossen and Carnine (1991) discuss four primary components of such instruction: (1) teaching letter–sound correspondence in isolation; (2) teaching the blending of sounds; (3) providing immediate feedback and corrections on oral reading errors; and (4) providing for extensive practice using sounds in isolation, word lists, and words in the context of reading passages. Students who develop fluent decoding skills are well prepared to become skilled readers who obtain meaning from text, as decoding skills are complemented with other forms of reading instruction.

Comprehensive reading instruction includes a great deal more than teaching phonics skills. For example, Sindelar, Lane, Pullen, and Hudson (2002) have suggested that students experiencing difficulty with reading may benefit from a variety of other strategies within three primary areas: (1) building fluency in reading/decoding, (2) building vocabulary, and (3) strengthening comprehension skills. A few of these strategies are noted here (for a more in-depth discussion of instructional strategies for reading comprehension, see the National Reading Panel Report published in 2000). Instruction for building reading and decoding fluency includes such strategies as repeated readings wherein passages are read several times (O'Shea, Sindelar, & O'Shea, 1987; Samuels, 1979) and previewing new readings (Rose & Sherry, 1984). Both interventions have been shown to enhance the reading fluency and comprehension of students with learning disabilities. Baker, Gersten, and Grossen (2002) also suggest that systematic instruction in vocabulary is warranted as part of comprehensive reading instruction. Sindelar and Stoddard (1991) note several research studies documenting the effectiveness of vocabulary-building strategies such as teaching synonyms via matching of printed words (Pany, Jenkins, & Shreck, 1982), teaching sets of words that belong within categories (Beck, Perfetti, & McKeown, 1982), and preteaching vocabulary words contained in a new reading assignment (Wixon, 1986).

Last, but certainly not least, we identify some instructional strategies to promote reading comprehension. First, as noted by Grossen and Carnine (1991), reading for comprehension assumes skill in decoding. Given fluent decoding skills, a number of instructional activities can be utilized to enhance reading comprehension (for a review, see Gersten, Fuchs, Williams, & Baker, 2001; Simmons et al., 2002). For example, prereading discussions of the assignment can help to put the reading into a context that the student can understand and relate to. Background knowledge or information related to the reading can be checked for and supplemented, as can necessary vocabulary. In addition to these prereading activities, several strategies to enhance comprehension can be used either during reading or following the completion of a passage. Students can be taught to understand readings and their structure by learning to ask a series of questions, known as "story grammar" or "story patterns" (Carnine & Kinder, 1985). Students also can be taught to draw diagrams or maps of the text that they are reading to help support their comprehension of material (Grossen & Carnine, 1991). Reading comprehension also can be facilitated by the development of writing and spelling skills (Anderson, Hiebert, Scott, & Wilkinson, 1985).

In addition to instruction in reading, language arts instruction typically focuses on the development of writing and spelling skills. Skills in both these areas are critical to the development of functional communication abilities. Stated differently, writing and spelling skills allow writers to have their intended effect on their reader(s). The treatment of this topic is beyond our scope here, and we direct readers to the excellent work of Graham, MacArthur, and Fitzgerald (2013) on writing/ spelling and interventions to improve these skills among low-performing students.

Clearly, this discussion of academic skills and instructional strategies is far from comprehensive. However, teachers and school psychologists with thorough knowledge of these and other procedures can utilize instructional interventions to build comprehensive and effective educational programs for students with ADHD who exhibit academic skills deficits.

For our purposes here, though, it is crucial to note that individualizing instruction successfully, for students with ADHD, often warrants and requires significant teacher support for designing and delivering interventions. In a series of recent related work, DuPaul and colleagues (2006), Jitendra and colleagues (2008), and Volpe, DuPaul, Jitendra, and Tresco (2009) detailed the content and delivery approaches of effective academic supports to students with ADHD and their teachers. Specifically, Jitendra and colleagues describe and discuss the use of explicit instruction in phonological awareness and word decoding, as well as collaborative strategic reading to support the development of reading and reading comprehension, respectively. In the area of math instruction, these authors also reviewed the use of cover–copy–compare fluency-building strategies, and schema-based instructional approaches to promote the development of higher-order skills in mathematics. Finally, DuPaul and colleagues and Volpe and colleagues provide evidence to support the use of consultation-based academic interventions to support both reading and math achievement for students with ADHD. It is interesting to note that the results of their research found similar, positive outcomes for both a generic collaborative consultation model, and a specific problem-solving behavioral consultation model.

Study and Organizational Skills

Children diagnosed with ADHD often present with a variety of academic performance problems in the areas of work completion, organization of desks and other materials, following directions, and studying for tests (Barkley, in press; Todd et al., 2002). Children experiencing such difficulties may benefit from direct instruction in study and organizational skills (for a review related to ADHD, see Evans et al., in press). An organized and thorough set of field-tested materials for teaching study and organizational skills to students in grades 3–6 has been published as *Skills for School Success* by Archer and Gleason (2002), with both elementary- and secondary-level materials. The goal of these authors was to prepare a curriculum to teach study skills for gaining, responding to, and organizing information. In this fashion, students would be encouraged to become more actively engaged in the classroom learning process. Similar work has been conducted at the University of Kansas by Donald Deshler, Jean Schumaker, and their colleagues, with a focus on strategies for use by secondary-level students (Lenz, Ehren, & Deshler, 2005; Schumaker & Deshler, 2010).

As discussed by Gleason, Archer, and Colvin (2010), students can be taught several strategies related to gaining information from written materials. These strategies involve previewing readings to identify main ideas and topics, reading text and concomitantly answering prepared questions about the reading, and utilizing strategies for taking careful and complete notes about the reading. In gaining meaning from text, children also must learn to read and understand the maps, graphs, pictures, and other visual aids that frequently accompany text. A second study skills area involves utilizing information gleaned from texts to respond to questions or other assignments based on the material. In this domain, the *Skills for School Success* (Archer & Gleason, 2002) curriculum contains lessons on carefully reading and answering end-of-unit questions, organizing and preparing written summaries of material that has been read, and taking quizzes and tests. For example, in learning to take quizzes and tests, students are taught how to anticipate the content of a forthcoming test, how to study and prepare for tests, and how to respond to particular types of questions, such as multiple-choice items.

Finally, Archer and Gleason (2002) have developed lessons for elementary-age children on how to manage time and materials in school. Three main topics are covered, including the organization of a school materials notebook, preparation and use of an assignment calendar, and the setup and completion of a neat, well-organized paper. For example, in setting up assignment papers, students are taught what is referred to as the HOW strategy. Here, the components and organization of a paper *heading* are learned, including name, date, and subject. Next, children are taught the components of a paper's *organization*, including the use of margins and blank lines. Finally, instruction focuses on what it means to produce a paper that is *written* neatly, including writing on lines and erasing neatly when necessary. Across each of these study skills areas, it is suggested that teachers first must provide appropriate models, then supply regular opportunities for the study and organizational skills to be practiced by students, and finally, give positive feedback and corrections as necessary. Few would disagree that these study and organizational skills are invaluable to all students, including those with ADHD. And recent investigations have documented the positive effects of direct instruction in these skills on children with ADHD (e.g., Abikoff et al., 2013). Other instructional strategies that have the potential to directly address the academic difficulties experienced by students with this disorder include peer tutoring, computer-assisted instruction, task and instructional modifications, and strategy training.

PEER TUTORING

According to Greenwood, Seals, and Kamps (2010), *peer tutoring* is an instructional strategy within which two students work together on an academic activity with one student providing assistance, instruction, and/or feedback to the other, and thus serving in the role of teacher or instructor. Several approaches to peer tutoring exist that share the characteristics of this definition, yet differ along the lines of instructional variables. For example, the range of models differs regarding instructional focus (e.g., skill acquisition vs. skill practice), tutoring structure (e.g., reciprocal vs. nonreciprocal tutoring), and procedural components (e.g., numbers of sessions per week, methods of pairing students, types of motivational systems used; for a review, see Ginsburg-Block, Rohrbeck, & Fantuzzo, 2006; Greenwood et al., 2010). Despite these differences, all models of peer tutoring share instructional characteristics that are known to enhance the sustained attention of students with ADHD. These characteristics include instruction that involves (1) a one-to-one student–teacher ratio/arrangement, (2) self-paced instruction determined by learner, (3) continuous prompting of academic responding, and (4) frequent immediate feedback about quality of performance (Pfiffner & DuPaul, in press).

Several research investigations have employed ClassWide Peer Tutoring (CWPT; Greenwood, Delquadri, & Carta, 1988; Greenwood, Maheady, & Delquadri, 2002) in general education classrooms that included students with ADHD. CWPT has been found to enhance the mathematics, reading, and spelling skills of students of all achievement levels (for a review, see Greenwood et al., 2010). This form of peer tutoring includes the following components: (1) division of the class into two teams, (2) formation of tutoring pairs among classmates within each team, (3) students take turns tutoring each other, (4) tutors are provided with academic scripts (e.g., math problems with answers), (5) praise and points are delivered contingent on correct answers, (6) errors are corrected immediately along with an opportunity for practicing the correct answer, (7) the teacher monitors tutoring pairs and provides bonus points for pairs who are following prescribed procedures, and (8) points are tallied by each individual student at the conclusion of each session. Tutoring sessions typically last 20 minutes with an additional 5 minutes for recording of student progress and putting materials away. Interestingly, earned points typically are not exchanged for backup reinforcers. Rather, at the conclusion of each week, the team with the most points is applauded by the other team.

A controlled case study of CWPT conducted with a 7-year-old boy with ADHD in a second-grade general education classroom found promising results (DuPaul & Henningson, 1993). The influence of CWPT, relative to baseline conditions, during instruction followed by independent seatwork was investigated, with a focus on on-task behavior, fidgeting, and math performance. CWPT was found to produce reliable increases in on-task behavior and similarly reliable reductions in fidgeting during math class relative to typical instructional conditions. Less consistent findings were obtained with respect to math performance, although the student did make measurable gains in this area.

In a replication and extension of this work with a larger group of students exhibiting significant ADHD-related behaviors, DuPaul, Ervin, Hook, and McGoey (1998) evaluated the effects of CWPT on the academic performance and behavioral control of 19 students (16 boys, 3 girls; median age = 7.5) with ADHD in first- through fifth-grade general education classrooms. Outcome measures included direct observations of ADHD-related behavior, teacher ratings, self-report ratings, and weekly pre- and posttests. CWPT was implemented for math, spelling, or reading depending on the academic area that each teacher identified as weakest for the student with ADHD.

The results of the DuPaul, Ervin, and colleagues (1998) study indicated that the active engagement of students with ADHD significantly increased from an average of 21.6% during baseline to an average of 82.3% when CWPT was implemented. Concomitant reductions in off-task behavior also were obtained. In addition, children's weekly posttest scores increased from an average of 55.2% during baseline to 73% for CWPT conditions, thus indicating that this intervention affected both attentional behavior and academic performance. Similar improvements in behavior and academic performance were exhibited by typically functioning classmates, thus attesting to the fact that peer tutoring can help *all* students, not just those with disabilities. Furthermore, the teachers and students in the DuPaul, Ervin, and colleagues study all reported CWPT to be effective and acceptable.

In general, these studies provide consistent evidence that peer tutoring is an intervention strategy that is able to improve the active engagement, academic performance, and, possibly, the social interactions of a wide variety of students, including those with ADHD. Given that students with ADHD have significant problems when asked to complete independent assignments, peer tutoring provides an alternative instructional mode providing for practice and refinement of academic skills.

COMPUTER-ASSISTED INSTRUCTION

The use of computer-assisted instruction (CAI) has been recommended for increasing the on-task and work production behaviors of students with ADHD. It has been suggested that the instructional features of CAI allow students with ADHD to focus their attention on academic stimuli (Lillie, Hannun, & Stuck, 1989; Torgesen & Young, 1983). That is, CAI has the potential to readily present specific instructional objectives, provide highlighting of essential material (e.g., with large print, color), use multiple sensory modalities, divide content material into smaller bits of information, and provide immediate feedback about response accuracy. In addition, CAI can readily limit the presentation of nonessential features that may be distracting (e.g., sound effects, animation). A few studies have shown positive effects of CAI with students diagnosed with ADHD.

As an example of a *computer-assisted academic intervention*, Ota and DuPaul (2002) examined the effects of using computer software with a game format (Math Blaster) to improve math achievement. The participants were three male, white, fourth- through sixth-grade students with ADHD. Following baseline (observation under normal classroom conditions), the math software was introduced sequentially in a multiple-baseline fashion for each participant. Observational data were collected during the baseline and experimental conditions along with a set of instructional-level math probes, which were administered several times per week throughout the study. All three participants showed some improvement in their performance on curriculum-based math probes; however, the strength of these improvements varied across individuals (i.e., effects were particularly pronounced for two of the three participants). Furthermore, all three participants showed substantial reductions in off-task disruptive behavior as a function of interacting with the computer software.

Research results provide preliminary evidence for school personnel that CAI may be an effective instructional alternative for at least some children with ADHD. Allowing students to receive CAI may result in improvements in work completion and attending behaviors. However, characteristics of the software packages may affect the attending behaviors of students with ADHD. Software packages that include game formats and animation may be more effective than drill and practice or tutorial programs. Clearly, there is a pressing need for continued research on CAI for students with this disorder.

The potential effectiveness of CAI for students with ADHD can be linked to previous non-computer-based research. Specifically, research involving children with ADHD has shown three task-related variables to be related to improved task performance. These variables are novel (as compared with familiar) stimulus conditions, immediate (as compared with delayed) feedback, and a one-to-one teacher–student ratio. Arranging these variables into the instructional conditions of a typical classroom on a regular basis is not feasible when considering the classroom teacher as the intervention agent. However, CAI can indeed deliver instruction infused with these variables. For example, recent work in the area of CAI has shown promise for improving academic skill development and performance for students with ADHD, presumably as a function of delivering instruction under conditions of one-to-one student–teacher ratio, novel stimuli, and immediate feedback.

Specifically, computers can promote the initial acquisition of skills and can enhance the mastery of already acquired skills via drill-and-practice software. For example, in the former area, Clarfield and Stoner (2005) demonstrated the promise of a computerized early reading instruction program, Headsprout, with young students identified with ADHD. Headsprout is an Internet-based instructional program (*www.headsprout.com*) that is highly interactive, entertaining, and attractive to young students. It also is designed to provide high rates of opportunities to respond and encouragement while delivering immediate feedback regarding accuracy of responding. In their study involving two first-grade students and one kindergarten student, Clarfield and Stoner compared individually delivered reading instruction using the Headsprout program with small-group reading instruction. Results indicated the computerized instruction produced significant reductions in off-task behavior and improvements in oral reading fluency rates, thus providing evidence of CAI effects on reading acquisition skills.

Similarly, two other research studies (Mautone, DuPaul, & Jitendra, 2005; Ota & DuPaul, 2002) have provided support for the effects of CAI on performance of already learned skills by students with ADHD. In both these studies, the Math Blaster Ages 6–9 software package (Knowledge Adventure, Inc., 2013) was used, as was single-subject research methodology with each participant serving as his or her own control. Results showed that relative to typical independent seatwork conditions, CAI math practice resulted in significant work completion/accuracy improvements as well as increases in academic engaged time.

Thus, a growing evidence base suggests the instructional features of CAI help students to focus their attention on academic stimuli. Although not always the case, CAI presents activities incorporating specific instructional objectives, provides highlighting of essential material (e.g., large print and color), utilizes multiple sensory modalities, divides content material into smaller bits of information, and provides immediate feedback about response accuracy. All told, however, more research is needed to determine the uses of specific software and its features to enhance the learning, concentration, and academic performance of students with attention problems.

TASK AND INSTRUCTIONAL MODIFICATIONS

Task Modifications

An educational accommodation that can improve the academic performance of students diagnosed with ADHD is TM. TM involves revising the curriculum or aspects of it in an attempt to reduce problem behaviors and increase appropriate classroom behaviors. In addition, TM is a proactive strategy, as changes are made before the curriculum is presented to the student. It has been argued that this type of positive academic modification is more responsive to the individual needs of the student (Meyer & Evans, 1989).

One type of TM, choice making, requires the student to choose activities from among two or more concurrently presented options. Previous studies examining the effects of choice making on students with developmental disabilities have demonstrated increases in social behavior and decreases in levels of disruptive behavior (Dyer, Dunlap, & Winterling, 1990; Koegel, Dyer, & Bell, 1987). The effects of classroom-based choice making were examined in a study conducted by Dunlap and colleagues (1994). In this study, the effects of choice making on the task engagement and disruptive behaviors of three students with emotional and behavioral disorders were examined. Of these three participants, one 12-year-old male was identified as having ADHD. This student was provided with a menu of academic tasks in English and spelling from which to choose. The results of the study indicated that choice making led to reliable and consistent increases in task engagement with concomitant reductions in disruptive behavior. Therefore, choice making may be a valuable TM for students with ADHD. Not only does allowing students to chose their assignments reduce disruptive behaviors and improve task engagement but this strategy promotes student initiative and independence. However, it is not clear whether this type of TM is effective at improving academic performance.

Based on the premise that children with ADHD have a greater need for cognitive stimulation than their nondiagnosed peers, a few TM studies have investigated the effects of modifying intratask stimulation (Zentall, 1989; Zentall & Leib, 1985). In one study conducted in a classroom setting, Zentall and Leib (1985) investigated the effects of added structure on the activity levels and performance of children using a repeated-measures design. Eight participants identified as hyperactive were randomly assigned to one of two experimental art conditions in which the structure of the task requirement was manipulated (explicit instructions combined with task materials vs. nonspecific instructions without task materials). Results indicated significant decreases in activity level of the participants, and suggested that modifying task requirements may affect activity levels of children identified as hyperactive.

In another classroom-based study, Zentall (1989) examined whether adding color to relevant cues in a spelling task improved the performance of children diagnosed as hyperactive. Participants included 20 hyperactive and 26 comparison boys who were preassessed on spelling achievement and randomly assigned to one of two condition-order groups. Results of this study indicated the participants identified as hyperactive demonstrated better performance than the comparison participants when relevant color was added to spelling tasks. Interestingly, the addition of color to irrelevant aspects of the task resulted in decreases in spelling performance. The educational implications of these results suggest that adding color to relevant components of a task may increase attention to detail and improve the academic performance of children with ADHD. However, the highly controlled spelling task and limited measures of academic achievement reduces the degree to which these findings can be generalized to classroom settings.

In one of the first studies to utilize classroom-based functional assessment procedures, Ervin and colleagues (1996) examined the effect of TM on the academic performance of children with ADHD. Based on the results of descriptive analyses and hypothesis development, it was purported that the task engagement of two male students diagnosed with ADHD would improve if a TM were conducted. Using a brief reversal design, the effects of an alternative writing method were examined with one male participant. This method included peer discussion, brainstorming of ideas, and the use of a computer for journal writing. Allowing the participant to modify his written assignments resulted in clinically significant decreases in off-task behavior. Specifically, the percentage of intervals in which off-task behavior was not observed was greater when the participant was able to use the computer ($M = 96.8\%$) than when the participant completed the written task by hand ($M = 64.8\%$). For the second male student diagnosed with ADHD, it was hypothesized that allowing him to take notes during a lecture would result in less frequent off-task behaviors than if he passively listened to the lecture. The results of a brief experimental manipulation indicated that the percentage of intervals without off-task behavior was consistently higher when the note-taking strategy was employed ($M = 97.8\%$) than when the participant did not use the strategy ($M = 54.5\%$). The results of this study are limited by the brief intervention period and the absence of academic performance data; however, they are intriguing and suggestive of future research directions.

Instructional Modifications

Similar to TM, specific instructional modifications can be implemented to improve the academic environments of students experiencing difficulties with inattention, impulsivity, or hyperactivity. As stated previously, few studies have examined this form of intervention with students displaying ADHD-related behaviors.

For example, Skinner, Johnson, Larkin, Lessley, and Glowacki (1995) examined the influence of two taped-words interventions, fast-taped words and slow-taped words, on word reading list performance. One of the three participating students was identified as having ADHD. Outcome measurement focused on reading accuracy rates across baseline conditions and the fast- and slow-taped-word procedures. Relatively higher rates of accurate reading were demonstrated in the slow-taped-word condition. Results of this study suggest that taped-words interventions can be effective procedures for improving reading accuracy rates for students with ADHD.

Results from the available research literature suggest that task and instructional modifications can lead to decreased disruptive behavior, increased task engagement, and increased academic performance. Furthermore, these types of modifications can occur within the context of the daily classroom routine, requiring minimal teacher preparation. However, it should be noted the results have been limited to immediate, short-term intervention effects. Again, this is an area in need of further investigation.

THE IMPORTANCE OF ONGOING TEACHER SUPPORT

Given evidence that students are not meeting the expectations of their current classroom, reasonable interventions and accommodations should be made in attempts to allow students to meet those expectations and achieve academic success. Interventions and accommodations might include matching instructional materials with current academic skills, providing more frequent positive and corrective feedback, enhancing motivation to engage in academic work, and increasing opportunities to learn and practice newly acquired skills. It also must be recognized, however, that teachers who are expected to make such accommodations or implement interventions should themselves be able to expect systematic assistance in the way of consultation and support services for the design, implementation, and evaluation of classroom-based strategies.

"Teacher support systems" have been identified as critical to the successful education of students with challenging behaviors (Simonsen et al., in press; Sugai & Horner, 2006). These researchers have noted that teacher support systems rely on instructional and behavioral programs that are grounded in three important commitments. These commitments are to (1) teaching students in those classrooms or schools in which they would be educated were they not exhibiting challenging behaviors; (2) providing student support in an ongoing fashion; and (3) producing positive and broad lifestyle outcomes, including preparing the student to participate successfully in the community and society.

Given these commitments for providing services to students identified with ADHD, in our view, teacher support activities at a minimum should consist of the following components: individualized consultation, differentiated education and coaching, assessment of the contextual fit of interventions and supports, and as appropriate, efforts to integrate interventions delivered by agents other than the teacher (e.g., computers, peers), as described in this chapter.

Mechanisms for providing teacher support are considered necessary components in the treatment of children with ADHD. Given the frequency and severity of disruptive behaviors that these students exhibit, it is not uncommon for teachers to express feelings of frustration and helplessness when attempting to manage their classrooms. These feelings should be expected and validated by professionals and parents who are interacting with classroom teachers. Furthermore, efforts should be made to help teachers deal with these feelings in a productive fashion (e.g., by providing instructional materials related to stress management). Second, the selection of treatment strategies should be made in view of each teacher's knowledge, skills, and contexts, based either on an assessment of contextual fit (see Horner, Salentine, & Albin, 2003, for a contextual fit rating scale) or based on teacher ability/willingness using a tool such as the School Supports Checklist (McKinley & Stormont, 2008), or based on a combination of such tools. Finally, Simonsen and colleagues (in press) have clearly demonstrated positive outcomes for coaching teachers in behavior management with difficult-to-manage students. These types of supports are critical to the success of interventions and supports in today's classroom, where with the advent of RTI-based services, teachers are often responsible for implementing multiple academic and behavior support plans across a number of students. The characteristics of the teacher support system enumerated previously are designed to address these practical issues in a proactive fashion rather than waiting for teacher complaints and frustration to occur.

Implementation of teacher support systems will require professionals with assessment and program development expertise, educators with supervisory or administrative rank and responsibilities for monitoring ongoing educational programs, and personnel to provide intervention assistance as needed in support of regular classroom staff. Ideally, this type of commitment to teacher support would be coupled with staff who are knowledgeable and skillful in the areas of instructional and behavioral support. In schools where such conditions exist, it is reasonable for parents and teachers to expect academic, behavioral, and social success for students with ADHD.

SUMMARY

Children with ADHD frequently experience difficulty in the areas of classroom behavior, academic performance, and scholastic achievement. Maximizing each child's likelihood for school success will require a variety of behavioral, instructional, and learning strategies aimed at the prevention and management of problems in these areas. This chapter has provided a review of effective behavior management interventions and instructional strategies, as well as review of promising instructional and self-management strategies. The need for systematic teacher support was also noted. In addition to further research on promising intervention approaches, the challenge before us is one of integrating the various strategies into treatment programs that are based on individual student needs such that all students with ADHD experience success in school.

CHAPTER 6

Interventions and Supports in Secondary and Postsecondary Schools

ADHD is a chronic disorder with most elementary school-age children continuing to exhibit significant symptoms into and beyond middle and high school. For example, Bussing, Mason, Bell, and Garvan (2010) followed an ethnically diverse sample of 94 children (5–11 years old) with ADHD for 8 years and found 56% of the children continued to exhibit clinically significant symptoms in adolescence with findings consistent across gender, race, and SES. Approximately 6.5% of 13- to 17-year-olds meet diagnostic criteria for ADHD based on findings from the large nationally representative sample participating in the National Comorbidity Survey Replication Adolescent Supplement Study (Kessler et al., 2012). Furthermore, there is growing evidence that a significant percentage of the college population has ADHD (DuPaul, Weyandt, O'Dell, & Varejao, 2009). Students with ADHD experience significant educational, social, and psychological challenges that may limit their successful completion of postsecondary education. Thus, middle school, high school, and college students with this disorder will require educational and behavioral supports that meet their unique developmental needs.

The purpose of this chapter is to describe intervention and support strategies that may enhance the psychological, behavioral, social, and educational functioning of secondary and postsecondary school students with ADHD. We begin with a brief overview of ADHD in adolescence (i.e., middle and high school) with specific emphasis on functional impairments experienced during this developmental phase. Next, we describe a variety of possible treatment strategies including school-based behavioral and academic interventions, home-based interventions, home–school communication, and transition programming for post-high school. Given that growing numbers of students with ADHD are pursuing postsecondary education, we provide an overview of what is known about the academic, social, and psychological functioning of college students with this disorder. Treatment strategies are described including psychosocial interventions (e.g., cognitive-behavioral therapy, coaching), psychotropic medication, and educational accommodations and support. The importance of coordinated care is emphasized given that college students with ADHD may struggle with newfound independence when they are on their own in the postsecondary education environment.

CHALLENGES EXPERIENCED BY ADOLESCENTS WITH ADHD

As students with ADHD move from elementary school to middle school and beyond, they face a plethora of developmental hurdles that are substantially higher for them than for their peers. Furthermore, secondary settings are characteristically more demanding with respect to student organizational abilities, academic skills, and self-directedness. Specifically, secondary school students are expected to be able to study for tests and display adequate organizational skills (e.g., keep a neat notebook), as well as plan for their future beyond high school. The interaction between typical impairments associated with ADHD and increasing demands for independence, self-control, organization, and time management in secondary schools significantly limits the chances for successful educational outcomes in this population.

As is the case for elementary school students with ADHD, middle and high school students with this disorder frequently experience significant academic impairment (Langberg et al., 2011). In one of the most comprehensive studies of academic functioning among high school students with ADHD, Kent and colleagues (2011) found students with this disorder to have significantly lower GPA, lower class placement (e.g., remedial- vs. honors-level classes), and higher rates of course failure than their typically developing peers. Furthermore, students with ADHD were reported by teachers to turn in a significantly lower percentage of assignments and were significantly more likely to be absent or tardy from class. As a result, adolescents with ADHD were over eight times as likely to drop out of school. Similarly, Barkley and colleagues (2008) and Galéra, Melchior, Chastang, Bouvard, and Fombonne (2009) found that adolescents with ADHD were more likely to experience one or greater grade retentions and fail to graduate from secondary school relative to students without ADHD.

In similar fashion, adolescents with ADHD typically experience difficulties with social interactions and peer relationships. For example, Sibley, Evans, and Serpell (2010) found middle school students with ADHD to exhibit significantly greater problems with peer relationships relative to their typically developing classmates based on parent report of social functioning and peer ratings of liking. Furthermore, these young adolescents with ADHD (*M* age = 12 years old) exhibited significantly more impairment in two important social cognitive skills, specifically social comprehension and problem-solving abilities. Secondary school students with ADHD also are more likely than their classmates to report bullying others and to be victimized by bullies (Timmermanis & Wiener, 2011).

In addition to impaired peer relationships, teens with ADHD may experience significant challenges getting along with teachers and adult authority figures. Although specific investigations of teacher–student interactions and relationships have not been conducted with the adolescent ADHD population, middle and high school teachers have been found to report significantly elevated behavioral and social difficulties for students with ADHD (e.g., Barkley, Fischer, et al., 1990). Furthermore, high school students with ADHD are at higher-than-average risk for school suspensions and expulsions (Barkley et al., 2008). Elevated behavior ratings and school disciplinary rates presumably indicate that teachers perceive students with ADHD to be significantly disruptive to classroom and school activities, which may negatively impact teacher–student relations.

A variety of other psychological difficulties and psychiatric comorbidities are associated with ADHD during adolescence. Among the most common associated problems are significantly higher levels of antisocial behavior, criminal activity, and substance use relative to non-ADHD controls (Langley et al., 2010). Furthermore, teenagers with ADHD are two times as likely as youth without ADHD to use nicotine and other substances and about two to three times more likely to develop substance abuse disorders involving nicotine, marijuana, and cocaine (Charach et al., 2011; Lee, Humphreys, Flory, Liu, & Glass, 2011). The risk for alcohol use disorder is lower wherein adolescents with ADHD are about 1.35 times as likely to exhibit this disorder than their typically developing counterparts (Charach et al., 2011). The increased risk of substance abuse is consistent across a range of demographic characteristics (e.g., age, sex, race; Lee et al., 2011) but is accounted for, in large part, by comorbid oppositional defiant disorder or conduct disorder

(Harty, Ivanov, Newcorn, & Halperin, 2011), as well as history of child-hood maltreatment (De Sanctis et al., 2008).

Adolescents with ADHD may also be at increased risk for inter-nalizing disorders. Chronis-Tuscano and colleagues (2010) conducted a longitudinal study examining risk for depression and suicidal behav-ior in adolescence in a large sample of 4- to 6-year-old children with ADHD and demographically matched comparison peers. Adolescents with ADHD were over four times as likely as comparison children to meet diagnostic criteria for depression by age 18 and were nearly four times as likely to have attempted suicide. Furthermore, the importance of comorbid disorders, especially symptoms of internalizing disorder, at an early age for predicting later emotional and behavioral outcomes has been supported relatively consistently across the literature. Harty, Miller, Newcorn, and Halperin (2009) found that children with ADHD and comorbid disruptive behavior disorders appear to be at higher risk for emotional dysregulation difficulties (e.g., anger, verbal and physical aggression) in adolescence than do children with ADHD in isolation.

In addition to risk for internalizing and externalizing disorders, adolescents with ADHD may experience disruptions with other impor-tant areas of functioning including precocious sexual behavior (Galéra et al., 2010), significantly higher frequency of motor vehicle accidents and moving violations (Barkley, 2004) and higher rates of parent–teen conflict (Barkley, Guevremont, Anastopoulos, & Fletcher, 1992). The combination of ADHD and associated functional impairments and/or comorbid psychiatric disorders present significant costs to the educa-tional system and community at large. In fact, the mean cost per stu-dent with ADHD to school districts is $5,007 annually (in 2010 dol-lars) above and beyond the cost associated with general education. This annual per student cost translates to a total national cost of $13.4 billion per year (Robb et al., 2011). Thus, efforts to identify and treat ado-lescents with ADHD are critical from mental health, educational, and economic standpoints.

ASSESSMENT OF ADHD IN ADOLESCENTS

As discussed in Chapter 2, school-based assessment of ADHD is best conducted in the context of a data-based decision-making model that is part of a three-tiered intervention program. Specifically, possible iden-tification of ADHD would commence for those students who do not exhibit a positive response to Tier 1 (universal) and Tier 2 (targeted) interventions implemented in the classroom or other school settings. The formal assessment of ADHD involves collection of multiple measures across several respondents to determine (1) whether an individual's behaviors are consistent with DSM criteria for the disorder (including the presence of functional impairment), (2) whether there are competing hypotheses (e.g., presence of another disorder) for the apparent ADHD behavioral symptoms, (3) whether any comorbid disorders are present, and (4) what treatment strategies are warranted to address the individual's difficulties. Multiple measures include diagnostic interview with a parent as well as possibly a teacher, behavior rating scales completed by parent(s) and teacher(s), and archival records related to academic and behavioral functioning (e.g., school records, reports of prior psychoeducational evaluations; Sibley, Pelham, et al., 2012).

Important modifications are necessary to account for developmental and contextual factors when evaluating secondary school students suspected of having ADHD (Sibley, Pelham, et al., 2012). First, an adolescent's motivation to participate in a diagnostic evaluation and, eventually, treatment, is enhanced by including measures that provide the teenager with input into the assessment process. For example, the adolescent could be asked to complete self-report behavior ratings. These measures not only provide input and enhance motivation but also could provide helpful insight into possible symptoms of internalizing disorders (e.g., depression, anxiety). As noted in Chapter 2, however, self-report ratings should be interpreted with caution because teenagers with ADHD do not typically provide accurate reports about their ADHD symptomatology or their self-esteem. In fact, several studies have demonstrated that children and adolescents with ADHD exhibit a positive illusory bias when completing self-appraisal ratings such that ratings of functioning are especially elevated in those areas of functioning most at deficit (Hoza, Pelham, Dobbs, Owens, & Pillow, 2002).

Some assessment methods used in elementary school, especially direct observations of behavior, are difficult, if not impossible, to conduct in high school settings. Collecting direct observation data in an unobtrusive fashion in a typical high school classroom is relatively disruptive to classroom ecology and most middle and high school students can readily determine that they are being observed and their behavior may change accordingly. Furthermore, collection of behavior ratings from multiple teachers may be unwieldy and they may be relatively unfamiliar with the specific student. Thus, it often is recommended to obtain ratings from teachers of two or three core academic subject areas (e.g., English, math, science) rather than an entire team of teachers (Evans, Allen, Moore, & Strauss, 2005).

Two typical challenges associated with adolescence are potentially problematic for teens with ADHD and should be considered during the assessment process. First, parents and teachers increasingly expect adolescents to function independently in terms of self-care, educational activities/assignments, and conformity with rules and legal obligations. Second, adolescents typically spend more time with peers than with family members or teachers; thus, peer acceptance and pressure to conform to peer group standards become increasingly important. Adolescents with ADHD may be even more likely than their non-ADHD classmates to experience significant challenges with independent functioning and peer acceptance given the self-regulation deficits and peer rejection often associated with the disorder. Thus, assessment measures should evaluate possible difficulties with organizational skills, homework completion, self-care, conduct problems, peer acceptance status, and social skills. In fact, Sibley, Pelham, and colleagues (2012) found assessment of functional impairment to be of greater value than evaluation of ADHD symptoms in identifying adolescents with the disorder. Functional challenges may be the primary areas of concern above and beyond ADHD symptoms and, thus, should be targeted directly by treatment strategies.

INTERVENTION CONSIDERATIONS WITH SECONDARY-LEVEL STUDENTS

Middle and high school students with ADHD present a significant challenge to educators, as a result of the interaction of the chronic nature of ADHD and the more general characteristics of adolescence. These include demands and expectations for increasing academic, social, and behavioral independence, judgment, and self-regulation. Furthermore, these expectations take place in the increasingly complex contexts of completing high school and planning for postsecondary work and/or education; negotiating within-family responsibilities surrounding automobile use, social engagements and activities, substance use, romantic and sexual interests/activities, and, ultimately, independent living.

Support for adolescents with ADHD in these endeavors is likely to take many forms. For example, intervention strategies discussed in Chapter 5 that warrant consideration with secondary students include contingency contracting, self-monitoring and self-reinforcement, CAI, and instruction in study and organizational skills. In addition, these students may need greater then typical amounts of support in planning for their educational and employment futures. Specifically, many colleges and universities have excellent support programs for students with disabilities; learning to explore such options is likely to be important for these students. Becoming an effective self-advocate also will be important, including understanding one's rights, one's disability, and one's skills/weaknesses. Such understanding will likely be critical to postsecondary academic success—as will availing oneself of accessible supports and resources.

One promising avenue for the support of adolescents with ADHD is that of being "coached" in a one-to-one relationship intended to support the adolescent in achieving his or her self-selected goals. In this regard, Dawson and Guare (1998) have developed a *Coaching the ADHD Student* resource workbook that provides guidelines organized into three brief chapters on the foundations, mechanics, and applications of coaching students with ADHD, as well as appendices with materials for use within coaching activities. Briefly, Dawson and Guare describe the following steps to coaching: do a needs assessment, obtain commitment from participants, select a coach, arrange an initial meeting between the student and the coach, and initiate regular coaching sessions (daily is recommended). Further suggestions are offered as to the focus of the coaching relationship on goal setting, developing plans for attaining goals, identifying and overcoming obstacles to goal attainment, and evaluation of progress.

This coaching model is based on correspondence training research (Paniagua, 1992; Risley & Hart, 1968) with its focus on promoting a match between what a person says he or she will do and what he or she actually does. The model and methods make good conceptual sense; however, empirical investigations are needed to further validate this approach to intervention.

In the context of the family, adolescents with ADHD and their parents are likely to benefit from some form of counseling support (Robin, 1998; see also Chapter 8 for further discussion). Such support may range from understanding ADHD and its influence on the family's interaction patterns to supporting and planning the education of an adolescent with ADHD to negotiating privileges and responsibilities in the context of the family. As with previous examples, individualizing the nature and type of academic, family, and individual support will be one of the keys to successful outcomes.

INTERVENTIONS FOR MIDDLE AND HIGH SCHOOL STUDENTS

Adolescents with ADHD receive treatment across a variety of settings (e.g., mental health specialty clinics, human service agencies, general medical practices) with the majority obtaining services in mental health specialty clinics (68.1%) and schools (63.2%) (Merikangas et al., 2011). Of those adolescents with ADHD receiving treatment, approximately 50% of these individuals obtain limited services with the equivalent of fewer than six visits (Merikangas et al., 2011). Given that schools are a primary intervention delivery site for this population, it is imperative that school personnel implement data-based, effective strategies. Unfortunately, very few empirical studies have examined the implementation and impact of interventions delivered in middle and high school settings for students with ADHD (DuPaul & Eckert, 1997; DuPaul, Eckert, & Vilardo, 2012). Nevertheless, we are able to provide an overview of possible school-based behavioral and academic interventions with the latter primarily focused on enhancing organizational and study skills or self-regulation strategies. In addition, home-based interventions, home–school communication strategies, and transition programming for post-high school (e.g., college or workforce) are discussed.

Organizational and Study Skills

In most secondary schools, minimal instruction in study and organizational skills is provided. Students are assumed to develop these skills as they progress through the grade levels as a function of their burgeoning cognitive and emotional maturation. Although this assumption may be valid for most adolescents, it is clear that many students with ADHD do not acquire adequate study skills and that their academic performance is compromised accordingly. As described in Chapter 5, direct instruction in study and organizational strategies is considered a well-established treatment for ADHD must be provided to these students as early as possible in their schooling (Evans et al., in press).

Despite the dearth of study skills intervention research with adolescents, those studies that have been conducted suggest certain guidelines that can be followed:

1. Initial instruction in how to study for tests and proper note taking should take place in the later elementary and early middle school years (i.e., fifth and sixth grades), when homework and long-term projects become more demanding. This instruction should be provided by either the general education classroom teacher or support personnel (e.g., guidance counselor, school psychologist) on an ongoing basis with ample opportunity for supervised practice.

2. Students with ADHD should be required to keep homework assignment books as soon as substantial amounts (i.e., more than 30 minutes per night) of such work are required. Both short- and long-term assignments should be recorded in this book. Initially, the teacher should check and initial the assignment book at the end of each school day to ensure that the proper assignments are recorded. Furthermore, parents

should review the assignment book prior to each homework session to make sure that the student understands what is required. Home-based contingencies (e.g., preferred free-time activities) should be directly linked to compliance with assignment book responsibilities. The latter component is crucial because many students with ADHD will not consistently write down their assignments unless there is a direct "payoff" for doing so. As the student demonstrates greater levels of individual responsibility in using the assignment book, the level of supervision by teachers and parents can be reduced. Nevertheless, students with ADHD should continue to be required to keep an assignment book throughout their schooling.

3. If necessary, compensations for the attentional and organizational deficits associated with ADHD can be made in the form of accommodations. First, students could be allowed to tape-record lectures as a supplement to note taking. This is particularly helpful when the child is taught how to take notes by making transcriptions of the audiotaped lecture under the supervision of a teacher, older student, or peer. Second, an extra set of textbooks should be kept at home during the school year to prevent missed opportunities to complete homework assignments due to "forgetting" appropriate texts.

4. Continued direct instruction and monitoring of study, note-taking, and organizational skills may be necessary across several grade levels and should be considered an integral component of school-based programming for many adolescents with ADHD.

The most comprehensive and widely studied organizational and study skills training program for middle school students with ADHD is the Challenging Horizons program (CHP) developed by Evans, Axelrod, and Langberg (2004; *www.oucirs.org*). The CHP was originally designed as an after-school program that provided training and support to middle school students with ADHD in study skills, social skills, and homework management. The study skills component focuses on organizational skills and note taking. One of the primary objectives of organizational skills training is for students to consistently use an assignment book. Thus, trainers (e.g., undergraduate or graduate students in psychology, school counselors, school psychologists, teachers) help students to check their use of an assignment book relative to a "gold standard" model and record the percentage of items entered correctly. Contingencies are provided based on criteria established for accuracy. Parents and teachers initial assignment books on a daily basis; however, they are urged to let students independently record and check assignments. The other primary focus of organizational skills training is on proper maintenance of notebooks, binders, book bags, and lockers. Again, a checklist is developed for students to provide guidance on how each of these items should be maintained. Trainers check each of these items on a daily basis and contingencies are provided if organization standards are met. If errors are made, these are corrected immediately with trainer guidance. As students make progress, the program is tapered toward random weekly checks.

The CHP note-taking component includes three phases: (1) training and guided practice in the note-taking process, (2) note-taking practice, and (3) promoting generalization to classroom setting. For the note-taking process, students are provided with a structured format for notes. Trainers model listening to presentation of information, thinking aloud regarding that information, and then taking notes. The next step is to have students help with the think-aloud process as well as identify main ideas and details that should be included in notes. Trainer prompts to follow these steps are faded over time until students engage in the process independently. The next phase involves trainers checking the quality of notes generated independently by students with contingencies provided for meeting specified accuracy criteria. The final and most challenging phase is to promote generalization of the note-taking process to the actual classroom. Teachers provide prompts and feedback to students as they practice the skills.

Implementation of CHP has been associated with significant gains in organizational skills and note taking at group and individual levels (e.g., Evans, Serpell, Schultz, & Pastor, 2007; Evans, Schultz, DeMars, & Davis, 2011). In recent years, CHP has been extended for use during the school day with implementation by school-based mentors, primarily general education teachers. Evans and colleagues (2007, 2011) found that relative to a control group, middle school students with ADHD receiving CHP showed greater improvement in inattention and social behavior. Furthermore, within-grade GPA decreased more for the control group indicating that CHP may be protective in relation to typical deterioration in academic progress experienced by middle school students with this disorder.

Similar to the CHP, the Homework, Organization, and Planning Skills (HOPS) program was designed for implementation by school personnel to address organizational skills difficulties experienced by middle school students with ADHD (Langberg, 2011). HOPS includes 16 sessions focused on organization of school materials, homework management, and a home-based reward system. Two parent meetings are included at key points in the 16-session program to encourage parent monitoring and reinforcement of child organizational skills and homework completion. This is a manualized program with extensive supporting materials for implementation by school psychologists and other school-based personnel. Initial outcome data for HOPS is promising with respect to improvements in student organization of materials, planning of school tasks, and completion of assignments (Langberg, Epstein, Becker, Girio-Herrera, & Vaughn, 2012; Langberg, Epstein, Urbanowicz, Simon, & Graham, 2008).

Several studies have examined organizational and study skills training at the high school level in the context of multicomponent psychosocial intervention protocols. For example, Sibley and colleagues (2011) conducted a pilot study of a package of psychosocial interventions (e.g., DBRC, behavior tracking system, academic instruction, and organizational skills training) to address academic, behavioral, and social functioning in 19 teenagers with ADHD (*M* age = 14.06) attending a summer treatment program that included classroom instruction. Nearly all (82.4–94.7%) participants were reported by parents, counselor, or teacher to have improved at least somewhat after completing the treatment program. Improvements were noted in multiple domains including conduct problems, adult-directed defiance, social functioning, inattention/disorganization, mood/well-being, and academic skills. Sibley, Smith, Evans, Pelham, and Gnagy (2012) found similar improvements for a separate sample of 34 adolescents with ADHD (*M* age = 13.88) wherein between 63 and 90.9% of participants showed improved functioning across academic, behavioral, and social domains following a summer treatment program. Unfortunately, these findings are limited by the lack of a comparison group to control for history, maturation, and treatment expectancy effects. Furthermore, given that multiple treatment components were included in the summer treatment program, it is unclear which component(s) including organizational skills training were causally related to improved outcomes.

Self-Regulation Strategies

As discussed in Chapter 5, self-regulation or self-management strategies can be effective in addressing the needs of students with ADHD. Presumably, this approach is especially well suited to adolescents with this disorder given their growing independence and reduced willingness on the part of teachers to implement behavioral interventions at the secondary level. Furthermore, middle and high school students with ADHD typically experience difficulties being prepared for class and completing homework on a timely basis. Presumably, these difficulties are related, in part, to poor attention to detail and low motivation to complete routine tasks. Thus, one approach to addressing class preparation and homework completion involves training students to monitor their own preparatory behaviors.

Gureasko-Moore, DuPaul, and White (2006) studied the effects of self-monitoring on the class preparation behaviors of three middle school students with ADHD. All of these students had significant difficulties with a variety of behaviors including arriving to class on time, having necessary materials (e.g., pen and paper), and having completed homework to turn in. The school psychologist developed a checklist of five or six preparatory behaviors in collaboration with classroom teachers for use by students in self-monitoring. The psychologist then met with students for a few minutes each day across 4 days to provide training and practice in self-monitoring. Self-monitoring was implemented for several weeks and then faded (i.e., written checklist removed) following at least 1 week of successful class preparation. All three students showed significant gains in class preparation behaviors (i.e., consistent 100% completion of assigned steps) that were maintained without treatment through the end of the school year (see Figure 6.1). These findings were replicated with a separate sample of six middle school students with ADHD who self-monitored both class preparation and homework completion (Gureasko-Moore et al., 2007).

Self-regulation strategies, either alone or in combination with academic strategy instruction or positive reinforcement, have also been evaluated for high school students with ADHD. Graham-Day, Gardner, and Hsin (2010) examined the effects of self-monitoring alone and self-monitoring plus reinforcement on the on-task behavior of three 10th-grade students with ADHD. All three students were taught to use self-monitoring in the context of a study hall specifically for students with disabilities. Participants were provided with 15 opportunities during a 20-minute period to indicate whether they were paying attention using an individual checklist (i.e., circle "yes" if paying attention or circle "no" if not paying attention). Students were prompted to self-monitor using a variable 2-minute schedule via audiotaped chimes. A self-monitoring plus reinforcement condition was also included wherein students compared their on-task checklist with that of an independent observer. If student and observer ratings were off by one or fewer responses, then the entire study hall class received reinforcement (e.g., candy). Two of the three students showed reliable increases in on-task behavior with self-monitoring alone while the third student only exhibited reliable improvement when group reinforcement was added to self-monitoring.

The self-regulated strategy development (SRSD) model of strategy instruction has been used to address deficits in reading recall and expository writing in high school students with ADHD. SRSD involves

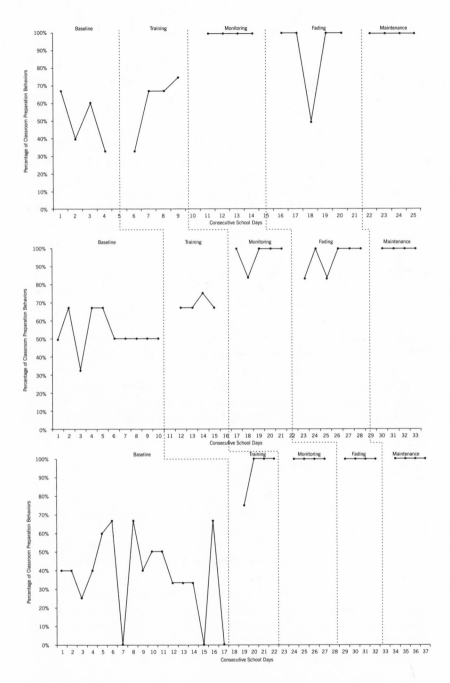

FIGURE 6.1. Percentage of classroom preparation behaviors for three adolescents with ADHD receiving self-monitoring training. From Gureasko-Moore, DuPaul, and White (2006). Copyright 2006 by Sage Publications, Inc. Reprinted by permission.

explicit instruction in cognitive strategies relevant to a specific skill area until mastery is achieved (Harris & Graham, 1996). Specifically, strategy instruction is scaffolded to enable students to use the strategy independently and effectively while also encouraging students to self-monitor and manage their use of the strategy on their own. Johnson, Reid, and Mason (2012) taught three ninth-grade students with ADHD to use a multicomponent reading comprehension strategy (i.e., Think Before Reading, Think While Reading, Think After Reading [TWA]) following the SRSD model. Prior to reading, students were taught to think about what they know and what they want to know about the specific subject matter covered in the text. They also were encouraged to consider the author's purpose in writing the text. Next, students were encouraged to link what they are reading to any prior knowledge they may have on the topic, to think about their reading speed, and to carefully reread any text that is unclear. Finally, after completing the reading assignment, students were taught to identify main ideas and to summarize the content of the reading by retelling what they have learned. The TWA strategy was taught across five lessons using the SRSD model. Steps to TWA were introduced and modeled by the instructor; followed by guided practice by the student. Scaffolded practice involved instructor prompts and feedback when needed. Finally, students independently practiced using the TWA strategy independently while self-monitoring their accurate use of the strategy. All three students in the Johnson and colleagues investigation showed improved social studies expository text recall, with specific improvement in the number of main ideas percentage of supporting details recalled. Recall gains were maintained 2 and 4 weeks following the end of intervention.

Jacobson and Reid (2010) obtained similar positive effects for the persuasive essay writing of three high school students with ADHD. SRSD was used to teach two strategies to plan and organize ideas for persuasive writing. For planning the essay, students were taught to STOP (suspend judgment, take a side, organize your idea, and plan more while you write). For organizing their ideas, students were instructed to use the mnemonic DARE (develop topic sentence, add supporting ideas, reject possible arguments for the alternative view, and end with a conclusion). Increases in number of essay elements, length, planning time, and holistic quality of the essays were noted across all three students with gains maintained 3 weeks after termination of instruction.

Home-Based Intervention

As is the case for school-based intervention, few controlled studies of home-based intervention for adolescents with ADHD have been conducted. Of those few investigations, most have evaluated upward extensions of treatments that are efficacious for younger children, such as parent education in behavior modification (see Chapter 8). In a seminal study of three family therapy approaches for teenagers with ADHD, Barkley and colleagues (1992) recruited sixty-one, 12- to 18-year-olds (*M* age = 13.6–14.2 depending on treatment group) who were randomly assigned to behavior management training, problem-solving and communication training, or structural family therapy. Treatments were delivered across 8–10 weekly sessions with assessment data on teen and family functioning collected prior to intervention, right after intervention sessions ended, and then at a 3-month follow-up. In contrast to hypothesized superiority for behavior management training and problem-solving and communication training relative to structural family therapy, significant improvements were found for all three treatment groups. Specifically, participants exhibited fewer symptoms of internalizing and externalizing disorders as well as improved school functioning, while mothers reported lower levels of depression, and mother–teen interactions improved with respect to conflict, negative communication, and anger. In general, these improvements were maintained 3 months after treatment ended. Alternatively, individual response to treatment was minimal, as only 5–30% of participants showed reliable change and even fewer (i.e., 5–20%) were normalized or recovered with treatment. The limited positive response to treatment is not surprising given the relative brevity of intervention and the multiple, chronic functional impairments exhibited by adolescents with this disorder. Thus, it is unclear whether behavioral interventions implemented by parents of teens with ADHD are as successful as similar treatment strategies with younger children.

Home-based self-regulation strategies have also been evaluated. For example, Axelrod, Zhe, Haugen, and Klein (2009) examined the effects of a self-regulation intervention on the on-task behavior of five 13- to 16-year-old adolescents with ADHD in the context of completing homework. The intervention involved self-monitoring in 3-minute or 10-minute fixed intervals that was paired with individual reinforcement (e.g., access to extra television or video game time) when student responses matched an independent observer with 80% or greater accuracy. Significant improvements in on-task behavior were found for all five participants.

Timely, accurate completion of homework often is challenging for adolescents with ADHD. Thus, several intervention programs have been developed to enhance homework performance in this population. The CHP and HOPS programs described earlier in this chapter include components designed to support homework completion. For example, the after-school version of CHP includes time for students to complete homework under the supervision of program facilitators (Evans et al., 2004). The HOPS program provides students with strategies to help them complete homework independently (Langberg, 2011). Both programs also involve parents in monitoring and reinforcing homework completion.

Meyer and Kelley (2007) designed and evaluated a homework and study skills intervention for middle school students with ADHD. Over the course of one or two sessions, students were trained to self-monitor homework completion and to implement the SQ4R method for social studies reading comprehension and test preparation. SQ4R involved surveying titles and headings before reading, formulating questions, reading to find answers to questions, reciting answers to questions in own words, writing answers to questions, and reviewing text and question answers. Parents also attended a training session wherein they were encouraged to support students in following homework management steps including prompting the student to begin homework, organize materials, and complete daily monitoring checklists. Parents did not participate in completing homework checklists or checking work accuracy. They did, however, provide contingencies (e.g., access to preferred activities) for completion of homework and self-monitoring checklists. Meyer and Kelley assessed the efficacy of this program with a sample of 42 sixth- to eighth-grade students (36 boys, 6 girls) all of whom were diagnosed with ADHD and exhibited homework completion problems. Teachers reported a significant reduction in homework problems with concomitant improvement in classroom preparedness for students who participated in training relative to students in a wait-list control group. These improvements were maintained at 4-week follow-up and were associated with high levels of parent and student satisfaction.

Home–School Communication

As discussed in Chapter 5, strategies to promote consistent and positive home–school communication are critical to school success for students with ADHD. Collaboration between home and school is particularly important for students at the secondary level given the greater complexity of material, increased task demands, and higher expectations for student independence. The most popular method of home–school communication has been a daily report card that provides teacher input on student completion of key academic and behavioral goals with follow-up reinforcement at home provided by parents (see Chapter 5; see also Figure 6.2 for an example of a daily report card for an adolescent).

SCHOOL–HOME NOTE

Name __Richard__   Date __10/20__

SUBJECT __Math__

    Was prepared for class (Yes) No NA   Homework assignment:
    Used class time well (Yes) No NA   *Test Friday on*
    Handed in homework (Yes) No NA   *Chapter 3*
    Homework (Test) Grade F   D (C) B A NA Teacher's Initials __WJ__

Comments: __Seems to be paying attention better and using__
              __his time well.__

SUBJECT __Social Studies__

    Was prepared for class Yes (No) NA   Homework assignment:
    Used class time well (Yes) No NA   *Answer questions*
    Handed in homework Yes (No) NA   *1–10, page 113*
    (Homework) Test Grade F (D) C B A NA Teacher's Initials __MS__

Comments: __Did not bring notebook; he talked a good bit__
              __during class.__

SUBJECT __English__

    Was prepared for class (Yes) No NA   Homework assignment:
    Used class time well (Yes) No NA   *None*
    Handed in homework Yes No (NA)
    Homework (Test) Grade F   D (C) B A NA Teacher's Initials __JL__

Comments: __Participated nicely in class.__

Parent Comments: __Ms. Sessions, Richard says he handed in__
              __his homework. Would you mind checking with him?__

FIGURE 6.2. Abbreviated school–home note used with middle and high school students. (This note was completed by Richard, his teachers, and his parents.) From Kelley (1990). Copyright 1990 by The Guilford Press. Reprinted by permission.

Unfortunately, very few, if any, empirical studies have examined the implementation and efficacy of daily report cards in secondary school settings to address the needs of students with ADHD. In our experience, daily report card systems can be more challenging to implement in secondary schools given the number of teachers involved, the reluctance of some teachers to participate in intervention for an individual student, and the resistance that students, particularly at the high school level, may have to close monitoring and communication between teachers and parents. Two possible modifications can be considered to at least partially address these issues. One option is to have communication occur on a weekly rather than daily basis (i.e., weekly report card system). The main advantage of this option is it places less demands on teachers and may be more palatable to resistant students. Alternatively, weekly home-based reinforcement is arguably less effective than daily contingencies associated with school performance. Another option is to incorporate self-evaluation procedures with the daily report card. Student ratings could be paired initially with teacher ratings with the latter phased out over time as described in Chapter 5 for classroom-based self-evaluation. Thus, eventually, daily reports to parents are based solely on student self-evaluation ratings. This option may address both teacher and student reluctance to participate in a daily report card system. Of course, the degree to which this option is effective awaits empirical study.

Supporting Transition to Postsecondary Education

As a function of their impulsivity, students with ADHD frequently do not consider the long-term consequences of their actions, nor do they plan ahead with any consistency. Thus, adolescents with this disorder often require greater guidance in planning for postsecondary school activities (i.e., entering the workforce or college). Although vocational and educational counseling are typically proffered to all secondary-level students at varying degrees of intensity, it is particularly crucial for individuals with ADHD to receive ongoing intensive advising in this area. The identification of interests and strengths at an earlier age than is common for other children may be necessary for students with this disorder. This should not be an effort to "pigeonhole" a child into one track (e.g., vocational education) versus another (e.g., college preparatory courses), but rather to encourage the student to develop a focus or interest area that will maintain his or her motivation for continuing schooling. One of the greatest risks facing this population is a loss of interest in education, resulting in leaving school prematurely. Thus, helping the student to look ahead and plan for the future may spur an interest in school, even if such interest is limited to selected subject areas. Beginning in middle school and continuing through each high school grade, students with ADHD should meet regularly with their guidance counselors or related personnel so that the latter can provide continuous assessment and programming related to vocational/collegiate aspirations.

Schwiebert, Sealander, and Bradshaw (1998) provide several suggestions, albeit in the absence of empirical support, for school counselors working with high school students with ADHD to aid in the transition to postsecondary education. Counselors should first advocate for students to have a comprehensive psychoeducational evaluation that focuses extensively on academic history and functioning. A report based on this evaluation should identify specific academic needs and provide detailed recommendations for how these would be addressed at the college level. This evaluation may be critical in obtaining necessary accommodations and related support services in college. Next, school counselors should assist students with ADHD in taking appropriate college-bound coursework. This will ensure that students will have taken all necessary courses, thus preventing possible roadblocks to college admission.

High school counselors should help students with ADHD to prepare a transition file that may be helpful in obtaining appropriate support services and accommodations in college (Schweibert et al., 1998). This transitional file should include, for example, high school transcripts, ACT and/or SAT scores, diagnostic report and treatment recommendations, copies of any IDEIA or 504 educational plans, student writing sample (e.g., personal statement, essay), evidence of participation in extracurricular activities and/or honors received, and copies of letters and applications to colleges completed by the student.

The student should also be assisted in evaluating possible colleges, particularly with respect to the availability and quality of support services for students with disabilities (Schweibert et al., 1998). The counselor may help the student investigate what documents will be needed to qualify for support services at various colleges along with other important information (e.g., how many credit hours will qualify for full-time student status). Specific support services that could be investigated include availability of special orientation sessions; alternative testing options; the degree to which disability staff advocate for student needs with faculty; availability and quality of tutoring and academic support; opportunity to use recorded textbooks; possible course substitution options; assistance with study, test-taking, and note-taking skills; availability of note-taking services; assistance with managing schedule and time; possible extensions of assignment deadlines; and technological assistance (Richard, 1992).

Finally, students should be assisted in developing self-advocacy skills (Schweibert et al., 1998). Counselors may guide students through practice exercises and role-play scenarios where students need to self-identify ADHD and request support or accommodations. Students may also be guided in writing letters requesting special considerations based on their ADHD. Counseling students in understanding their ADHD and its impact on their lives, particularly on educational functioning, may motivate students to accept training in time management and self-care skills that will be critical to success in college.

ADHD IN COLLEGE STUDENTS

The impact of ADHD on the functioning and success of college students has received increased attention in recent years as growing numbers of high school students with ADHD are pursuing postsecondary education (Weyandt & DuPaul, 2013; Wolf, Simkowitz, & Carlson, 2009). Although precise prevalence figures are not available, approximately 2–4% of the college student population reports clinically significant levels of ADHD symptoms (e.g., DuPaul et al., 2001; Pope et al., 2007; Weyandt, Linterman, & Rice, 1995). Furthermore, 5% of a large, nationally representative sample of first-year college students reported having ADHD (Pryor, DeAngelo, Palucki, Blake, Hurtado, & Tran, 2010). Approximately 25% of college students who receive disabilities services are identified with ADHD (Wolf, 2001).

Given the increasing numbers of students with ADHD pursuing postsecondary education, research has examined the degree to which the academic, psychological, social, and behavioral functioning of college students with ADHD is compromised relative to their classmates. First, college students with ADHD typically earn lower GPAs, are more likely to be on academic probation, and are less likely to graduate from college (Weyandt & DuPaul, 2013). Second, preliminary findings suggest that college students with ADHD are more likely to report difficulty in relations with parents and peers, lower levels of social skills and social adjustment, and diminished levels of self-esteem (e.g., Shaw-Zirt, Popali-Lehane, Chaplin, & Bergman, 2005). Third, college students with ADHD are more likely than nondiagnosed peers to exhibit symptoms of one or more comorbid disorders, such as mood (depression and anxiety), substance, and eating disorders (e.g., Heiligenstein & Keeling, 1995). Finally, college students with ADHD are at greater risk than peers for using alcohol and illicit substances, including marijuana and other drugs (e.g., Upadhyaya et al., 2005). Given that ADHD is associated with multiple important risks that may significantly limit successful outcomes in the college environment, it is imperative that students with this disorder receive effective intervention and support services throughout their postsecondary education.

INTERVENTIONS FOR COLLEGE STUDENTS
WITH ADHD

Because college students with ADHD may experience difficulties across one or more areas of functioning, a multimodal treatment approach typically is necessary (Weyandt & DuPaul, 2013). Unfortunately, very few controlled investigations have examined the effects of various treatment strategies for college students with ADHD. Nevertheless, it is important to be aware of those strategies that have solid conceptual underpinnings and/or initial outcome data with the ADHD postsecondary population. Psychosocial treatment may include cognitive-behavioral therapy and/ or coaching of organizational skills and time management. Educational support (e.g., tutoring) and accommodations (e.g., extra time on exams) often are recommended. Finally, psychotropic medication, particularly central nervous system (CNS) stimulants, may be used to reduce ADHD symptoms. Given that services will involve multiple providers both on and off campus, coordination of care will be critical particularly because students will presumably manage their own care with minimal supervision by parents or other caregivers.

Psychosocial Intervention Strategies

A variety of psychosocial interventions have been suggested for treating ADHD symptoms in college students including cognitive-behavioral therapy, individual counseling, stress reduction strategies, anger management, and promotion of self-care (e.g., proper sleep and nutrition habits; Wolf et al., 2009). These approaches could comprise a comprehensive college-based support program provided by university- and/or community-based service providers (Wolf et al., 2009). Regardless of setting or provider, psychosocial treatment is designed to accomplish three goals: (1) increasing motivation to complete college-related responsibilities in a timely fashion; (2) improving self-regulation skills in academic, social, and occupational contexts; and (3) reducing or preventing significant symptoms of comorbid emotional or behavioral disorders (e.g., mood disorder; Weyandt & DuPaul, 2013).

The most widely recommended psychosocial treatment for college students with ADHD is cognitive-behavioral therapy (Weyandt & DuPaul, 2013). The primary goals of cognitive-behavioral therapy are to help students recognize maladaptive coping patterns (e.g., procrastination of challenging assignments due to anxiety and faulty beliefs) and implement effective problem-solving strategies to circumvent this maladaptive process. Ramsay and Rostain (2006) describe detailed steps for clinicians to follow in implementing cognitive-behavioral therapy across an academic semester for college students with ADHD. At the beginning of the semester, practitioners should help students identify relevant goals for therapy including both academic challenges (e.g., increase timely completion of difficult assignments) and nonacademic life activities (e.g., decrease alcohol use). Students are helped to understand the linkages among cognitions, emotions, and behaviors that may present challenges in reaching stated goals. For example, when given a challenging assignment students may experience maladaptive thoughts ("I always fail on difficult, long-term assignments") that are associated with aversive feelings (e.g., anxiety). Anxiety, in turn, may cause students to use maladaptive compensatory strategies such as procrastination. The clinician helps students to recognize these patterns and then guides them in using an adaptive, problem-solving approach to making small, realistic changes in their routines and activities. As students practice problem-solving strategies, practitioners provide feedback regarding the relative success of therapeutic homework and support continued use of problem solving in anticipating midsemester challenges (e.g., midterm exams, increased workload). Given the increased academic (e.g., final exams) and social (e.g., end-of-year events) demands that typically occur at the end of a semester, clinicians should support students in increasing efforts to use coping strategies. Students are also prepared for termination of cognitive-behavioral therapy by helping them to appreciate the successes achieved during the course of the semester, as well as plan for possible relapse by empowering them to seek additional help during the semester break and/or in subsequent semesters. Although cognitive-behavioral therapy has substantial face validity as a treatment for ADHD in the college population, there are no controlled studies of this intervention currently available (Weyandt & DuPaul, 2013).

Coaching, another commonly recommended psychosocial intervention for college students with ADHD, "involves helping students deal with aspects of their disability that interfere with academic performance and coping with aspects of the college experience, such as procrastination, lack of concentration, ineffective self-regulation, poor planning, anxiety, social incompetence, or time management" (Swartz, Prevatt, & Proctor, 2005, p. 648). According to Swartz and colleagues (2005), coaching involves an initial meeting to set expectations, structure meeting content and schedule, as well as formulate long-term goals. Weekly objectives (i.e., short-term, attainable outcomes) related to each long-term goal are set at the end of each coaching session and evaluated at the beginning of each subsequent meeting. Coaches record outcomes for weekly objectives so that students can visually track progress toward goal attainment. Students and coaches agree on rewards and consequences for session attendance and progress toward goals (e.g., payment to coach if session is missed or weekly objective is not attained). Similar to cognitive-behavioral therapy, coaches guide and support students in using a systematic problem-solving approach toward attaining goals that involves discussion of challenges or obstacles to goal attainment, identifying possible strategies for circumventing challenges or obstacles, changing consequences for actions, evaluating the effectiveness of strategies on a weekly basis, and, if needed, making changes to strategies. As is the case for cognitive-behavioral therapy, there are no controlled treatment outcome studies of coaching with the college ADHD population. Thus, practitioners must exercise caution in presuming that psychosocial treatments alone will be successful (Weyandt & DuPaul, 2013).

Educational Interventions and Accommodations

Educational interventions are focused on providing students with training in specific content-area skills (e.g., quantitative skills taught in a math course); teaching ways to organize course materials and tasks, study for exams, and/or take class notes; and supporting the implementation of strategies or practice of newly acquired academic skills (Weyandt & DuPaul, 2013). The most commonly recommended educational interventions for college students with ADHD involve instruction in study/organization skills as well as methods to improve comprehension of lecture and reading assignments. In one of the few controlled studies of educational intervention for college ADHD, Allsopp, Minskoff, and Bolt (2005) developed a model for delivering course-specific strategy instruction for college students with disabilities that was evaluated with a sample including students with ADHD some of whom also had learning disabilities. Students received individualized strategy instruction based on their specific learning needs as well as prior empirical support for a strategy designed to meet those needs. For example, to address a student's reading comprehension skills, the RAP paraphrasing strategy was used with the following steps: R—read a paragraph; A— ask what the main ideas are; and P—put the ideas into your own words (Schumaker, Denton, & Deshler, 1984). One- to 2-hour strategy sessions were conducted several times over the course of a semester with results indicating significant increases in GPA. Academic improvement was particularly noteworthy for those students who independently practiced strategies between training sessions, as well as those who reported a supportive relationship with their instructor. Alternatively, those students who had additional cognitive or emotional difficulties beyond ADHD were less likely to show improvement with training.

Educational accommodations are changes to educational practice that mitigate the impact of a disability, in this case ADHD, on student access to the curriculum (Harrison et al., 2013). As such, accommodations differ from interventions in that the former do not involve training to improve skill or knowledge. Although specific accommodations are tailored to the needs and impairment experienced by individual students, typical recommendations for students with ADHD include providing extra time or breaks during tests, allowing use of spell-check for word processing during examinations, placing students in distraction-free environments during tests, providing someone to take notes during class lectures, and extending assignment deadlines (Wolf et al., 2009). Unfortunately, empirical studies evaluating the efficacy of these and other educational accommodations for college students with ADHD have not been conducted. Thus, practitioners should use caution in assuming that accommodations will result in academic improvement for this population.

Pharmacotherapy for College Students with ADHD

As is the case for children and adolescents with ADHD, pharmacotherapy is a frequently recommended treatment for college students with this disorder (Weyandt & DuPaul, 2013). A variety of psychotropic medications could be considered; however, CNS stimulants are the drug of choice for adults with ADHD (Barkley, 2006). Although the effects of stimulants on the symptoms and associated impairments experienced by college students is presumed to be similar to the impact of stimulant treatment for children and adolescents, only one controlled study has specifically examined medication effects in a college sample. DuPaul, Weyandt, and colleagues (2012) examined the effects of a prodrug stimulant (lisdexamfetamine dimesylate [LDX]) on the behavioral, psychosocial, academic, and executive functioning of 24 college students with ADHD. Students participated in a 5-week double-blind, placebo-controlled medication trial that included the following weekly phases administered in a counterbalanced fashion: no-drug baseline, placebo, or 30, 50, and 70 mg of LDX per day. The same measures were collected over the course of 1 week for college students without ADHD who were not receiving medication. LDX was associated with large, statistically significant improvements in ADHD symptoms and executive functioning (e.g., task management and organizational skills) for 86% and 73% of participating students, respectively. Significant, but smaller improvements were found for psychosocial and academic outcomes. Very few adverse side effects were reported by participants. Alternatively, although substantial behavioral improvements were found, college students with ADHD did not improve to the point of "normalization" and remained at a significant disadvantage relative to the non-ADHD control participants. Thus, it is critical that pharmacotherapy be augmented with effective psychosocial and academic interventions as multimodal treatment may lead to larger and more comprehensive change (Weyandt & DuPaul, 2013).

SUMMARY

ADHD is a chronic disorder associated with long-standing academic, behavioral, and social impairments for most individuals diagnosed with this condition. Thus, it is critical for school psychologists and other school personnel to use empirically supported assessment and intervention strategies in secondary and postsecondary educational settings. The good news is that reliable and valid assessment measures are available for initial identification and ongoing monitoring of symptoms and impairment for middle school, high school, and college students with ADHD. Alternatively, far fewer studies have been conducted to establish the effectiveness of various intervention options particularly for high school and college students with the disorder. That said, research conducted thus far has provided solid support for various psychosocial and educational support strategies at the middle school level. In addition, studies are increasingly focusing on interventions that may reduce ADHD symptoms and enhance functioning among high school and college students with the disorder. Thus, practitioners have a growing number of strategies for addressing the needs of this population with the hopes that greater research attention in the coming years will yield more intervention options with solid empirical support.

CHAPTER 7

Medication Therapy

The prescription of psychotropic medication is the most common treatment for ADHD. For example, more than 4% of children and adolescents are treated with psychostimulant medications (e.g., MPH) in the United States (Safer & Zito, 2000; Zito et al., 2008). The highest rates (approximately 7% of the population) of stimulant treatment are for children between 5 and 14 years old (Zito et al., 2008). Psychostimulant medication use has grown steadily over the last few decades, particularly among preschool and secondary school populations (Olfson, Marcus, Weissman, & Jensen, 2002; Safer & Zito, 2000). The average duration of medication use is between 2 and 7 years, depending on the age of the child (Safer & Zito, 2000). Furthermore, more research has been conducted on the effects of stimulant medications on the functioning of children with ADHD than any other treatment modality for any childhood disorder (Connor, 2006b).

Numerous studies have consistently demonstrated short-term enhancement of the behavioral, academic, and social functioning of the majority of children being treated with stimulant compounds. In fact, several meta-analyses indicate that effects on behavioral and social functioning are in the moderate to large range with improvements over placebo conditions varying from 0.5 to over 1.0 standard deviation units (Faraone & Buitelaar, 2010; Van der Oord, Prins, Oosterlaan, & Emmelkamp, 2008). Smaller effects in the range of 0.33 standard deviation units have been found for academic functioning (Van der Oord et al., 2008). Despite these positive treatment effects, the limitations of pharmacotherapy (e.g., possible adverse side effects, lack of evidence of long-term efficacy) have led to the adoption of multimodal intervention approaches for ADHD (Barkley, 2006). Stimulants appear to exert greater effects on problems associated with ADHD symptoms (e.g., academic underachievement) when combined with other effective treatment approaches, such as behavior modification (MTA Cooperative Group, 1999). But given the demonstrated efficacy and widespread use of psychotropic medications in treating ADHD, it is important for school-based personnel to become familiar with (1) the types of medications used to treat ADHD, (2) possible behavioral and adverse side effects associated with these medications, (3) factors to consider in recommending medication trials for individual children, (4) methods to assess treatment response within school settings, (5) how to communicate assessment data to physicians and other medical professionals, and (6) the limitations of pharmacotherapy.

TYPES OF PSYCHOTROPIC
MEDICATIONS EMPLOYED

CNS Stimulants

Psychostimulant medications are so named because of their demonstrated ability to increase the arousal or "alertness" of the CNS. Their effects on children with ADHD are not "paradoxical," as they exert similar physiological and behavioral effects with the normal population (Rapoport et al., 1980). Given the structural similarity of psychostimulants to certain brain neurotransmitters (e.g., dopamine), they are considered sympathomimetic compounds (Donnelly & Rapoport, 1985). The most commonly employed CNS stimulants are MPH (Ritalin, Concerta, Metadate, Quillivant XR), dextroamphetamine (Dexedrine), mixed amphetamine (Adderall), and LDX (Vyvanse). Of the three medications, MPH is the most widely employed: It is used in over 80% of children treated with stimulants (Safer & Zito, 2000). There is evidence that lisdexamfetamine may be somewhat more effective in symptom reduction than MPH presumably due to differences in enhancing dopamine transmission in the brain (Faraone & Buitelaar, 2010). Other types of stimulants (e.g., caffeine) are not discussed here because they have not been found to be as effective as the above medications nor are they typically used clinically.

Dose Ranges

The CNS stimulants, their available tablet sizes, and typical dose ranges are displayed in Table 7.1. Fixed dose ranges, as opposed to those based on body weight (i.e., mg/kg), are given to reflect typical prescribing practice. Also, research indicates that neither gross body weight nor body

TABLE 7.1. Stimulant Medications, Tablet Sizes, and Dose Ranges

Brand name[a]	Tablet sizes	Dosage regimen	Dose range[b]
Ritalin (methylphenidate)	5–20 mg SR, 20 mg	Twice daily Once daily	2.5–25 mg 20–40 mg
Concerta (methylphenidate)		Once daily	
Metadate (methylphenidate)		Once daily	
Quillivant XR (methylphenidate oral suspension)	NA; liquid	Once daily	
Dexedrine (d-amphetamine)	5-mg spansule 10-mg spansule 15-mg spansule 5-mg tablet	Once daily	2.5–25 mg
	5 mg/5 ml (elixir)	Twice daily	2.5–25 mg
Adderall (mixed amphetamine)	5–20 mg	Once daily	5–20 mg
Vyvanse (lisdexamfetamine dimesylate)	30–70 mg	Once daily	30–70 mg

[a]Generic name in parentheses.
[b]Dose range for each administration is provided.

area is a significant predictor of dose–response to MPH in the pediatric age range (Rapport & Denney, 1997). Once a child's "optimal" dose is established, as discussed later in the chapter, medication is usually dispensed once per day (in the case of sustained-release preparations) or twice per day (at breakfast and lunch for standard preparations).

Given the relatively short behavioral half-lives of these compounds, school personnel have a greater opportunity to observe the child with ADHD when medicated than do parents and therefore must be included in the assessment of treatment response. Both MPH and dextroamphetamine are available in short-acting and sustained-release forms. Because the behavioral effects of the sustained-release compounds purportedly last longer (i.e., 8 hours postingestion) than the short-acting derivatives, they (along with Adderall and Vyvanse, which are also long-acting preparations) have several advantages, including the preclusion of noontime medication administration at school and greater confidentiality of treatment (Connor, 2006b). Thus, at present, sustained-release medications are preferred over short-acting preparations for treating most children and adolescents. MPH is also available in liquid form (Quillivant XR), which may be easier to administer to children particularly those who have difficulty swallowing pills, while not sacrificing efficacy in symptom reduction (Wigal, Childress, Belden, & Berry, 2013).

Antidepressant Medications

Several antidepressant medications have been evaluated for treatment of ADHD including desipramine (Norpramine), imipramine (Tofranil), bupropion (Wellbutrin), and nortriptyline. Although these medications may reduce ADHD symptoms and related difficulties (e.g., aggression), their effects, particularly in the cognitive area, are not as strong as CNS stimulants (Connor, 2006a). Furthermore, desipramine and imipramine have been associated with rare but serious cardiac side effects and thus are not recommended for clinical use.

Antihypertensive Medications

Clonidine, an antihypertensive agent, is moderately effective in reducing ADHD symptoms (for a meta-analysis, see Connor, Fletcher, & Swanson, 1999). For example, Hunt, Mindera, and Cohen (1985) obtained clonidine-induced enhancement of teacher and parent ratings of hyperactivity and conduct problems in 70% of children treated. But it should be noted that when the effects of clonidine are directly compared to those of MPH, the latter is found to be superior (Connor et al., 1999). Alternatively, clonidine may be preferred in certain situations due to continued effects in the evening and an absence of the sleep or appetite disturbance that is sometimes found with MPH. In fact, the combination of clonidine and MPH may be helpful in those cases where MPH alone has led to side effects such as insomnia (Connor, Barkley, & Davis, 2000; Hunt et al., 1985). The most frequent adverse side effects of clonidine are sedation, irritability, and a drop in blood pressure (Connor et al., 1999). Guanfacine (Intuniv, Tenex) is another antihypertensive agent that has been found to lead to similar behavioral effects as clonidine in both short-term placebo-controlled trials (e.g., Biederman et al., 2008; Sallee, Lyne, Wigal, & McGough, 2009) and long-term open trials (Sallee, McGough, et al., 2009). Adverse side effects appear to be less frequent and severe than those found with clonidine (Connor, 2006a) and may diminish as children acclimate to the medication (Faraone & Glatt, 2010). Given their modest efficacy and association with relatively benign adverse side effects, it appears that clonidine and guanfacine are viable second-tier treatments for ADHD.

Atomoxetine

Atomoxetine (Strattera) is a nonstimulant compound that affects nor-epinephrine in a similar manner to stimulants. Short-term placebo-controlled trials have shown atomoxetine to significantly reduce ADHD symptoms (e.g., Dittmann et al., 2011; Kelsey et al., 2004) and improve the quality of childrens' and parents' quality of life (Escobar et al., 2009) in the majority of treated children. Possible adverse side effects are relatively benign and include loss of appetite, nausea, nervousness, and abdominal pain (Yildiz, Sismanlar, Memik, Karakaya, & Agaoglu, 2011). Furthermore, this medication appears to be safe and well toler-ated by nearly all children receiving treatment across several years (Don-nelly et al., 2009). Although short-term reduction of ADHD symptoms is similar to that obtained with MPH (Hazell et al., 2011), few studies have examined the effects of atomoxetine on areas of functioning (e.g., academic, social) directly impacted by ADHD. Nevertheless, atomox-etine is considered the most viable alternative to stimulant medication in cases where stimulants are ineffective or are associated with significant adverse side effects.

Summary

Although these and other initial results are promising, most of the avail-able research with medications other than stimulants have only exam-ined effects on symptoms with minimal data regarding treatment effects on important areas of functioning. Thus, effects on academic perfor-mance and cognitive functioning are critically needed. In addition, the magnitude of treatment effects associated with alternative drugs and stimulants need to be compared directly within large samples of children with ADHD. For these reasons and given that stimulants are the most frequently prescribed medication for this disorder, the remainder of this chapter will focus on CNS stimulants, primarily MPH.

BEHAVIORAL EFFECTS OF STIMULANTS

Based on the empirical literature, approximately 75% of elementary school-age children with ADHD treated with stimulant medications respond positively to one or more doses (see Rapport & Denney, 2000).[1]

---

[1] Effects of stimulants for preschool-age children, based primarily on the PATS study (Greenhill et al., 2006), are discussed in detail in Chapter 4.

Remaining children either exhibit no change or their ADHD symptoms worsen with treatment, thus implicating the need for alternative medications or treatment approaches. Thus, it is not guaranteed that a given child with ADHD will respond to a particular stimulant nor should medication response be used as a confirmation of diagnosis (i.e., a positive response does not confirm an ADHD diagnosis, nor does a negative medication response indicate that a child does not have ADHD). Furthermore, a lack of response or adverse effects associated with one of the stimulants does not rule out the possibility of a positive response to one of the remaining medications in this class (Elia & Rapoport, 1991). Historically, MPH is by far the most commonly employed stimulant (Safer & Zito, 2000). Several investigations have delineated that the behavioral effects of MPH, dextroamphetamine, and mixed amphetamine compounds are quite similar (e.g., James et al., 2001), although lisdexamfetamine may be moderately more efficacious (Faraone & Buitelaar, 2010).

The effects of stimulant medications upon nearly every area of behavioral, emotional, and physical functioning of children with ADHD have been investigated (for meta-analytic reviews, see Faraone & Buitelaar, 2010; Van der Oord et al., 2008). The areas of greatest potential concern to school professionals will be reviewed briefly below.

Effects on Behavioral Control and Attention

Stimulant medications have been found to have positive effects on the ability of children with ADHD to sustain attention to effortful tasks (Barkley, DuPaul, et al., 1991; Douglas, Barr, O'Neill, & Britton, 1986; Rapport et al., 1987) and to inhibit impulsive responding (Brown & Sleator, 1979; Rapport et al., 1988). In many cases, attention to assigned classwork is improved to the extent that the child's behavior appears similar to his or her typically developing classmates (Abikoff & Gittelman, 1985; DuPaul & Rapport, 1993). Furthermore, these medications significantly reduce disruptive motor activity, especially task-irrelevant movements during work situations (e.g., Cunningham & Barkley, 1979). Problems with aggression (Hinshaw, 1991; Klorman et al., 1988), classroom disruptive behavior (Barkley, 1979), persistence with frustrating tasks (Milich, Carlson, Pelham, & Licht, 1991), and noncompliance with authority figure commands (Barkley, Karlsson, Strzelecki, & Murphy, 1984) also have been shown to improve with these medications. A meta-analysis conducted by Connor, Glatt, Lopez, Jackson, and Melloni (2002) found moderate to high effect sizes for stimulant-induced improvements in overt and covert aggression. In fact, effects on aggressive behavior were equivalent to effect sizes obtained for ADHD symptoms. In general, improvements in behavior control and sustained attention are strongest at the higher doses and are ubiquitous across home, clinic, analog classroom, and school settings. Similar behavioral effects have been obtained for adolescents with ADHD; however, the percentage of positive responders is lower (i.e., 50–70%) than among elementary school children (Evans & Pelham, 1991; Pelham, Vodde-Hamilton, Murphy, Greenstein, & Vallano, 1991).

Behavioral effects of stimulants are, in part, moderated by environmental factors. Northup and colleagues (1997, 1999) have conducted several studies explicating the relationship between environmental contingencies and MPH response. These investigations demonstrated that MPH effects vary across situations as a function of contingencies operating in the environment. For example, in a laboratory situation where children were asked to complete tasks under differing conditions, MPH effects on disruptive behavior were strongest when an adult was present in the room and weakest when the child was alone (Northup et al., 1999). Although MPH operates directly on biological factors (i.e., brain functioning), the effects of this and similar drugs are dependent on prevailing contingencies and the rates of behavior that the latter elicit (Murray & Kollins, 2000; Rapport, DuPaul, & Smith, 1985). Thus, Northup and Gulley (2001) have recommended that school psychologists evaluate medication effects in the context of functional behavioral assessments, wherein MPH dosage and environmental factors are systematically manipulated to find optimal combinations of each treatment approach. The applicability of this laboratory paradigm to school settings awaits investigation; however, it is clear that the behavioral effects of stimulants do not occur in a vacuum and environmental factors must always be considered when evaluating medication response.

Effects on Cognitive and Academic Performance

Stimulant medication effects on the cognitive performance of children with ADHD traditionally have been studied using laboratory-based paradigms such as the Paired Associates Learning test (Swanson & Kinsbourne, 1975) and tests of short-term recall (Sprague & Sleator, 1977). Salutary effects of MPH on children's cognitive functioning have been found on tests of verbal retrieval (Barkley, DuPaul, et al., 1991; Evans, Gualtieri, & Amara, 1986), paired associates learning (Rapport et al., 1985), stimulus equivalence learning (Vyse & Rapport, 1989), and short-term recall of visual stimuli (Sprague & Sleator, 1977). In general, the dose–response effects of MPH on cognitive performance have been found to be linear, with the greatest enhancement occurring at the highest doses (Rapport & Kelly, 1991; Solanto, 2000). It is important to note, however, that these dose–response effects have been delineated at the group level and there are substantial differences in dose responsivity across individual children, as will be explicated later in this chapter.

Reviews of stimulant medication effects on the academic performance of children with ADHD have generally concluded that this area of functioning is impacted minimally by pharmacotherapy over the *long term* (Scheffler et al., 2009). For example, Barbaresi, Katusic, Colligan, Weaver, and Jacobsen (2007) followed 370 children with ADHD from school entry to high school graduation and found a statistically significant but small correlation ($r = .15$) between medication dose and reading achievement test scores. Powers, Marks, Miller, Newcorn, and Halperin (2008) obtained more promising findings in a sample of 169 children with ADHD followed over 9 years. Specifically, students treated with stimulants obtained significantly higher achievement test scores and high school GPA than untreated students. These findings are limited by the lack of experimental procedures to control for possible confounding variables (e.g., SES, quality of instruction). Studies examining long-term academic effects have primarily utilized traditional academic achievement tests (e.g., Wechsler Individual Achievement Test) or report card grades. Such measures may not be sensitive enough to detect short-term or more subtle changes in cognitive functioning associated with treatment. Several additional factors limit the utility of norm-referenced achievement tests for treatment evaluation purposes, including (1) a failure to adequately sample the curriculum in use, (2) the use of a limited number of items to sample various skills, (3) the use of response formats that do not require the student to perform the behavior (e.g., writing) of interest, and (4) an insensitivity to small changes in student performance (Shapiro, 2011a).

Research studies conducted by several independent research teams have found acute MPH-induced improvements in academic productivity and accuracy among large samples of children (Douglas et al., 1988; Pelham, Bender, Caddell, Booth, & Moorer, 1985; Rapport et al., 1987, 1988; Wigal et al., 2011) and young adolescents with ADHD (Evans & Pelham, 1991; Evans et al., 2001; Pelham et al., 1991). Attention to teacher lectures, completion of study hall assignments, and quiz and test scores among middle school students with ADHD also are enhanced by MPH (Pelham et al., 1991). As with other domains, these effects have been strongest in the higher dose range when analyzed at the group level. Rather than standardized achievement tests, these investigators employed written tasks assigned by each child's classroom teacher to assess academic performance. Although such measures may be more sensitive to treatment-related change and presumably possess greater ecological validity than do published, norm-referenced instruments, their reliability (i.e., stability over time) must be established prior to evaluating intervention effects. It is somewhat puzzling why short-term improvements in academic performance have not translated to greater scholastic success in the long run (i.e., relatively small effects on academic achievement across several years; Barbaresi et al., 2007; Scheffler et al., 2009). However, the probability of obtaining enhanced long-term academic outcomes may be increased if medication dosage is initially determined based on the enhancement of academic functioning rather than simply on behavioral control, as has been done in the past (Rapport & Kelly, 1991).

Several studies emanating from independent investigative teams have delineated MPH effects on the trajectory of academic skill acquisition. Specifically, dose–response effects are evident on curriculum-based measures of reading and math that parallel findings with other academic measures (Roberts & Landau, 1995; Stoner, Carey, Ikeda, & Shinn, 1994). However, findings typically show a wide range of individual responsivity to medication for this area of functioning relative to behavior change. As discussed in Chapter 2, CBM probes are an efficient and sensitive means for evaluating intervention effects on academic skills. As such, greater use of these measures is strongly recommended for both clinical practice and research.

Effects on Social Relationships

MPH has been found to significantly improve the quality of social interactions between children with ADHD and their parents, teachers, and peers. For example, several studies have shown that stimulants increase children's compliance with parent or teacher commands and enhance their responsiveness to the interactions of others (Connor, 2006b). These same investigations found that negative and off-task behaviors are reduced in compliance situations, resulting in a decrease in the frequency of authority figure commands and an increase in positive adult attention to child behavior. In fact, the effects of stimulants on both overt and covert aggression are nearly of the same magnitude as medication effects on ADHD symptoms (Connor et al., 2002).

Similar results have been obtained for the peer relations of children with ADHD. When treated with MPH, children with ADHD are found to be less aggressive with others, behave more appropriately with other children, and to be accepted to a greater degree by their peers (Cunningham, Siegel, & Offord, 1985; Gadow, Nolan, Sverd, Sprafkin, & Paolicelli, 1990; Hinshaw, 1991). Salutary effects on social behavior appear to maintain for at least 2 years (Abikoff, Hechtman, Klein, Gallagher, et al., 2004). Alternatively, King and colleagues (2009) found children with ADHD to generate more hostile responses to provocation in peer interaction scenarios than did children receiving a placebo. Thus, the impact of MPH on children's aggression appears equivocal. Although not studied extensively, the social behavior of adolescents with ADHD is improved with MPH, particularly at lower dosages (Smith et al., 1998). The effects of MPH on the prosocial behavior of children with ADHD remains unclear. Some studies have found no change in the frequency of initiating interactions with others (Hinshaw, Henker, Whalen, Erhardt, & Dunnington, 1989; Wallander, Schroeder, Michelli, & Gualtieri, 1987), while others have found a reduction in positive interactions with peers (Buhrmester, Whalen, Henker, MacDonald, & Hinshaw, 1992). Beyond direct effects on social behavior, MPH has been found to enhance other areas of functioning that may indirectly impact social status. For example, a group of children with ADHD was found to pay attention better during softball games (e.g., greater recall of the game score) when receiving MPH versus a placebo (Pelham et al., 1990).

Dose–Response and Individual Responsivity

Beyond a delineation of specific behavioral effects, the results of empirical investigations of stimulants with children with ADHD have led to a number of important conclusions regarding the general properties of these drugs. First, MPH-induced changes in a specific behavioral realm vary across dose in a systematic fashion, at least at the group level of analysis (e.g., Barkley, Anastopoulos, Guevremont, & Fletcher, 1991; Pelham et al., 1985; Rapport & Denney, 2000; Rapport et al., 1985; Sprague & Sleator, 1977). For most areas of functioning (i.e., cognitive, social, behavior control), these dose–response effects have been linear, with higher doses leading to the greatest change. Second, at an individual level of analysis, separate classes of behavior may be affected differently by MPH even at the same dose (Rapport & Denney, 2000; Sprague & Sleator, 1977). For instance, a given child may show the greatest improvement in academic performance at a different dose than that level of medication that was "optimal" for impulse control or sustained attention. Finally, although linear dose–response effects are consistently found at the group level of analysis, individual children vary considerably with respect to behavior change across doses (Douglas et al., 1986; Pelham et al., 1985; Rapport & Denney, 2000). Even when children share similar characteristics (e.g., diagnosis, age, and body weight), there may be considerable variability in dose responsivity presumably due to individual differences in CNS functioning (Rapport & Denney, 2000).

To illustrate the idiosyncratic nature of MPH effects, Figure 7.1 presents school-based, dose–response data for three individual children with ADHD who were participants in a study conducted by Rapport, DuPaul, and Kelly (1989). Behavioral changes for three measures are presented, including percentage of on-task behavior during independent work, percentage of academic work completed correctly (i.e., Academic Efficiency Score [AES]), and teacher ratings on the Abbreviated

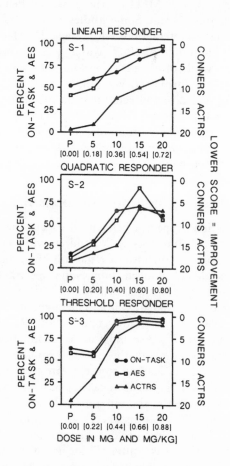

FIGURE 7.1. Dose–response curves of three dependent measures for three individual children of similar body weight (M = 25 kg). Percentage of on-task frequency and Academic Efficiency Score (AES) are plotted along the left-hand ordinate. Total score on the Abbreviated Conners Teacher Rating Scale (ACTRS) is plotted on the right-hand ordinate. Improvement for all three measures is indicated by an upward movement on the axis. From Rapport, DuPaul, and Kelly (1989). Copyright 1989 by M. D. Rapport. Reprinted by permission.

Conners Teacher Rating Scale (ACTRS; Werry, Sprague, & Cohen, 1975). A double-blind, placebo-controlled experimental design was employed wherein each child received four active MPH doses (i.e., 5, 10, 15, and 20 mg) and an inert placebo in a randomly determined sequence. The children were of similar age and body weight, but exhibited rather dramatic differences in MPH response. For example, S-1 (Figure 7.1, top) evidenced attentional and behavioral improvement as a direct function of increasing dose, peaking at the highest dose of 20 mg (i.e., linear dose–response effects). Alternatively, improvements in S-2's classroom behavior and performance were obtained up to the 15-mg dose, where peak effects were evidenced, followed by a decrement at the 20-mg dose. The latter is referred to as a "quadratic response" since there was one change in the slope of the dose–response curve. Finally, S-3 did not exhibit academic or behavioral change until a "therapeutic threshold" was attained at 10 mg, with little in the way of further enhancement at the higher doses (i.e., a threshold response). Thus, the dose–response profile and "optimal" or therapeutic dose differed for the three children.

Normalization of Classroom Functioning

Although the *statistical* significance of the behavioral effects of MPH have been demonstrated reliably, the *clinical* significance of behavioral changes for individual children with ADHD has been demonstrated less frequently. Some investigations have indicated that the task-related attention (Loney, Weissenburger, Woolson, & Lichty, 1979; Rapport, Denney, DuPaul, & Gardner, 1994; Whalen et al., 1978; Whalen, Henker, Collins, Finck, & Dotemoto, 1979) and aggressive behaviors (Hinshaw et al., 1989) of children receiving MPH is statistically indistinguishable from that of their normal peers. Abikoff and Gittelman (1985) found that 60% of children treated with MPH evidenced "normalized" behavior in attention span and impulse control in the classroom. In similar fashion, Pelham and colleagues (1993) found that approximately 60% of children receiving 0.6 mg/kg MPH were rated by teachers to behave "very much like a normal child" when interacting with peers and adults. Alternatively, in the large-scale Multimodal Treatment of ADHD (MTA) study (MTA Cooperative Group, 1999), children with ADHD who received intensive treatment, including MPH, for 14-months showed significantly inferior behavioral, social, and academic functioning at 6- and 8-year outcomes relative to a normative comparison group (Molina et al., 2009).

As is the case with other outcomes, the degree to which functioning is normalized by stimulant medication varies across individuals.

Rapport and colleagues (1994) examined the degree to which MPH normalized the classroom behavior and academic functioning of 76 children with ADHD based on comparisons with a normal control group of 25 children. Children with ADHD participated in a double-blind, placebo-controlled trial in which they received each of four doses (5, 10, 15, and 20 mg) of MPH and a placebo. Dependent measures included teacher ratings of social conduct, direct observations of classroom on-task behavior, and accuracy on independent academic tasks. Between 53 and 78% of the sample obtained scores within the normal range of functioning at one or more doses of MPH depending on the specific measure employed (see Figure 7.2). Notably, teacher ratings of behavior control showed the most prominent improvements and normalization, followed by direct observations of task-related attention and academic efficiency. Approximately 47% of the sample did not show improvement in academic efficiency. Although these results provide further evidence of the strong therapeutic effects of stimulant medication, concomitant interventions (particularly those targeting academic performance) will be necessary for many children with ADHD, even for those whose classroom behavior is normalized by MPH.

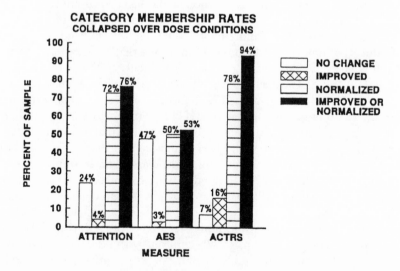

FIGURE 7.2. Percentage of 76 children with ADHD exhibiting no change, clinically significant improvement, and normalized school behavior across three classroom variables as a function of placebo and MPH dose. From Rapport, Denney, DuPaul, and Gardner (1994). Copyright 1994 by the American Academy of Child and Adolescent Psychiatry. Reprinted by permission.

Combination of Medication and Behavioral Therapy

The two most common interventions for ADHD are stimulant medication and behavioral intervention strategies (Barkley, 2006). Several large- (e.g., Abikoff, Hechtman, Klein, Weiss, et al., 2004) and small-scale (e.g., Abramowitz, Eckstrand, O'Leary, & Dulcan, 1992) studies have examined the individual and combined effects of stimulants and behavioral interventions. The results of these investigations have indicated that stimulants in isolation are associated with moderate to large reductions in ADHD symptoms that are superior to behavioral interventions. Alternatively, in most studies, behavioral interventions lead to greater improvements in functional impairments associated with ADHD such as academic achievement, peer relationships, and family interactions. Furthermore, the combination of stimulants and behavioral interventions lead to superior effects, particularly regarding functional impairments, than do either treatment in isolation.

The largest-scale and most comprehensive investigation of these two treatments was the MTA study completed at multiple sites in North America (MTA Cooperative Group, 1999). A sample of 579 children, 7- to 10-years-old diagnosed with ADHD, was randomly assigned to one of four treatment groups. One group received stimulant medication that was titrated using state-of-the-art, multimethod, controlled trials, while a second group received multiple behavioral interventions across home, school, and summer camp settings. The school component of the latter protocol included (1) ongoing consultation with classroom teachers regarding behavioral interventions, and (2) a paraprofessional working with the student with ADHD for half the school day on a daily basis for 12 weeks in the fall of the school year. The paraprofessional implemented behavioral interventions such as token reinforcement for appropriate classroom behavior. A third group received both carefully titrated medication and comprehensive behavioral intervention. Finally, a fourth group of participants received treatment as delivered in the community (community-care control group). Approximately 67% of control group participants were receiving stimulant medication that was titrated using less controlled and more typical procedures than was the MTA medication group. Dependent measures across multiple areas of functioning were collected at three time points during and immediately following the 14-month treatment protocol.

Participants in all four groups showed significant reductions in ADHD symptomatology during and following treatment. Significantly greater reductions in symptoms were obtained for the medication management and combined intervention groups relative to the behavioral-only and community-care control groups. Although carefully titrated stimulant medication clearly was the superior unimodal treatment, additional analyses shed light on the contribution of behavioral interventions. Specifically, the greatest improvement, particularly for problems associated with ADHD (e.g., oppositional behavior, social performance difficulties), was evidenced by children who received the combined intervention protocol (Conners et al., 2001; Swanson et al., 2001). Children in the combined intervention group required a lower mean dosage of medication than did the medication-only group. Using a relatively conservative definition of treatment "success," Swanson and colleagues (2001) found that 68% of combined intervention children were successfully treated relative to 56%, 34%, and 25% of the medication-only, behavioral intervention-only, and community-care control group children, respectively. Although, the effect size separating the behavioral intervention and community-care control group was small (Conners et al., 2001), it is important to note that most of the control group participants received stimulant medication as typically prescribed in the community. Thus, intensive behavioral programming appears equivalent to "medication as usual."

Interestingly, the initial comparative advantage for medication relative to behavioral intervention has diminished over subsequent follow-up assessments at 24-months (MTA Cooperative Group, 2004), 36-months (Jensen et al., 2007), and 6–8 years (Molina et al., 2009). In fact, the best predictors of outcome at 8 years was not type or intensity of treatment during the 14-month MTA trial, but rather children with better sociodemographic status at treatment entry, milder initial ADHD symptoms, and exhibited optimal response to any treatment had the best outcomes. It is likely that combined treatment approaches may be the best way to optimize initial treatment response and thereby enhance long-term outcomes.

Given the findings of the MTA study and prior less comprehensive investigations, the combination of stimulant medication and behavioral interventions is now considered the "optimal" approach to treating ADHD for many children (Barkley, 2006). There are important shortcomings of each treatment when used alone, including a limitation of effects to the times when the interventions are "active," each is ineffective for a significant minority of children with ADHD, and the long-term effectiveness of both treatments has not been documented (Hoza, Pelham, Sams, & Carlson, 1992; Pelham & Murphy, 1986). Alternatively, the combination of behavioral and pharmacological treatments may minimize the limitations of each treatment while maximizing the chances of obtaining clinically significant changes (Pelham & Murphy, 1986).

Research has shown that "dosage" is an important variable in determining the response of children with ADHD to the combination of behavioral interventions and stimulant medication. For example, Fabiano and colleagues (2007) evaluated changes in the classroom behavior and academic productivity of 48 children with ADHD as a function of varying dosages of MPH (placebo, 0.15, 0.30, and 0.60 mg/kg) combined with three "dosages" of behavior modification (no, low, and high intensity). The results, displayed in Figure 7.3, indicate that both treatments in isolation substantially reduced classroom rule violations (top panel) and enhanced classwork productivity (bottom panel) as a function of increasing dosage. However, the combination of the low dosage of both treatments (i.e., low behavior modification plus 0.15 mg/ kg MPH) yielded effects that were equivalent or superior to the high dosage of either treatment alone. Thus, an apparent synergistic interaction between MPH and behavioral strategies may yield successful outcomes at lower dosages of both treatments, thus minimizing effort and resources for behavioral interventions and lowering the probability of adverse side effects for MPH.

It is important to note that Fabiano and colleagues (2007) reported findings at the group level and that it is likely that responses to combined interventions will vary across individual children (Abramowitz et al., 1992). For example, some children will require a "low dose" of behavioral intervention (e.g., home-based daily report card) in combination with a low dose of MPH, while the ADHD symptoms of another child may be severe enough to warrant a high dose of MPH along with a "high dose" of behavioral intervention (e.g., classroom-based response cost system). Furthermore, the addition of one treatment may result in an adjustment in dosage of a previously implemented intervention. For example, the implementation of a behavioral intervention program may allow for a reduction in the amount of medication that a child may require. The titration of various strengths of each intervention must be conducted on an individual basis because the response to the combination of treatments will vary according to child (e.g., severity of ADHD-related behaviors) and environmental (e.g., classroom placement) factors (Pelham, 1989).

POSSIBLE ADVERSE SIDE EFFECTS OF CNS STIMULANTS

The most frequently reported acute adverse side effects to MPH and other stimulants are appetite reduction (particularly at lunch) and insomnia (American Academy of Child and Adolescent Psychiatry, 2007). The primary attribute of sleeping behavior affected by stimulants appears to be a delayed onset of sleep rather than disturbance

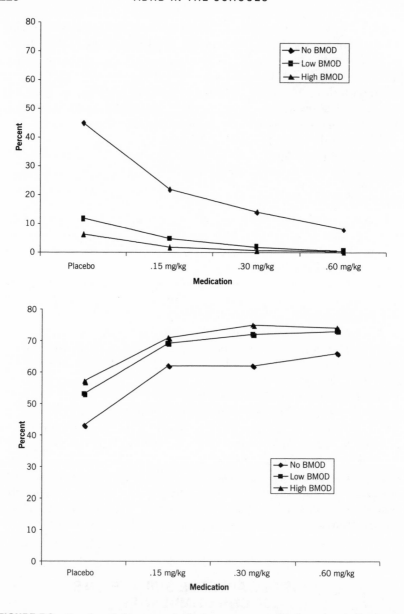

FIGURE 7.3. Graphs of classroom behavior measures. The top panel illustrates frequency of classroom rule violation at each level of behavior modification and medication and the bottom panel represents percentage of assigned seatwork completed at each level of behavior modification and medication. BMOD, behavior modification. From Fabiano et al. (2007). Copyright 2007 by the National Association of School Psychologists. Reprinted by permission.

of sleep per se (Stein & Pao, 2000). Other treatment emergent effects reported in the literature include increased irritability, headaches, stomachaches, and, in rare cases, motor and/or vocal tics (American Academy of Child and Adolescent Psychiatry, 2007). Several research studies have explicated the percentage of cases experiencing possible adverse side effects across a dose range of MPH (for a review, see Rapport & Moffitt, 2002). For example, Barkley, McMurray, Edelbrock, and Robbins (1990) examined the prevalence of parent- and teacher-reported side effects to two doses (i.e., 0.3 and 0.5 mg/kg) of MPH in a large sample of children with ADHD. These investigators found that over 50% of the sample exhibited decreased appetite, insomnia, anxiousness, irritability, or proneness to crying with both doses of MPH. It should be noted that many of these apparent side effects (especially those associated with mood) were present during the placebo condition and may represent characteristics associated with the disorder rather than its treatment. Stomachaches and headaches were reported in about 33% of the participants. The severity of these side effects was mild in most cases, increased as a function of dose, and did not necessarily result in the discontinuation of treatment.

The frequency and severity of possible adverse side effects should be assessed during nonmedication or pretreatment conditions to establish whether they are truly associated with drug ingestion. Rapport and colleagues (2008) examined possible side effects in 65 children with ADHD who participated in a double-blind, placebo-controlled, crossover study wherein they received a placebo and four MPH doses following baseline (i.e., nonmedication phase) assessment. Interestingly, parent ratings of children's "side effects," including both behavioral and physical complaints, were significantly *higher* in baseline relative to placebo and MPH conditions. Rapport and colleagues conclude that some apparent side effects of MPH may actually be an artifact of assessment measures that include scale items reflecting core or secondary characteristics of ADHD, as well as behavioral/physical complaints (e.g., stomachaches) that are common to all children. Thus, the inclusion of a nonmedication assessment phase is critical to establishing whether "true" adverse side effects are present.

Perceptions regarding the presence and severity of adverse side effects may vary across parents, teachers, and students. DuPaul, Anastopoulos, Kwasnik, Barkley, and McMurray (1996) collected adverse side-effect ratings from a sample of parents, teachers, and adolescents in the context of a multiple dosage trial of MPH. Although teacher ratings of side-effect severity did not vary systematically from placebo to active medication, parents reported side-effect severity to be greatest during the *placebo* condition. Conversely, adolescents reported a greater severity of side effects during the two highest dosage conditions relative to placebo. Thus, side effects have to be considered from the "eye of the beholder." Several respondents should be consulted to provide different perspectives on this phenomenon. In our experience, parents will be the best reporter of the most common adverse side effects such as appetite reduction and insomnia. Teachers can provide information regarding possible overfocused behavior, particularly during academic task conditions. Finally, children themselves may be the optimal reporters of possible medication effects on internalizing symptoms (e.g., anxiety) and are perhaps most sensitive to the overall severity of side effects.

Other possible treatment emergent effects that should be monitored include a "behavioral rebound" in the late afternoon and the onset or exacerbation of motor and vocal tics (American Academy of Child and Adolescent Psychiatry, 2007). The "behavioral rebound" phenomenon is typically described as deterioration in conduct (exceeding that which is observed during baseline or placebo conditions) that occurs in the late afternoon and evening following daytime administrations of medication (Johnston, Pelham, Hoza, & Sturges, 1987). Studies that have examined this phenomenon have indicated that it occurs in about 33% of children treated with MPH and that the magnitude of the rebound varies considerably across days for individual children (Johnston et al., 1987). Furthermore, a late afternoon administration of a small dose of MPH may reduce the severity of rebound effects (Connor, 2006b).

The degree to which stimulants induce motor tics and Tourette syndrome symptoms in children remains controversial. Some early studies indicated that a small minority of children may develop tics following stimulant treatment, and that tic frequency and severity did not diminish following termination of treatment (Bremness & Sverd, 1979). Alternatively, multiple investigations have indicated that the majority of children with ADHD and tic disorders will respond positively to stimulant treatment both in terms of behavior control and tic reduction (e.g., Castellanos et al., 1997; Gadow, Sverd, Nolan, Sprafkin, & Schneider, 2007). A minority of children may show exacerbation of tics, thus necessitating caution in prescribing stimulants for children exhibiting both ADHD and tic disorders. However, if monitored carefully, this class of medication may be viable for children with ADHD who have a personal or family history of tics.

Clinical observations have documented an increase in "overfocused" behavior among some children with ADHD treated with MPH (Solanto, 1984). This constriction of cognitive functioning may be demonstrated in a variety of ways, including persistence at a task for an abnormally long period of time, a disregard for relevant peripheral stimuli, or an inability to shift cognitive set to adapt to situational demands

(Solanto & Wender, 1989). Empirical investigations have failed to document the occurrence of this phenomenon at a group level of analysis. However, at least one study has indicated that a subgroup of children with ADHD may demonstrate overfocused performance as a function of MPH (Solanto, 2000). This subgroup may include children who are less hyperactive and who demonstrate better baseline performance on cognitive testing relative to other children with ADHD. In similar fashion, Rapport and colleagues (1994) found that 47% of a large sample of children treated with MPH did not show improvement in academic efficiency at any dose. Presumably, the academic performance of some of these children was compromised by MPH-induced overfocused behavior, although direct measurement of the latter was not conducted. These findings provide a strong rationale for individualized assessment of academic and cognitive performance across doses when evaluating response to psychotropic medications. In fact, Rapport and Denney (2000) recommend that stimulant dosage be titrated on the basis of improvements in academic efficiency rather than the more typical reliance on changes in behavioral control. This argument is bolstered by the fact that when MPH improves academic performance, behavioral control tends to improve as well; however, the converse is rarely true.

The only long-term adverse side effect of stimulant medication that has been well documented is suppression of height and weight gain. Studies examining this phenomenon have indicated that the probability of growth suppression increases with higher doses, is greater with dextroamphetamine than with MPH, and is higher during the first year of treatment (see American Academy of Child and Adolescent Psychiatry, 2007). Furthermore, preschool-age children may be more prone to growth suppression with annual growth rates 20% below expectations for height and 55.2% less than expected for weight (Swanson et al., 2006). A rebound in growth following discontinuation of treatment or habituation to this effect seems to occur thereafter, with little appreciable alteration in eventual adult height or weight (Greenhill, 1984; Reeve & Garfinkel, 1991).

Another possible long-term adverse side effect that has been examined extensively is whether stimulant treatment increases the risk for adolescent or adult substance use and abuse. Some studies (e.g., Biederman et al., 1997) have indicated that early stimulant treatment may actually reduce the risk for later substance use disorders, while others (e.g., Lambert, 2005) indicate increased likelihood of substance use (for a review, see Golden, 2009). Alternatively, more recent findings suggest that childhood stimulant treatment neither increase nor decrease the risk for substance abuse among adolescents and adults with ADHD (Biederman et al., 2008; Mannuzza et al., 2008; Molina et al., 2013). Perhaps the most prudent conclusion is that the risk for substance use disorders should be assessed among adolescents and adults with ADHD who receive or previously received stimulant treatment. Furthermore, integrated treatments that address symptoms of both ADHD and substance abuse need to be developed to address this complex comorbidity and/ or prevent the development of substance abuse in children with ADHD (Molina et al., 2013; Volkow & Swanson, 2008).

WHEN TO RECOMMEND A MEDICATION TRIAL

School psychologists and other educational professionals are in an ideal position to advocate for the appropriate treatment of a child with ADHD, given their opportunity to observe the student's functioning in a setting where the greatest problems with inattention, impulsivity, and high activity level typically occur (i.e., the school). The decision to initiate a trial of medication should not be an automatic response following the diagnosis of ADHD and obviously must be made in concert with a number of individuals, including the child's physician and parents. Prior to reaching this decision point, comprehensive physical and psychological examinations should be conducted to establish the presence and severity of ADHD symptomatology (see Chapter 2), as well as to identify any factors (e.g., heart condition) that may compromise the use of stimulant medication. Furthermore, in many cases, students should be exposed to foundational classroom strategies (e.g., effective classroom behavior management) and interventions to increase academic, behavioral, and social competencies (e.g., academic interventions, individualized parent education) prior to use of medication (Evans, Owens, Mautone, DuPaul, & Power, 2014). In concert with the child's physician, the psychologist should consider the following factors (DuPaul, Barkley, & Connor, 1998) prior to recommending a trial of medication:

1. *Professional guidelines for treatment of ADHD.* Several prominent professional organizations (e.g., American Academy of Pediatrics, American Academy of Child and Adolescent Psychiatry) provide detailed guidelines for the treatment of children and adolescents with ADHD with particular emphasis on when and what medications should be used. Treatment recommendations typically vary by age. For example, the American Academy of Pediatrics (2011) recommends parent- and/or teacher-administered behavioral therapy as a first-line treatment prior to psychotropic medication for preschool-age children. Alternatively, American Academy of Pediatrics (2011) guidelines indicate medication

as a first-line treatment along with behavioral interventions for school-age children.

2. *Severity of the child's ADHD symptoms and disruptive behavior.* As would be expected, the greater the severity of attention and behavior control difficulties, the more likely a medication trial will be necessary as a supplement to other treatment modalities (e.g., behavioral intervention strategies).

3. *Prior use of other treatments.* If other interventions (e.g., classroom behavioral intervention strategies, parent education) have not been implemented, a trial of medication may be postponed, particularly if the severity of the child's ADHD is relatively mild. If other interventions are currently implemented, one would want to assess their success and whether there is room for improvement (Power et al., 2003). Several questions must be considered including (a) Have symptoms of the disorder improved as a function of the current intervention plan? (b) Is the improvement considered sufficient by key individuals in the child's life? (c) Are any adverse side effects present that would indicate discontinuation or modification of current treatments? (d) What are the effects of the current intervention on key areas of functioning? and (e) What is the likelihood that adding medication to the treatment plan will result in further, clinically significant, improvement? If limited success has been obtained with other interventions, then medication should be considered as an adjunctive treatment.

4. *Empirical support for medication.* The specific medication to be employed should be determined, in part, based on prior empirical studies of this treatment. As has been discussed in this chapter, CNS stimulants have a strong track record of success in treating this disorder. Alternatively, other medications (e.g., atomoxetine, guanfacine, clonidine) may be used when stimulants are ineffective or result in notable adverse side effects (American Academy of Pediatrics, 2011).

5. *Parental attitude toward use of medication.* Parents who are strongly "antimedication" should be offered the opportunity to research the advantages and disadvantages of pharmacotherapy. Specifically, they should be provided with literature that clearly describes the behavioral effects, adverse side effects, and treatment-monitoring practices associated with medication (see Barkley, 2013b). They *should not be coerced* into a medication trial given the higher likelihood of low treatment compliance in such cases.

6. *Adequacy of adult supervision.* The parents must be functioning at a level where they will adequately supervise the administration of the medication and guard against its abuse. Furthermore, all adults

ADHD IN THE SCHOOLS

associated with the child's treatment program (i.e., physician, teacher, psychologist, parents) must make an ongoing investment of time necessary to determine the short- and long-term efficacy of the medication regimen.

7. *Child's attitude toward medication.* It is important that the use of medication is discussed with the child and that the rationale for treatment be fully explained, particularly with older children and adolescents. In cases where children are "antimedication" or oppositional, they may sabotage efforts to use it (e.g., refuse to swallow the pill).

Regardless of whether stimulant medication treatment is employed and successful, the school psychologist is in a singular position to implement additional therapies for the child with ADHD. It is imperative that other interventions (e.g., behavioral and/or academic strategies) are utilized prior to or in addition to medication in an effort to optimize the child's classroom functioning (American Academy of Pediatrics, 2011; Barkley, 2006). In fact, as mentioned previously, the concomitant use of behavioral strategies and stimulant medication may lead to additive behavioral effects, particularly on classroom behavior and academic productivity, thus minimizing the medication dose and/or the intensity of employed contingencies (Fabiano et al., 2007).

HOW TO ASSESS MEDICATION EFFECTS IN CLASSROOM SETTINGS

The methods used to monitor medication response in children with ADHD vary widely in content and quality. The results of the MTA study (MTA Cooperative Group, 1999) strongly indicate that controlled trials using multiple objective measures of drug response are optimal for titrating stimulant dosage. Unfortunately, all too frequently, titration of dosage and long-term assessment of efficacy are based solely on the subjective reports of parents, thereby increasing the chances of erroneous decisions (Connor, 2006b). School professionals can have an impact on this practice to a large degree by communicating with physicians regarding changes in children's school performance associated with pharmacotherapy. In fact, clinical guidelines published by the American Academy of Pediatrics (2011) and the American Academy of Child and Adolescent Psychiatry (2007) emphasize (1) the use of multiple outcome measures, (2) inclusion of school personnel in providing information about drug response, and (3) the need for ongoing monitoring via communication with schools and families. Furthermore, a survey of 700 randomly selected members of the National Association of School Psychologists indicates that approximately 55% of school psychologists engage in medication monitoring for students with ADHD with the sample as a whole agreeing that medication monitoring is an important role for school psychologists (Gureasko-Moore, DuPaul, & Power, 2005).

Because the response to stimulant medication is frequently idiosyncratic and dose specific, it is imperative to collect objective behavioral data across several doses, including a period of time when the child is not receiving active medication. Under ideal circumstances, a child's optimal dose should be established in the context of a double-blind, placebo-controlled assessment paradigm that includes multiple measures collected across several settings (e.g., home, school). This type of evaluation not only involves the aggregation of objective, quantitative data regarding a child's treatment response but also controls for the biases inherent in some assessment measures (e.g., parent and teacher rating scales).

In many instances, professionals do not have the resources and time to conduct elegant, placebo-controlled medication evaluations. Nevertheless, the school psychologist and physician can, as a team, collect objective data in a cost-effective fashion that would aid greatly in making medication-related decisions. Several steps are involved in this process including (1) designing a dosage sequence wherein the child receives one of several doses (including a baseline or nonmedication condition) every day for a week at each dose; (2) collecting objective measures of treatment response across dosage conditions; (3) assessing parent, teacher, and child perceptions of possible adverse side effects across doses (including when the child is not medicated); and (4) communication between the physician and the psychologist both during and after the medication trial to determine whether a child responds positively, which dose optimizes his or her performance, and whether the severity of a possible adverse side effect warrants discontinuing the trial. If possible, those adults who are directly evaluating changes in the child's performance (e.g., teachers) should be kept "blind" to the medication condition. For instance, even during a nonmedication phase the child may continue to go to the nurse's office for his or her noontime administration (and take a vitamin instead of short-acting MPH), thereby keeping the medication condition unknown from the teacher's perspective. With routine use of sustained-release stimulant compounds, it is easier to keep teachers and other school personnel "blind" to medication dosage.

Although the teacher is kept "blind" to the child's medication status, it is important to provide some information to the teacher about the positive effects and adverse side effects usually associated with stimulants. A handout for teachers regarding stimulant treatment of ADHD is provided in Appendix 7.1. This information will help the teacher to focus on those behavioral changes that are most relevant to this treatment.

Measures of Medication Response

Several objective measures should be collected across medication conditions to assess treatment-related change, including teacher and parent ratings of behavioral control and adverse side effects, as well as direct observations of classroom behavior and academic performance. For students with ADHD, predominantly inattentive presentation, ratings and observations of changes in attention span and work productivity will suffice, as these children do not typically exhibit significant problems with behavior control (Carlson & Mann, 2000). The core components of a school-based medication trial are listed in Table 7.2 and discussed below. It is important to note that practicing school psychologists report many of these measures (e.g., teacher and parent rating scales, direct observations of classroom behavior, and review of academic work samples) to be effective, acceptable, and feasible medication monitoring methods (Gureasko-Moore et al., 2005).

Teacher Rating Scales

A plethora of teacher rating scales have been found to be useful in evaluating the effects of stimulant medication, including the Conners 3rd Edition (Conners–3; Conners, 2008) and the ADHD Rating Scale–IV (DuPaul, Power, et al., 1998). The inclusion of one of these questionnaires can provide a measure of treatment-induced reductions in the frequency and/or severity of behavioral control difficulties from the teacher's perspective. These brief rating scales are preferred to more comprehensive, broadband measures (e.g., Child Behavior Checklist [CBCL]; Achenbach & Rescorla, 2001), as the former provide more circumscribed information about medication response and are more practical for teachers to complete on a repeated basis. Measures such as the School Situations Questionnaire (SSQ; Barkley, 1990) and the School Situations Questionnaire—Revised (SSQ-R; DuPaul & Barkley, 1992) can be included to assess changes in the pervasiveness of behavior problems and attentional difficulties across situations. Treatment-induced changes in academic productivity and accuracy can be assessed, in part, by using the Academic Performance Rating Scale (APRS; DuPaul, Rapport, & Perriello, 1991), the Academic Competency Evaluation Scale (DiPerna & Elliott, 2000), or the Impairment Rating Scale (IRS; Fabiano et al., 1999). All of these questionnaires have been found to possess

TABLE 7.2. Measures to Assess Medication Response

1. Teacher rating scales
   a. Conners–3 (Conners, 2000)
   b. ADHD Rating Scale–IV (DuPaul, Power, Anastopoulos, & Reid, 1998)
   c. School Situations Questionnaire (Barkley, 1990) or School Situations Questionnaire–Revised (DuPaul & Barkley, 1992)
   d. Academic Performance Rating Scale (DuPaul, Rapport, & Perriello, 1991)
   e. Academic Competency Evaluation Scale (DiPerna & Elliott, 2000)
   f. Impairment Rating Scale (Fabiano et al., 1999)
   g. Side Effects Rating Scale (Barkley, 1990)

2. Parent rating scales
   a. Conners–3 (Conners, 2008)
   b. ADHD Rating Scale–IV (DuPaul, Power, Anastopoulos, & Reid, 1998)
   c. Home Situations Questionnaire (Barkley, 1990) and/or Home Situations Questionnaire–Revised (DuPaul & Barkley, 1992)
   d. Impairment Rating Scale (Fabiano et al., 1999)
   e. Side Effects Rating Scale (Barkley, 1990)

3. Direct observations of school performance
   a. Classroom Observation Code (Abikoff, Gittelman-Klein, & Klein, 1977)
   b. ADHD Behavior Coding System (Barkley, Fischer, Newby, & Breen, 1988)
   c. Behavior Observation for Students in Schools (Shapiro, 1996, 2011b)
   d. On-Task Behavior Code (Rapport & Denney, 2000)
   e. ADHD School Observation Code (Gadow, Sprafkin, & Nolan, 1996)

4. Academic performance measures
   a. Percentage of assigned work completed correctly
   b. Curriculum-based assessment

5. Self-report rating scale
   a. Conners–3 Self-Report (Conners, 2008)

adequate levels of reliability and validity. However, it is recommended that teacher questionnaires be administered twice during baseline conditions to assess possible "practice" effects that are frequently obtained with these measures (Barkley, 2006).

Parent Rating Scales

There are several parent questionnaires that have been documented to be sensitive to stimulant medication effects with this population such as the Conners–3 (Conners, 2008) and the ADHD Rating Scale–IV (DuPaul, Power, et al., 1998). The Home Situations Questionnaire (HSQ; Barkley, 1990) and/or the Home Situations Questionnaire–Revised (HSQ-R;

DuPaul & Barkley, 1992) could be used to assess the situational pervasiveness of behavior control and attentional difficulties, respectively. As with the teacher questionnaires, all of these instruments have demonstrated reliability and validity for the purpose of assessing intervention effects (Barkley, 2006). Parents can also complete the IRS (Fabiano et al., 1999) to document any perceived changes in academic or social functioning. Given the short-term behavioral effects of stimulant compounds, it is possible that parents will have limited opportunities to directly observe medication-induced changes in ADHD symptoms. Thus, teacher ratings may provide more sensitive treatment outcome data than do parent ratings.

Direct Observations of School Performance

School professionals are in a unique position relative to other mental health professionals because they have the opportunity to observe children in one of their most important natural environments. Thus, questionnaires completed by parents and teachers can be supplemented with behavioral observations that are presumably not subject to the possible biases associated with rating scales. A variety of coding systems have been developed for observing the behavior of students with ADHD (see Chapter 2) including the ADHD Behavior Coding System (Barkley, 1998; Barkley et al., 1988), the Hyperactive Behavior Code (Jacob et al., 1978), the Classroom Observation Code (Abikoff et al., 1977), the Behavior Observation of Students in Schools (BOSS; Shapiro, 1996, 2011b), and the ADHD School Observation Code (ADHD SOC; Gadow et al., 1996). The use of such systems can provide valuable information regarding the frequency (usually in the form of percentages) of occurrence of various behaviors (e.g., on-task behavior, fidgets) over the course of the observation period. One alternative to the above coding systems is the simple recording of off- versus on-task behavior (i.e., visual attention to task materials) that has been found to be quite sensitive to the dose effects of MPH (see Rapport & Denney, 2000). The latter requires very little training and is likely to engender more than adequate levels of interobserver reliability.

Medication effects on children's social interactions should also be investigated. A variety of observational coding systems have been developed for this behavioral domain and have been adapted for evaluating stimulant medication effects (e.g., Pelham & Milich, 1991). For example, direct observations of social behavior using the ADHD SOC could be conducted in relatively unstructured settings such as the school lunchroom and/or playground. A variation of this observation code has been found to be sensitive to the effects of stimulant medication (e.g., Gadow et al., 1990) and allows one to document changes in both aggressive (e.g., physical aggression) and prosocial (e.g., appropriate social interaction) behaviors as a function of treatment.

Academic Performance Measures

Information regarding student's academic performance should be gathered in conjunction with behavioral observations. For example, the percentage of work that the child completes relative to the amount assigned and the percentage accuracy of work could be calculated following the observation session. Such data are highly sensitive to MPH dose effects and can indicate when a medication-induced "cognitive decrement" or "overfocusing" phenomenon has occurred (Rapport & Denney, 2000). Under the latter conditions the child may show behavioral improvements but a diminishment of academic productivity and/or accuracy. Baseline stability and interobserver reliability should also be assessed for these measures. Curriculum-based assessment strategies (Shinn, 1998) are potentially appropriate techniques to assess medication-related changes in this functioning area as well. Several CBM probes per medication condition could be collected to determine treatment effects on the trajectory of skill acquisition (Roberts & Landau, 1995; Stoner et al., 1994). The collection of at least 10 data points per condition allows for more reliable estimation of CBM slope and is highly recommended (Shinn, 1998).

Self-Report Ratings

For older children (e.g., over the age of 9 years old) and adolescents, it may be helpful to obtain self-report ratings of treatment-related changes in behavioral control, academic performance, and self-esteem. Although the reliability of self-report data in this population may be suspect (Barkley, 2006), self-report ratings may serve two purposes. First, these data provide information about areas of functioning (e.g., depressive symptoms, self-esteem) that is not available through other modalities. Second, the student is directly involved in the medication evaluation process, thus increasing the chances of cooperation and compliance with the treatment regimen. For example, the student could complete self-report of ADHD symptoms using the Conners–3 Self-Report (Conners, 2008). Self-report ratings of medication effects on ADHD symptoms appear to be sensitive to MPH effects, albeit less so than are parent and teacher ratings (DuPaul et al., 1996).

Assessment of Possible Adverse Side Effects

Teachers and parents should be asked to complete a brief Side Effects Rating Scale (Barkley & Murphy, 2006) on a weekly basis. Older children (i.e., those over the age of 9 years old) should be asked to complete this questionnaire as well. These ratings provide information regarding the number and relative severity of possible treatment emergent effects (e.g., irritability, insomnia, appetite reduction). Parents can provide the most useful information in this domain because they have the greatest opportunity to observe the activities most likely to be affected (e.g., eating, sleeping). Sometimes, self-report ratings can be particularly critical in revealing adverse side effects that are not observed directly by parents and teachers (DuPaul et al., 1996). As mentioned previously, it is crucial to obtain such ratings during a nonmedication condition as many behaviors that are possible adverse side effects (e.g., irritability) could be occurring in the absence of treatment as well.

Medication Evaluation Procedure

Prior to the initiation of the medication evaluation, comprehensive physical and psychological evaluations are conducted to establish the need for a trial of stimulant medication, as outlined previously. The major steps to a school-based medication evaluation are presented in Table 7.3. Once a medication trial has been agreed upon, the school psychologist should contact the child's physician to discuss and establish the sequence of dosages that can vary as a function of the age of the child. Using MPH as an example, the doses used would vary for preschoolers (2.5, 5, 7.5 mg), elementary schoolchildren (5, 10, 15 mg), and middle and high school students (10, 15, 20 mg). The dosage sequence should be randomized with the stipulation that the highest dose is never administered as the first dose. A nonmedication condition, preferably a placebo, is also included in this sequence. Both the physician and the school psychologist record the dosage sequence and store this information in a safe place until after the medication assessment is completed.

The physician prescribes 1 week's worth of medication at each of the doses, including a placebo, if possible. The parent then has the prescription filled at the pharmacy; if possible, the medication should be packaged in opaque, gelatin capsules. If this packaging is possible, the capsules are dispensed in vials that are labeled by week of the medication trial rather than by dosage to maintain the "blind." The parent and, in the case of short-acting preparations, school nurse dispense the medication according to the schedule determined previously. Although daily changes in dosage are recommended by some researchers in this

TABLE 7.3. Steps to School-Based Medication Evaluation

1. Parent obtains prescription (e.g., Ritalin, 5 mg) from pediatrician.
2. Staff member not involved directly with evaluation (e.g., school nurse) and physician determine order of administration of several doses (i.e., 5, 10, 15, 20 mg), including a nonmedication trial.
3. Parent (or school nurse) administers dose according to predetermined schedule on a daily basis.
4. Assessment measures collected on a weekly (daily) basis:
   a. Teacher ratings
   b. Parent ratings
   c. Side-effects ratings
   d. Observations of classroom behavior by independent observer during individual seatwork.
5. Assessment measures must be taken to reflect the child's behavior during the active phase of the medication (i.e., 2–4 hours postingestion for short-acting preparations; 2–6 hours for extended release compounds).
6. Are there "significant" changes in behavior (especially academic) at any dose?
7. If so, what is the lowest dose that brings about the greatest change with the fewest side effects?
8. Report results to child's pediatrician.

---

area (e.g., MTA Cooperative Group, 1999), it is often more practical to make these changes on a weekly basis. For instance, this would preclude asking teachers to provide behavior ratings on a daily basis.

Parent, teacher, and self-report ratings are completed on a weekly basis throughout the medication evaluation. Dosage changes should occur on Saturdays so that all ratings are completed on the last day of each dosage week (i.e., Fridays). If dosage changes occur on Saturdays, the parent is able to observe for possible adverse side effects and contact the physician in a timely fashion. If observed adverse side effects are severe enough, further administration of this dose would be omitted. It is optimal for the ratings to be completed with the parents, teacher, and child remaining "blind" to the medication dose to minimize measurement error due to rater bias. The best way to accomplish this is for the pharmacist to package the medication in opaque capsules and to use an inert placebo (e.g., lactose powder) during one of the "medication" weeks. If this is not possible, then the teacher and child may be kept "blind" by having the nurse dispense a vitamin tablet during the placebo or nonmedication week. Of course, the use of a sustained-release compound (e.g., Concerta) would preclude the need for "blinding" procedures at school; this is a chief advantage of such preparations. Pill counts should be used, whenever possible, to document compliance with medication administration. If the medication is not being dispensed in a consistent fashion at home, then both doses should be administered at school, if possible.

Regardless of the coding system employed, behavioral observations should be conducted at a time of the school day when the child is engaged in independent seatwork, because this is typically one of the more problematic situations for students with ADHD. Observations of social behavior in the school lunchroom and playground also may be helpful. Furthermore, observations should take place on as many days as possible during each dosage condition approximately 1.5–3 hours after medication ingestion to coincide with the time of peak behavioral effects. Observation periods should be between 15 and 20 minutes each. Also, observations should be conducted several times during baseline conditions to establish a stable "trend" (i.e., consistency in the data) prior to introducing treatment conditions. Interobserver reliability checks (e.g., conducted by a teacher aide or guidance counselor) should be obtained as frequently as possible, ideally at least once per dosage condition, throughout the medication trial to ensure the integrity of the data.

Academic performance data should be collected following each observation period. For example, the amount and accuracy of work completed during the observation session could be calculated before leaving the classroom. In addition, brief curriculum-based assessment probes could be conducted following an observation session. Care should be taken to collect such data from several students in the classroom so that the child with ADHD is not aware that he or she is being singled out for observation.

Although most practicing school psychologists view medication monitoring as acceptable and feasible, limited time and resources may prevent widespread implementation of our proposed medication assessment procedures. Volpe, Heick, and Gureasko-Moore (2005) have proposed a more agile behavioral assessment model that represents a compromise between internal validity and feasibility concerns. Specifically, the Agile Consultative Model of Medication Evaluation (ACMME) involves medication monitoring in the context of a behavioral consultation model (Bergan & Kratochwill, 1990). ACMME begins with an assessment of acceptability and feasibility of various measures and procedures from the perspectives of parent, teacher, physician, school staff, child, and pharmacist. This is an essential first step in helping the school psychologist decide whether a medication evaluation is even possible (i.e., in the case where all participants view assessment as unacceptable or unwieldy) and what measures can reasonably be included. Next, the school psychologist works with teacher(s) and parent(s) to identify target behaviors and arrange for baseline (i.e., nonmedication) data collection. This is similar to the problem identification (Bergan & Kratochwill, 1990) or needs identification (Sheridan & Kratochwill, 2008) stages of the behavioral consultation and conjoint behavioral consultation models, respectively. The third ACMME stage involves problem analysis wherein baseline data are reviewed and goals for behavior change are established. Finally, in the treatment implementation and evaluation stage, target behaviors and possible adverse side effects are assessed in the context of a relevant single-case experimental design. For example, a series of AB designs could be used to compare performance in baseline (A) and low-dosage (B) conditions. Or an alternating treatments design (Kazdin, 2011) could be used to evaluate the effects of multiple doses. Once an optimal dose is identified, maintenance probes are conducted periodically to assess whether medication effects are sustained and/or whether dosage adjustments are necessary. Volpe and colleagues provide a case example to illustrate the implementation of this model. Although the ACMME model has not been examined empirically on a wider scale, given its emphasis on acceptability and feasibility as well as its foundation in well-established behavioral consultation principles, this model has great potential for use in school-based practice.

COMMUNICATION OF RESULTS WITH THE PRESCRIBING PHYSICIAN

Throughout the course of the medication trial, the school professional should be in communication with the prescribing physician, especially when questions arise concerning possible adverse side effects. At the conclusion of the treatment evaluation, it is best if a written summary of the results is forwarded to the physician to facilitate discussion during a follow-up telephone conversation (see Chapter 9 for additional discussion of communication with physicians). Two major questions should be addressed in the report: (1) Are there clinically significant changes in the child's behavior control and academic performance at any active dose of the medication? and (2), If so, what is the lowest dose (i.e., the minimal effective dose; see Fielding, Murphy, Reagan, & Peterson, 1980) that brings about the greatest change with the fewest side effects? These questions are addressed by systematically comparing assessment data collected during active medication conditions to those data obtained during nonmedication conditions. Significant changes are indicated when there is a change of 1 standard deviation from placebo to active dose conditions. Alternatively, reliable change indices (Jacobsen & Truax, 1991;

Speer, 1992) could be calculated for each variable to determine statistical significance. Finally, comparison to a normative sample or to normal peers from the same classroom is helpful in determining the clinical significance of obtained treatment effects.

A sample summary of results for a 9-year-old girl with ADHD, Judy, who participated in a 4-week trial of MPH is presented in Table 7.4. Data are summarized across four dosage conditions (i.e., placebo and 5-, 10-, and 15-mg MPH) that were administered under double-blind conditions in a randomly determined sequence. Significant changes in objective ratings and direct observations of classroom behavior are identified by scores that are underlined (i.e., representing a change of 1 standard deviation from placebo or, in the case of direct observations, 10% change from placebo values). Judy evidenced appreciable improvement in behavioral control across settings during both the 10- and 15-mg conditions, with no apparent increase in possible side effects. Her academic

TABLE 7.4. Sample Summary of Results for a Trial of Methylphenidate

Measure	Placebo	Dose		
		5 mg	10 mg	15 mg
Parent ratings				
Conners–3[a]	7.0[b]	6.0	3.0[c]	2.0
Side effects—total	11.0	9.0	8.0	2.0
Side effects—severity	3.4	3.3	1.1	1.0
Teacher ratings				
Conners–3[d]	14.0	15.0	9.0	4.0
SSQ[e]—problem settings	8.0	8.0	3.0	0.0
SSQ—mean severity	5.1	4.9	1.3	0.0
APRS[f]	49.0	51.0	58.0	67.0
Behavioral observations				
Percent on task	60.3	68.9	80.0	89.7
Academic completion[g]	49.7	59.8	95.0	98.0
Academic accuracy[h]	62.0	61.0	78.0	88.5

[a]Conners–3 Impulsivity Hyperactivity Factor.
[b]Values are raw scores for all variables.
[c]Underlined values represent change of greater than 1 standard deviation relative to placebo.
[d]Conners–3 Hyperactivity Index.
[e]School Situations Questionnaire.
[f]Academic Performance Rating Scale Academic Productivity Score.
[g]Percentage of work completed relative to classmates.
[h]Percentage correct on academic work.

performance was optimally affected at the latter dose, which resulted in a recommendation for her to receive MPH at a 15-mg dose twice per day for the remainder of the school year.

The report to the physician should include a brief table of assessment results, with a one- to two-page report highlighting the changes in each area of functioning at each dose level. A summary paragraph should be used to indicate the dose, if any, that school personnel felt was most helpful in enhancing the child's school performance (see Chapter 9). Obviously, the physician and child's parents determine the ultimate course of treatment. A week or two after sending the report to the physician, a follow-up phone call should be made in case the physician has any questions about the report or if additional school-based information is necessary before a final medication decision can be reached. Finally, a postassessment feedback session should be conducted with the child's parents and teachers to discuss the results of the medication evaluation and to answer questions about further treatment with medication (Gadow, Nolan, Paolicelli, & Sprafkin, 1991).

ONGOING MONITORING OF MEDICATION RESPONSE

Once a student's optimal dosage is established, the measures described previously should be collected periodically throughout the school year to evaluate the need for dosage adjustments or the onset of adverse side effects (see Powell, Thomsen, Frydenberg, & Rasmussen, 2011). The vast majority of the measures need to be readministered only every several months or so. It is usually a good idea for parents to complete the Side Effects Rating Scale on a monthly basis and submit this information to the physician.

Approximately every 6 months that a child is taking medication, the physician usually conducts a brief physical examination. During this time, the child's height, weight, blood pressure, and heart rate are recorded to determine potential side effects. The school psychologist should attempt to collect relevant parent and teacher ratings prior to the 6-month checkup and relay any anecdotal information related to medication response to the physician.

When parents or teachers report that a previously effective dose "doesn't work anymore," the psychologist and the physician should work in tandem to determine possible factors for this apparent deterioration in response before making dosage adjustments. Behavioral changes could be related to medication factors (e.g., a switch from trade name to generic forms of the medication, poor compliance with treatment) or environmental events (e.g., family stress events, increase in difficulty of

academic material). It is important to carefully assess possible nonmedication factors that could account for a decline in functioning. Often,
parents and teachers of children with ADHD may be unrealistic in
their expectations regarding the amount and consistency of behavioral
improvements associated with pharmacotherapy. Thus, they should real-
ize that even when medicated, children may experience occasional "bad
days" regardless of the dosage being employed.

LIMITATIONS OF STIMULANT
MEDICATION TREATMENT

As with most treatment regimens, there are factors associated with
psychotropic medications that limit their overall effectiveness. Some of
these factors have been discussed previously, especially possible short-
and long-term adverse side effects. Furthermore, these medications do
not "teach" children to compensate for symptoms of their disorder and
thus must be supplemented by skill-building strategies such as behavioral interventions (O'Leary, 1980). Of greatest concern are equivocal
data regarding the long-term efficacy of stimulant medication treatment.
Early longitudinal studies did not show significant differences between
groups of children with ADHD who had or had not been treated with
stimulants (e.g., Weiss, Kruger, Danielson, & Elman, 1975). Although
early studies have been rightly criticized for myriad methodological
shortcomings (e.g., insensitive outcome measures), similar findings
regarding lack of long-term differences between medicated and nonmed-
icated students were found with the MTA study (Molina et al., 2009),
which used state-of-the-art research methodology. These results reinforce the fact that no single treatment modality, even one with demonstrated short-term efficacy, is sufficient in bringing about durable reductions in ADHD symptomatology.

Given the relatively brief intervals of behavior control resulting
from a single or twice-daily dose of stimulant medication, much of the
drug's influence has dissipated by the time the child is home from school.
Furthermore, the family will witness the brunt of any adverse side effects
(e.g., insomnia) resulting from pharmacotherapy. As a result, families of
children with ADHD will need more professional help to deal with the
child's behavior problems at home (see Chapter 8). School professionals
should be knowledgeable about the professional resources in the mental
health community so that appropriate referrals on behalf of the family
can be made (Barkley, 2006).

Although objective data are used to determine medication response,
treatment decisions often rely heavily on "clinical judgment" (Gadow

et al., 1991). For example, there may be times where treatment-related changes vary across areas of functioning or sources of data (e.g., parents, teachers). In such situations, the psychologist and the physician must decide which measures are most important to the decision. This can vary as a function of treatment priorities and children's strengths and weaknesses. Specifically, those domains that address children's greatest pretreatment difficulties are given the most weight in reaching decisions regarding dosage (Pelham et al., 1993). In addition, children's response to other interventions and the degree to which additional improvement is necessary to move children into the normal range of functioning is also taken into account (Pelham et al., 1991).

SUMMARY

Various psychotropic medications have been used to enhance the attentional, behavioral, and academic functioning of children with ADHD. CNS stimulant medications are the most effective medication for the symptomatic management of children with ADHD. Among positive treatment responders, stimulant medications significantly enhance the attention span, impulse control, academic performance, and peer relationships of children with ADHD, although effects on the latter two functioning areas must be replicated further. Adverse side effects (e.g., insomnia, appetite reduction) are relatively benign and are more likely to occur at higher dose levels. Given that the behavioral effects of stimulants are moderated by dose and individual responsivity, each child's treatment response must be assessed in an objective manner across a range of therapeutic doses. School professionals can play a major role in evaluating stimulant-induced changes in the classroom performance of children with ADHD and providing objective outcome data to the prescribing physician. Because the overall efficacy of stimulant medication treatment is limited by a number of factors, other interventions (e.g., behavioral strategies and academic support) are likely necessary to optimize the probability of long-term improvements in the behavioral and academic status of children with ADHD.

APPENDIX 7.1. Stimulant Medication Treatment of ADHD:
A Teacher Handout

Children with ADHD exhibit significant problems with inattention, impulsivity, and overactivity. One of the most effective interventions for this disorder is the use of central nervous system (CNS) stimulant medications. The latter include Ritalin, Concerta, Metadate, Quillivant (all four are methylphenidate [MPH]), Dexedrine (dextroamphetamine), Adderall (mixed amphetamine), and Vyvanse (lisdexamfetamine). Of these medications, MPH is by far the most commonly prescribed. CNS stimulants purportedly increase the availability of certain neurotransmitters (i.e., dopamine and norepinephrine) in specific parts of the brain. This results in a greater level of CNS arousal, and hence increased attention and behavior control. It was once believed that these medications exerted a paradoxical (i.e., sedating) effect in children with ADHD and that this response was diagnostic. On the contrary, these medications act to stimulate brain activity not only in youngsters with ADHD but most other children and adults as well. Thus, one cannot diagnose a child as having ADHD based on his or her response to stimulant medication.

BEHAVIORAL EFFECTS

The primary behavioral effects of stimulants include enhanced attention, decreased impulsivity, and reduced task-irrelevant motor activity. Students are more likely to complete assigned tasks accurately, are more compliant with classroom rules, and exhibit fewer aggressive behaviors. They may also show improved handwriting and fine motor skills, as well as greater acceptability by their classmates. In fact, some studies have shown that for a majority of treated children, stimulant medication can lead to changes in attention span and academic productivity such that levels of functioning in these areas are no different from those of their peers. It is important to note, however, that these medications do not "cure" ADHD and that a child with ADHD should be expected to evidence the usual "ups and downs" of behavior control even when a positive response has been obtained. Furthermore, these medications are never to be used as the sole treatment for ADHD. Often, when combined with other interventions (e.g., classroom behavioral strategies), medication effects on behavior control are enhanced.

The behavioral effects of short-acting stimulants usually last between 3 and 4 hours after ingestion. Thus, most children take these medications twice per day (i.e., in the morning before school and at lunchtime). This effectively "covers" the school day, but teachers should be aware of a possible dropoff in effectiveness toward the latter stages of the morning. Longer-acting or extended-release stimulants typically are taken once per day, with behavioral effects lasting up to 8 hours. Some children do not respond as well to these sustained-release medications, however.

Approximately 70–80% of children with ADHD between the ages of 5 and 12 years old who receive stimulant medication evidence a positive response. For adolescents, the percentage of positive responders is somewhat lower (i.e., 60%). Thus, it can be assumed that the majority of students with ADHD who are treated with a stimulant will respond positively. Response to these medications varies as a function of the dose. Some children will respond to lower doses, while others will require higher doses to achieve the same effects. Dose–response to stimulants varies widely across individual children and cannot be predicted on the basis of a child's age or body weight. Specifically, the strength of obtained behavioral effects can range across children and doses from mild (i.e., minimal positive change in behavior) to strong (i.e., "normalization" of behavior control). Thus, most physicians will try a range of doses of a specific stimulant in an effort to determine a child's "optimal" dose.

In those instances when a child with ADHD does not respond to a particular stimulant, this is indicated by no change or, in some cases, a worsening of the core characteristics of ADHD (i.e., inattention, impulsivity, and overactivity). Usually, the physician will try an alternative stimulant when this occurs. For instance, some children who do not respond to Ritalin can be successfully treated with Adderall. If none of the stimulants work, some physicians may prescribe other medications such as Strattera (atomoxetine) or antihypertensives like Intuniv (guanfacine). Thus, when a child's behavior is not affected by the first medication prescribed, there are other alternatives.

ADVERSE SIDE EFFECTS

The primary, acute side effects of stimulant medications are insomnia and appetite reduction. One of the latter side effects is likely to occur in about 50% of children treated with MPH, particularly at higher doses and during the initial stages of treatment. In most cases, however, effects on sleep and appetite are quite mild and do not require discontinuing treatment. Other less common adverse side effects include stomachaches, headaches, and increased anxiety or sad mood. Some children treated with MPH will experience a "behavioral rebound" effect in the late afternoon when the medication is wearing off. The rebound effect is indicated by a worsening of the child's behavior and mood to an extent beyond what was evident prior to taking medication. The latter can be dealt with by reducing the dosage or by adding a late-afternoon administration of the medication. A very small number (i.e., less than 5%) of children treated with stimulants will exhibit motor and/or vocal tics (i.e., repetitive motor movements or vocal noises). Usually, these will disappear after reducing the dosage or discontinuing the medication. In some cases, albeit very few, these tics will continue even when treatment is terminated.

One potential side effect that may be most prominent in school settings is an "overfocusing" effect. The latter refers to instances when a child may be exhibiting exemplary behavior control, but appears to be concentrating too hard on tasks with minimal output. In some children, this overfocused effect may be indicated by appearance (e.g., "glassy" eyes, restricted emotional expressions), while in others this may be signaled by a dropoff in academic performance (e.g., reduced amount of work completed correctly). This reaction is usually a result of the child receiving a dose of medication that is too high.

Teachers and other school professionals should be cognizant of the possible side effects of stimulant medications. When these are noted to occur, the child's parents, physician, and/or the school nurse should be informed. This is especially the case when the child begins to exhibit tics or overfocused behavior. Care should be taken to evaluate possible side effects in comparison with the child's behavior without medication. In other words, sometimes what appears to be a side effect of medication is actually a behavior associated with ADHD that was evident prior to the initiation of treatment. For instance, some children with this disorder are prone to irritable moods regardless of whether they are receiving stimulant medication or not.

ROLE OF SCHOOL PROFESSIONALS IN TREATMENT

It is quite important that teachers and other school professionals are in communication with a child's parents and/or physician whenever stimulant medication is prescribed. This is true for at least two reasons. First, these medications are most active in affecting a child's behavior during the school day. In fact, many parents do not have the opportunity to see medication effects on their children's behaviors. Second, children with ADHD evidence their greatest problems in school settings, and thus the success of treatment is determined, in large part, by changes in a child's school performance.

School professionals can play a role in three stages of treatment. First, teacher input should be sought prior to initiating medication treatment. This is necessary to address whether the child has ADHD and, if so, whether medication treatment is needed. If the child's physician does not actively seek this information, then someone from the school should contact the physician to provide school data. Second, changes in the student's behavior control and academic performance should be among the primary measures used to determine the best dose of medication. Objective information (e.g., rating scales completed by the teacher) about the child's classroom performance is invaluable in making medication-related decisions. Third, once a child's dosage is determined, teachers should communicate any significant changes in student performance that may occur during the school year. Although such changes are not always related to medication, sometimes a dropoff in behavior control may indicate that an adjustment in dosage is necessary. Thus, the school and the physician should be communicating throughout the various stages of medication treatment.

CHAPTER 8

Adjunctive Interventions for ADHD

Children and adolescents with ADHD often display problems with inattention, impulse control, and activity level across home, school, and community environments. Beyond the core behaviors that define ADHD, youth may exhibit difficulties in peer relationships, frequent noncompliance with authority figure commands, and conduct problems such as lying and stealing, as well as poor homework completion and study skills. Unfortunately, no single treatment modality, including psychostimulant medication, is sufficient for ameliorating the myriad problems related to ADHD. The chronic and potentially debilitating nature of difficulties associated with ADHD requires the use of multiple interventions implemented across settings over a long time period. In addition, treatment strategies should focus on multiple target behaviors to maximally impact the child's overall functioning. For many children with this disorder, a "prosthetic" environment must be engineered over the long term both at school and at home (Barkley, 2006). In keeping with this conclusion, the largest treatment outcome study conducted to date with this population (i.e., the MTA study; MTA Cooperative Group, 1999) included multiple components (parent training, school intervention, and summer treatment program) as part of its psychosocial intervention protocol.

Previous chapters have detailed the use of classroom-based behavioral procedures and psychotropic medications in the treatment of ADHD. Certainly, the combination of these therapeutic modalities represents the "optimal" intervention approach for many students with ADHD at the current time. Nevertheless, adjunctive interventions will be necessary in many cases as a function of the severity of ADHD symptoms and the presence of additional behavioral difficulties. In this chapter, several therapeutic strategies that can supplement classroom behavioral programming and pharmacotherapy are delineated. First, school-based training of social skills is discussed. Peer coaching strategies also are described briefly. Next, home-based interventions such as parent education and behavioral family therapy are detailed, especially in relation to their impact on school performance. Strategies to promote success in completing homework assignments also are reviewed. In the final section of the chapter, we discuss treatments for ADHD that have minimal or no demonstrated efficacy, yet often are touted as effective in the popular media. The implementation of these latter interventions can reduce the time and resources available for proven treatments. Thus, it is important to make parents, teachers, and other school personnel aware of the relative support in the research literature for each of the therapies discussed in this book.

SCHOOL-BASED INTERVENTIONS

A variety of classroom-based interventions have been described previously for elementary (Chapter 5) and secondary (Chapter 6) students. Several other treatment strategies can be useful in addressing problems related to ADHD. Social skills training techniques such as modeling, behavioral rehearsal, and reinforced practice have been proposed to ameliorate the social relationship difficulties often exhibited by children with ADHD. Although empirical support for social skills training with this population is somewhat limited, we feel it is important for school practitioners to know what procedures might be most effective based on available research.

Social Skills Training

As discussed in Chapter 1, children and adolescents with ADHD frequently have difficulties getting along with their peers and sustaining close friendships with others. Their problems with inattention and impulse control disrupt the "social performance" of youth with this disorder in several areas. First, individuals with ADHD may enter ongoing peer activities (e.g., board or playground games) in an abrupt, disruptive manner that ultimately may lead to peers becoming dissatisfied with the activity. For example, a child with ADHD is not likely to ask permission before trying to join a game and then may participate in a manner contrary to established rules. Second, students with ADHD frequently do not follow the implicit "rules" of good conversation. Youth with this disorder are likely to interrupt others, to pay minimal attention to what others are saying, and to respond in an irrelevant fashion (i.e., non sequitur) to the queries or statements of peers. Third, children and adolescents with ADHD are more likely than their typically developing counterparts to "solve" interpersonal problems in an aggressive manner. The use of aversive control is not surprising, given the strong association between ADHD and physical aggression. Thus, arguments and fights with peers are common. In a related manner, students with ADHD are prone to losing control of their temper and becoming angry quite easily. Teasing and other forms of provocation that might be ignored or dealt with in an appropriate fashion by most children may be reacted to in a swift and violent manner by many youngsters with this disorder.

Given the variety of social performance problems that children and adolescents with ADHD may display, they are more likely than their typically developing classmates or even aggressive children to be rejected by their peers (Barkley, 2006). Of greater concern is the well-established finding that a child's rejected status often is stable over the course of development (Parker & Asher, 1987). Thus, interventions designed to address these myriad difficulties must be implemented for a sufficient duration to counteract the high risk for problematic outcome. What makes attempts to intervene in this area so difficult, however, is that children and adolescents with ADHD do not appear to have deficits in social *skills* per se. They are able to state the "rules" for appropriate social behavior as well as their peers. What sets them apart from their typical peers is that they often do not act in accord with these rules. This performance deficit is consistent with the assumption that youth with ADHD are impaired in delaying responses to the environment. Thus, in many interpersonal situations, they've behaved before they've had a chance to think about the consequences of their actions.

These deficits in social *performance* are more difficult to ameliorate than skills problems for two primary reasons. First, most currently available social relationship interventions target deficits in skills rather than problems with performance. Furthermore, because social performance problems occur across settings (e.g., classroom, playground, neighborhood), interventions addressing these difficulties must be implemented by a variety of individuals in a cross-situational fashion. Behavioral peer relationship interventions implemented at the point of performance are considered a well-established treatment for ADHD based on available empirical evidence (Evans et al., in press).

In similar fashion, interventions that target social knowledge and the acquisition of prosocial behaviors in group therapy formats (i.e., "traditional" social skills training) have not been found to lead to durable changes in interpersonal functioning for children with ADHD in "real-world" environments. Although impressive gains in conversation skills, problem solving, and anger control have been obtained during training sessions themselves, rarely do these improvements continue once the child leaves the therapy room (Pelham & Fabiano, 2008).

The lack of maintenance and generalization of social skills training effects has led investigators to design more comprehensive approaches to social relationship intervention for children with disruptive behavior disorders. For example, Sheridan (1995) has developed the Tough Kids Social Skills program for use in school settings. This program includes three possible levels of social skills training: small group, classwide, and schoolwide. Although all three training levels may be helpful for students with ADHD, it is likely that children with this disorder will require small-group (i.e., Tier 2) training given their protracted relationship difficulties. Twelve 60-minute group sessions are organized into three units: social entry, maintaining interactions, and problem solving. Training in social entry addresses conversation skills, joining peer activities, and expressing emotions. Two sessions are focused on maintaining interactions, including carrying on a conversation and playing cooperatively. Several problem-solving sessions are conducted to promote dealing with anger, maintaining self-control, and solving arguments. One or more booster sessions are used to promote maintenance of gains in social performance. Sheridan, Dee, Morgan, McCormick, and Walker (1996) have established preliminary empirical support for using the Tough Kids Social Skills program with students with ADHD.

Each Tough Kids session is conducted in a similar fashion. First, "homework" from the previous session is reviewed and discussed by the group. Group rules are also reviewed at the beginning of each session. Next, the specific social behavior targeted by that session is reviewed verbally and modeled by the group leader. Third, students role-play the specific social behavior using scenarios generated by participants and the group leader. It might be helpful to videotape role plays to facilitate review and feedback. The fourth component of the session is to have group members review each role play and provide feedback to participants. Students also can be asked to review their own performance before hearing feedback from other group members. Next, snacks are provided for those students who earned reinforcement by behaving in accord with group rules. Finally, each student is asked to set a goal for the coming week that is related to the specific social behavior covered during that week's session. These goals should be individualized as much as possible. A behavioral contract is then used to identify reinforcers that will be available contingent upon students' reaching their stated goals.

Generalization Programming

Although the skills training package described previously may lead to appreciable gains in socially appropriate behaviors exhibited in the training setting, such changes do not necessarily transfer spontaneously to the real world (e.g., playground, neighborhood, classroom). Thus, a comprehensive peer relationship intervention program must include direct steps to promote maintenance and generalization of acquired social behaviors. Generalization programming can entail within-training strategies as well as structuring the environment to support enactment of prosocial behaviors (Hoff & Robinson, 2002).

Various procedures should be incorporated into the social skills training sessions themselves to increase the probability of generalization to real-world settings. As exemplified in the Tough Kids Social Skills program, these strategies include (1) using real-life vignettes generated by the group participants for role plays, (2) employing multiple exemplars and diverse training opportunities during modeling and role plays, (3) assigning homework that incorporates self-monitoring and self-reinforcement procedures, and (4) having periodic booster sessions to reinforce and extend previous training.

One of the major reasons that appropriate social behaviors do not generalize to real-world environments is that adults (e.g., parents, teachers) and peers do not necessarily prompt and/or reinforce the desired behaviors on a consistent basis. Under typical circumstances of infrequent reinforcement, continued use of newly acquired skills is unlikely to occur. Therefore, changes must be made to the child's natural environment such that the latter supports the ongoing use of appropriate interpersonal behaviors. Components of environmental programming might include (1) instructing parents and teachers to prompt children to enact the behaviors trained in the social skills sessions; (2) developing contingency management programs at home and at school to reinforce trained skills and decrease the probability of verbal and physical aggression (e.g., token reinforcement plus response cost for specific social behaviors); and (3) teaching children to elicit reinforcement from others in the environment, based on their engaging in prosocial behaviors (DuPaul & Eckert, 1994).

Consistent with this approach, Pfiffner and McBurnett (1997) found that parents in social skills intervention for children with ADHD resulted in improvements in children's social interactions that were maintained several months after treatment ended. Furthermore, when parents collaborated with teachers to target children's peer interactions on a DBRC, significant gains over time were found in this area in the school setting. Several studies have shown that when social skills training is supplemented by coached group play in recreational settings, as well as contingent reinforcement of positive social behaviors at school and home, that significant gains are made that can be maintained over time (for a review, see Pelham & Fabiano, 2008). Thus, parents and teachers are integral members of the "social skills intervention team" by serving as agents for generalization.

Strategic Peer Involvement

In addition to parents and teachers, peers should be enlisted to support the generalization of prosocial behaviors across settings. The inclusion of peers is quite important, as they often are present in settings where adult monitoring and attention is remote (e.g., neighborhood games). Moreover, peers are the crucial determinants of whether changes in social behaviors are clinically significant (i.e., enhanced social acceptance and increased friendships). Peers could be involved in all phases of social skills intervention. First, typically developing peers can participate as "role models" in the skills training sessions. Through their participation in role plays and providing feedback, they could serve in a "cotherapist" role. In fact, behavior change is significantly greater in social skills training programs that include a diverse peer group relative to the use of groups of children who all have antisocial behavior difficulties (Ang & Hughes, 2002).

Second, peers could serve as social skills "tutors" in the natural environment by prompting and reinforcing the enactment of social behaviors that have been targeted in the training sessions. Once again, this would require training typically developing peers in the parameters of acting as cotherapists. Cunningham and Cunningham (2006) have developed a student-mediated conflict resolution program that involves peers acting as playground monitors. The use of peer-mediated programs is associated with schoolwide reductions in playground violence and negative interactions. As another example of this approach, Grauvogel-MacAleese and Wallace (2010) examined the impact of peer-implemented differential reinforcement for three children with ADHD. The typically developing peers were trained to ignore target students when the latter engaged in off-task behavior and to praise or provide assistance when target students were appropriately engaged. This peer-mediated intervention led to significant gains in task engagement for the students with ADHD.

Third, typically developing peers can be directly trained to include students with ADHD in their social interactions. Mikami and colleagues (2013) investigated peer inclusion training (Making Socially Accepting Inclusive Classrooms [MOSAIC]) as an adjunct to contingency management in enhancing the social behaviors and peer acceptability for a sample of elementary school-age children with ADHD. Results indicated that both contingency management alone and contingency management plus MOSAIC led to significant improvements in social behavior problems. Contingency management plus MOSAIC was associated with significantly greater enhancement of sociometric preference, reciprocated friendships, and positive messages from classmates relative to the contingency management alone condition. Thus, strategies to increase peer group inclusiveness may provide incremental benefits in social functioning beyond direct targeting of social difficulties using behavioral procedures alone.

Finally, parents can structure home-based friendship training experiences by supervising their child with ADHD in the context of highly structured, noncompetitive activities with a small group of peers. In many cases, this would be preferable to encouraging children with ADHD to participate in community-based activities such as athletic teams or scouting, which may be less closely supervised and inherently more competitive. For example, Mikami, Lerner, Griggs, McGrath, and Calhoun (2010) implemented a Parental Friendship Coaching (PFC) intervention with 32 families of children with ADHD. Parents participated in eight, 90-minute training sessions focused on teaching children how to interact with peers in the context of a playdate. Behavioral interventions such as prompting, frequent feedback, and contingent reinforcement were emphasized along with collaborative problem solving among parents and children prior to and following playdates. Relative to a no-treatment control group, PFC led to significant improvements in children's social skills on playdates and enhancement of peer acceptance as reported by teachers. In addition, parents receiving the PFC facilitated peer interactions through corrective, noncritical feedback as was taught in the treatment program.

Coaching Teens with ADHD

Students with ADHD frequently experience difficulties planning their activities and completing tasks within reasonable amounts of time. For this reason, they may benefit from support strategies that promote goal setting, self-monitoring, and timely task completion. One possible way to accomplish this is through the use of coaching strategies wherein an adult or peer works with the student with ADHD to prompt and reinforce appropriate goal-setting and time management behaviors. Dawson and Guare (1998, 2012) have developed a program for coaching teens with ADHD and/or executive skill deficits. There are two major phases to their coaching program. In the first phase, the adolescent with ADHD works with a coach to (1) identify possible long-term goals, (2) determine criteria that define successful goal attainment, and (3) delineate potential barriers to reaching a goal. For example, a student may wish to obtain a successful grade in a particular subject area. The criterion for success would be the specific grade (e.g., a B or better) and, perhaps, teacher judgment that the student has mastered the material. Possible barriers to success could include a lack of understanding of some of the subject matter, distractions present in the home environment (e.g., smartphone, video games) that could get in the way of studying, and poor note-taking skills.

In the second phase of the coaching program, the student and coach meet on a regular basis to design strategies and review progress toward goals. These sessions include four components (denoted by the acronym REAP): (1) *r*eview, (2) *e*valuate, (3) *a*nticipate, and (4) *p*lan. The coach and student review what the latter has accomplished between sessions and evaluate whether progress is being made toward the long-term goal. Many times, this process is aided by setting interim short-term goals to provide reinforcement for successive approximations toward the long-term goal. Possible hurdles toward further goal attainment are antici-pated and a plan is developed for how the student will negotiate these hurdles while implementing strategies designed to help with goal attain-ment. Sessions are conducted on at least a weekly basis and are relatively brief (30 minutes).

Although Dawson and Guare (1998, 2012) do not present extensive outcome data regarding their coaching model, it is a promising approach to helping adolescents with ADHD. In particular, students who have made significant behavioral improvement through other treatment strat-egies (e.g., stimulant medication and behavior contracting) may be ame-nable to taking the next step toward self-control. A student needs to be motivated and willing to work with an adult or peer in order to profit from the coaching program. Thus, school practitioners should consider the match between the student and the program approach, as well as who might best serve as a coach for the student. In some cases, an adult (e.g., teacher, counselor, or older sibling) might be the best "fit," whereas in other situations a student may work best with a peer or a higher-achieving classmate.

HOME-BASED INTERVENTIONS

Parent Education

It often is important for parents of children with ADHD to receive supportive instruction in behavior management strategies designed to enhance their children's attention to household tasks and rules. In some instances, school psychologists or social workers provide parent edu-cation services in the school setting, especially when these services are not available in the community (e.g., with a clinical child psychologist).

When school-based parent education is provided, there usually is an emphasis on helping parents to supervise the completion of academically relevant tasks such as homework and studying for tests. Several programs for providing parent education in behavior modification strategies have been developed (e.g., Eyberg et al., 2001; Sonuga-Barke, Daley, Thompson, Laver-Bradbury, & Weeks, 2001; Webster-Stratton, 1996) and behavioral parent education is considered a well-established treatment for ADHD based on available empirical evidence (Evans et al., in press).

For example, Barkley (1997b) developed a parent education program to more specifically address the core problems related to ADHD. This education program can be conducted with individual parents or in a group format. Usually the child does not participate in the education program, except in cases where the therapist wants the parent to practice management skills in vivo. Education sessions last 1–1.5 hours for an individual family and 1.5–2 hours for groups of parents.

In the Barkley (1997b) *Defiant Children* program, each education session follows a similar sequence of activities, including a review of the information covered the previous week, a brief assessment of whether any critical events occurred since the previous meeting, and a discussion of homework activities that were assigned at the end of the last session. The therapist then provides instruction with respect to particular management methods that the parents are to practice during the subsequent week. Following didactic instruction, the therapist models the appropriate behavior(s). The parents rehearse the management strategies and receive feedback and further guidance from the therapist. At the end of the session, additional practice of management skills is assigned as homework for the coming week. Written handouts detailing the session's techniques and procedures are distributed for review.

Parent education is usually provided over the course of nine weekly sessions. Session topics include a discussion of why children engage in disruptive behavior, strategies for attending to child behavior, methods to increase compliance and independent play, development of a token reinforcement program, use of response cost and time-out from positive reinforcement, strategies to manage child behavior in public places, use of a home–school communication program, and how to handle future behavior problems. At the conclusion of the initial course of parent education, follow-up meetings are scheduled every several months to provide "booster" sessions in management techniques and to support maintenance of acquired skills.

The Barkley (1997b) parent education program involves primarily didactic (i.e., one-way) communication of information regarding behavior modification procedures. Other parent education programs (e.g., Webster-Stratton, 1996) involve more interaction and participation by parents. For instance, parents view brief videotaped vignettes of parents interacting with children and are then asked to identify both appropriate and inappropriate disciplinary procedures. Parents may also be asked to engage in role plays to practice procedures being taught in sessions. It is believed that participatory parent education may enhance family engagement with and adherence to prescribed strategies. In fact, parent attendance and engagement with treatment can be challenging particularly for parents with their own mental health issues or for families from economically disadvantaged and/or ethnic/linguistic-minority backgrounds (Chronis, Chacko, Fabiano, Wymbs, & Pelham, 2004). For that reason, investigators have explored methods to increase family engagement and make the treatment process as acceptable and feasible as possible. For example, Chacko and colleagues (2008) developed the Strategies to Enhance Positive Parenting (STEPP) program that involves specific components (e.g., preintervention motivational interviewing) to improve family engagement. Relatively high levels of parent attendance and concomitant child behavior improvements have been found for the STEPP program (Chacko, Wymbs, Chimiklis, Wymbs, & Pelham, 2012).

As summarized in comprehensive reviews of the literature (e.g., Pelham & Fabiano, 2008) and meta-analyses (e.g., Fabiano et al., 2009), multiple research investigations have established the efficacy of behavioral parent education for enhancing outcomes for children with ADHD particularly with respect to compliance with household rules and directives, completing assigned responsibilities, and positive parent–child interactions. Thus, parent education is considered an empirically supported intervention in the context of multimodal treatment for ADHD (Pelham & Fabiano, 2008) as is noted in recommended treatment guidelines (American Academy of Pediatrics, 2011). Nevertheless, research remains necessary to establish the durability over time and the generalization across settings of obtained treatment effects with this population.

Behavioral Family Therapy for Adolescents

Teenagers with ADHD often exhibit higher rates of disruptive noncompliant behavior, conduct problems, and conflicts with family members than non-ADHD adolescents (Barkley, 2006; Barkley & Robin, 2014). Interpersonal conflict is particularly prominent in families of adolescents with both ADHD and oppositional defiant disorder because these families are more likely to exhibit aversive behaviors (e.g., insults, complaints) in discussions than are parent–teen dyads in groups of ADHD only or normal control adolescents (Edwards, Barkley, Laneri, Fletcher, & Metevia, 2001). Possible treatment approaches to address parent–adolescent conflict include the most common interventions for ADHD (i.e., stimulant medication and contingency management) and various forms of family therapy (e.g., structural family therapy; Minuchin, 1974).

A behavioral family therapy approach known as "problem solving and communication training" (PSCT; Robin & Foster, 1989) combines elements of contingency management training and structural family therapy. Specifically, PSCT involves skill-building techniques such as instruction in problem solving and appropriate communication behaviors, as well as prescribed changes in family systems and coalitions. In many cases, cognitive therapy procedures are employed to restructure the irrational belief systems of family members (Robin & Foster, 1989).

Two investigations have evaluated the effectiveness of PSCT in treating adolescents with ADHD and oppositional defiant disorder. Barkley and colleagues (1992) found PSCT to be as effective as contingency management training and structural family therapy in reducing the number of conflicts and the intensity of anger during conflict discussions at home. In addition, PSCT significantly improved the quality of parent–adolescent communication according to the independent reports of 21 teenagers with ADHD and their mothers. Improvements also were reported by parents with respect to their adolescent's school adjustment and in the broadband dimensions of both internalizing (e.g., depression) and externalizing (e.g., conduct problems) symptomatology. This treatment was rated positively by all family members on consumer satisfaction questionnaires and obtained improvements were maintained at a 3-month follow-up. Unfortunately, treatment effects were not obtained on direct observations of parent–adolescent conflict, did not result in clinically significant change for most of the sample, and PSCT appeared to worsen the degree of irrational beliefs that some mothers held about their teenagers' conduct problems.

Barkley and colleagues (2001) replicated these findings while also determining whether combining PSCT with contingency management procedures would enhance outcomes. Behavioral effects were equivalent for PSCT alone and in combination with contingency management training, although families were more likely to drop out of the PSCT alone group. Family functioning was normalized in up to 70% of the families across the two treatment conditions. These findings provide at least preliminary support for the use of PSCT for treating adolescents with ADHD and their families. More research is needed to determine which families are most likely to profit from this treatment approach and whether other intervention components (e.g., contingency management) are necessary for a given family.

Homework Interventions

Given the academic and behavior difficulties experienced by students with ADHD, it is not surprising that many of these students have problems completing homework in a timely successful fashion (Power, Werba, Watkins, Angelucci, & Eiraldi, 2006). Specific difficulties include not writing down assignments, not bringing assignments home, not completing assignments in an accurate fashion, arguing with parents about completing homework, and failing to turn in assignments on time (Power et al., 2001). Problems with homework completion are critical because of the connection between homework and academic achievement (Cooper, Robinson, & Patall, 2006). Thus, over the years, intervention programs have been developed to address homework difficulties (e.g., Olympia, Jenson, & Hepworth-Neville, 1996).

Power and colleagues (2001) have developed and pilot tested a very promising homework intervention program specifically for students with ADHD. Their Homework Success program involves seven 90-minute sessions conducted with parent groups. As such, this program could be incorporated into an ongoing parent education program (as described previously) or could be a stand-alone program. There is a strong collaborative component to this program, in which teachers and children are also included at appropriate points in treatment. For example, a parent–teacher conference is facilitated at the outset of the program to identify specific homework problems and emphasize the importance of home–school collaboration.

The core component of this program is the use of goal-setting and contingency management procedures to encourage more consistent homework performance. Topics of the Homework Success sessions include introducing the program, establishing a homework ritual, providing positive reinforcement, managing time and goal setting, using aversive procedures appropriately, anticipating future homework problems, and providing follow-up support. This is a skills-based program wherein parents are instructed in new strategies during each session. Parents are expected to complete their own homework between sessions and their success in implementing strategies is reviewed at the beginning of each session. Power and colleagues (2001) emphasize the use of data to track changes in homework performance over time and they provide several measures to facilitate feasible data collection. Although extensive controlled research has yet to be conducted with this program, controlled case study data indicate that Homework Success leads to improvements in homework completion and accuracy (e.g., Resnick & Reitman, 2011).

Multisetting Interventions

Because ADHD symptoms impact children's functioning across settings, most prominently home and school, efforts have been made to design, implement, and evaluate treatment strategies that involve collaboration between parents and teachers. For example, the Collaborative Life Skills program (CLS; Pfiffner, Villodas, Kaiser, Rooney, & McBurnett, 2013) incorporates multiple behavioral interventions that are used in school and home for elementary school-age children with ADHD. CLS is composed of three components (classroom behavioral intervention, group-based behavioral parent training, and child skills group) delivered simultaneously over 12 weeks by school-based mental health professionals. The classroom component includes a school–home daily report card, homework plan, and individualized accommodations (e.g., preferential seating). Group-based behavioral parent training includes 10 1-hour sessions teaching behavior management skills (e.g., contingent reinforcement) as described previously for parent education. Children also participate in ten 40-minute group sessions during the school day to learn social skills (e.g., good sportsmanship) and independence (e.g., establishing and following routines) through didactic instruction, behavior rehearsal, and practice role plays. Pfiffner and colleagues (2013) found CLS to be associated with statistically significant, moderate to large improvements in ADHD symptoms, homework problems, task engagement, achievement test scores, and report card grades. Academic improvements were partially mediated by CLS improvements in student organization skills. Although the effects of CLS need to be evaluated relative to a control condition, initial findings are quite promising in relation to improvement in a critical area of functioning for students with ADHD (i.e., educational performance).

In similar fashion, Family–School Success (FSS) was designed to improve family and educational functioning for elementary school students with ADHD (Power et al., 2012). FSS is composed of 12 sessions with six simultaneous, separate parent and child group sessions, four individualized family therapy sessions, and two family–school consultation sessions including parents and teachers. In these sessions, clinicians guide participants through standard behavioral parent education procedures (as described previously), daily report cards, homework interventions, and conjoint behavior consultation. The FSS is manualized and implementation is associated with high levels of integrity. When compared with a comparison condition providing education and support to parents, FSS was found to have statistically significant, small to moderate effects on the quality of the family–school relationship, homework performance, and parenting behavior (e.g., reduction in negative/ineffective discipline) with effects on the latter maintained at 3-month follow-up (Power et al., 2012). Given these promising results, school professionals should consider partnering with community-based clinicians to implement multisetting interventions like CLS and FSS to address the multiple, cross-situational needs often exhibited by students with ADHD.

Parent Support Groups

It usually is quite helpful for parents of children with ADHD to interact with other parents of similar children to share their frustrations, successes, and advocacy strategies. Several national parent organizations have been founded to play a supportive role, to serve as a clearinghouse for information relative to ADHD, and to lobby political groups to supply greater services for this population. One of the most prominent national parent organizations is the Children and Adults with Attention-Deficit/ Hyperactivity Disorder (CHADD; *www.chadd.org*) organization based in Landover, Maryland. CHADD was founded in 1987 and has local chapters in virtually every state. In addition to publishing a quarterly magazine, this organization sponsors an annual conference on ADHD that draws a national audience. CHADD members include not only parents but teachers and health care professionals working with children with ADHD. Organizations such as CHADD serve an important role in the overall treatment of ADHD as they provide valuable information about the disorder as well as guidance for its members in advocating for proper educational and therapeutic intervention for their children.

INTERVENTIONS WITH LIMITED OR NO EFFICACY

Many treatments for ADHD have been proposed and promoted over the years that have been found, via controlled research, either to have minimal efficacy in ameliorating attention deficits or have not been subjected to controlled empirical investigation. Examples include relaxation training, play therapy, megavitamins, amino acid supplementation, herbal medicines, and ocular motor exercises. Despite a lack of demonstrated efficacy, many of these interventions (e.g., dietary management) are quite popular and are commonly employed. Although some alternative or complementary treatments have gained empirical support in recent years (for a review, see Arnold, Hurt, Mayes, & Lofthouse, 2011), continued support for these treatments is typically derived from theory, "expert opinion," and/or face validity (i.e., the approaches appear to make great intuitive sense and consequently have tremendous consumer appeal). Although ineffective treatments are rarely physically harmful, their use diverts valuable time, energy, and resources from the implementation of more effective therapies. Thus, it is important for school practitioners to be aware of ineffective treatment modalities and to discourage their use whenever necessary. Of course, this should be done in a sensitive manner, while offering alternative, better-supported, interventions.

Factors to Consider before Recommending a Treatment

Due to the plethora of proposed treatments for ADHD, it is not possible to discuss the relative merits of every one of these techniques. Nevertheless, it is important to enumerate several guidelines that can be employed when considering the use of a new or alternative therapy for ADHD because the use of the latter may detract from treatment efforts in more effective directions (Ingersoll & Goldstein, 1993).

1. If the developer or a proponent of a particular therapy states that the treatment "cures" ADHD or that it can be used alone to treat this disorder, then an automatic red flag should be raised. Even empirically documented, effective treatments for ADHD (e.g., stimulant medication) do not lead to irreversible improvements in children's functioning and must be supplemented by a variety of treatments implemented across settings. Thus, claims for "cures" must be met with a high degree of caution.

2. Treatments that are touted as effective and potentially curative for a variety of disorders (e.g., ADHD, learning disabilities, autism, depression) should be met with caution. It is highly unlikely that one specific therapy would lead to clinically significant results in treating children with a variety of disorders. Such claims should lead to an automatic red flag and further information regarding the empirical underpinnings of the therapy should be obtained.

3. It is incumbent upon the developer or proponent of a novel treatment to demonstrate its therapeutic efficacy in the context of a controlled, experimental design using reliable and valid dependent measures. It is not sufficient to offer case study data or testimonials from

satisfied clients. Furthermore, data should be available that allow direct comparison of the effects of novel therapies relative to those associated with established effective interventions. Thus, one of the first questions to ask proponents of a new treatment for ADHD is "Where are the data?"

4. In some circumstances (e.g., when response to established interventions is minimal), treatments that are safe, easy, cheap, and sensible may be considered even with limited empirical evidence as opposed to treatments that are risky, unrealistic, difficult, or expensive. The latter should definitely be avoided without compelling, supportive evidence (Arnold et al., 2011).

5. Several questions can be asked to assess the quality of experimental research investigating a novel treatment. Were the participants classified as ADHD using reliable and valid indices of the disorder? Were the dependent measures collected in such a fashion as to reduce possible biases (e.g., behavioral observations conducted by individuals who were unaware of the clinical population being studied and the treatment being investigated)? Are threats to the internal validity (e.g., maturation) of the treatment controlled for? How generalizable are the obtained results to other children with ADHD? Was the clinical significance (e.g., normalization) of the obtained findings assessed? Did the investigators examine the generalization of treatment effects across settings (e.g., home and school) and over time (e.g., follow-up assessment)?

6. Whenever school professionals encounter novel treatments that are not substantiated by empirical evidence, it is important to communicate their skepticism to parents and educators of children with ADHD. Parents of these children may be particularly prone to adopting new therapeutic approaches given their frustrations in dealing with ADHD-related difficulties and their knowledge of the limitations of currently available treatments. Furthermore, in our experience, these parents often lack a clear understanding of the necessity and requirements of the scientific study of treatments.

SUMMARY

The chronic exhibition of ADHD-related behaviors across settings and caretakers necessitates the implementation of a multimodal treatment program over several years or longer. Several adjunctive intervention approaches can supplement the use of classroom behavior support strategies and psychotropic medications. Additional school-based treatments may include social skills training and peer coaching. Home-based treatments include parent education in behavior modification techniques, behavioral family therapy for adolescents with ADHD, homework interventions, and parental participation in support organizations (e.g., CHADD). Multi-setting interventions like CLS and FSS should be strongly considered as part of a muiltmodal treatment program. Over the years, many therapies for ADHD (e.g., Feingold diet) have been proposed that either have not been subjected to empirical investigation or have been found ineffective in the treatment of this disorder. Given the popularity of some of the latter therapies, it is important that school-based professionals are cognizant of both empirically sound and less efficacious interventions in order to more effectively advocate for the appropriate treatment of students with ADHD.

CHAPTER 9

Communication with Parents, Professionals, and Students

Clear and accurate communication is a foundation of all professional service delivery in education, psychology, medicine, and related professions, and is a cornerstone of high-quality service delivery in support of students with ADHD, their parents, and their teachers. There are several reasons as to why clear and accurate communication is so critical. The first is that assessment of ADHD and related problems is a process involving multiple informants and multiple methods across multiple settings. This process involves the communication of information, observations, opinions, and professional judgments among parents, teachers and other school-based professionals, students, psychologists, and physicians—with great potential for differences in perspective and experiences with the child in question. Similarly, the design, implementation, and evaluation of interventions for children and adolescents with ADHD involve comparable processes and communications. Additionally, the variability in behavior across time, settings, and students with ADHD requires careful ongoing monitoring and adjustments to support systems, thus creating the need for ongoing collaborative discussions. As a result, clear and ongoing communication with parents, teachers, and other professionals involved with identified children is warranted, and will necessarily involve discussions of issues critical to assessment, diagnosis, instructional planning, intervention management, and professional service delivery in general.

For example, concerns regarding a child's problem behavior(s) typically are raised first by school professionals and/or parents. Furthermore, it is often the case that medical professionals (e.g., pediatricians, psychiatrists) are involved with students who are diagnosed with ADHD. Together, these persons will make screening, referral, classification, and intervention selection and outcome decisions. Productive interactions among these persons rely on clear and specific communications despite differing vocabularies, perspectives, and backgrounds.

Consider also that the diagnosis of ADHD is based on a psychiatric classification system (DSM-5; American Psychiatric Association, 2013), yet the identified children and their parents interact most frequently with school-based education professionals, while also being served in many cases by community-based physicians and mental health professionals. Education professionals typically are less familiar with DSM criteria than they are with the special education classification system contained in the IDEIA 2004 (Public Law 108-446). Equivalent understanding of these two classification systems across involved individuals cannot be assumed, thereby necessitating explanatory communications (and, in some cases, professional training) regarding the systems and their foundations (e.g., research, policy), terminology, implications for treatment planning, and related issues.

Clearly, effective design, implementation, and evaluation of medical, behavioral, and educational interventions for children with ADHD rely a great deal on effective communication, given the inherent differences of beliefs, opinions, and knowledge of the professional literature across the persons involved. Of particular concern here is that the development of interventions often is a clinic-based or office-based activity, while an intervention's implementation, positive behavioral effects, and any undesirable effects are experienced in home, classroom, and community settings. Thus, the evaluation of interventions and their effects requires communication among physicians, parents, teachers, students, and other professionals.

Last but not least, the ethical principles and standards for practice of the National Association of School Psychologists[1] (2010b) indicate that professional communication with parents, students, and other professionals is an expected component of appropriate school psychology practice. These guidelines for professional conduct specify that the purpose(s) and possible consequences of the professional's involvement, as well as intervention options and alternatives, be discussed with parents and students in a manner that is understandable to them. Guidelines also are provided regarding the development of relationships between professionals (e.g., school psychologists and pediatricians) when such relationships are in the best interest of the students being served. In the latter sections of this chapter pertinent examples of these guidelines are provided as introductory statements for those sections.

---

[1]The American Psychological Association, the Council for Exceptional Children, and other professional organizations have similar ethical guidelines.

The purpose of this chapter is to identify and discuss several important issues related to ADHD for communication among and between school professionals and others involved with identified students, including parents, other professionals, and the students themselves. Although each topic in this volume is worthy of discussion and consideration, primary attention here is given to (1) the relationship between a diagnosis of ADHD and educational services; (2) the responsibilities of education professionals; (3) issues surrounding stimulant medication treatment; and finally, (4) issues specific to communication with parents, physicians and other professionals, and students. Perhaps we are stating the obvious; however, we believe that by discussing and attempting to clarify these issues, professional and parental decision making and actions can be facilitated, resulting in improved outcomes for children.

DSM DIAGNOSES AND EDUCATIONAL SERVICES

When ADHD is a concern, professionals and parents will need to discuss a range of answers to the question "How does a DSM diagnosis or other classification relate to educational service delivery?" The usefulness of diagnostic classification systems of childhood problems has been debated for decades (Cipani & Schock, 2011; Garmezy, 1978; Mayes, Bagwell, & Erkulwater, 2008; Schact & Nathan, 1977; Szasz, 1960), yielding a wide range of professional opinions. In fact, DSM-5 (American Psychiatric Association, 2013) states that a diagnosis is merely a starting place for planning services, and that more information about the individual and contextual issues and variables of concern will be need to effectively provide professional supports.

From an *educational* decision-making standpoint, it must be recognized that the DSM system of classification is tied to assessment tools and procedures that are *nomothetic* in their foundations and assumptions. In psychology and education, reliable and valid nomothetic assessment yields information useful for comparing children with one another along the measured dimension or construct (e.g., intelligence). For example, a child who earns a score at the 37th percentile on an intelligence test has performed less well than a peer who earns a score at the 78th percentile. Developing an instructional intervention or planning an educational program for either child based solely on this information is not defensible. However, information based on nomothetic assessment procedures can be used in a reliable and valid manner for making screening, referral, and classification decisions.

By comparison, intervention planning and effectiveness decisions are more readily linked to other types of assessment tools and procedures that are *idiographic* in their foundations and assumptions. Idiographic assessment does not focus on the relative classification of individuals vis-à-vis their behavioral presentations (e.g., Anna meets criteria for ADHD, while James does not), but rather is concerned with relative comparisons of the behavior of an individual over time (e.g., Sam's reading achievement in March is much improved relative to his reading achievement in November) as a result of intervention, development, change in programs, and the like.

When the idiographic assessment measure possesses the technical characteristics of accuracy and utility, it can yield information useful for the development of effective instructional and intervention programs. For example, accurate assessment information regarding a child's ongoing and differential performance in two different reading curricula could be directly relevant to instructional planning decisions (for a thorough comparison of nomothetic and idiographic approaches to assessment, see Cone, 1986; Haynes, Mumma, & Pinson, 2009; Merrell, Ervin, & Gimpel Peacock, 2012). Based on the child's reading performance, a decision to provide instruction within the curriculum yielding higher rates of success would seem warranted. Intervention outcome evaluations, that is, comparing a child's behavior or performance over time, also need to be grounded in idiographic assessment information, although supplemental information regarding peer comparisons might also be useful.

A primary limiting factor preventing direct linkages between diagnosis and intervention is the large degree of variability in the behavior of children diagnosed with ADHD (Barkley, 2006). That is, all children diagnosed with ADHD do not display the same problem behaviors, nor do they experience the same difficulties, if any, in school. In assessment terms, Haynes (1986) has referred to the variability among persons classified in the same manner as an issue of "diagnostic homogeneity." Specifically, Haynes noted that "if individuals placed in a particular classification category . . . are homogeneous on dimensions of topography, etiology, and response to treatment, categorization is sufficient for description and intervention design, and the benefits of additional pre-intervention assessment are reduced" (p. 391). Given the variability in behavioral topography and response to treatment of children with ADHD (Barkley, 2006), intervention design, implementation, and evaluation will require even more professional effort than that required for diagnosis or classification. In part, the focus of this effort must depend on professional training and responsibilities.

These issues should be discussed openly at various stages of the assessment process. When a child is exhibiting significant attention and/or behavior control problems, the first step is to collect screening information (see Chapter 2). Sometimes, at this stage, the child's parent or teacher specifically questions the presence of ADHD, as though this is all that needs to be determined. This situation provides an opportunity to put the diagnostic process into perspective. Specifically, it should be communicated clearly that evaluation data are being collected not simply to derive a diagnosis, but also to gather information that will lead to effective intervention. Similarly, when the multimethod assessment of ADHD is concluded, it is helpful to reiterate that a diagnosis is actually a "way station" between the referral and the design of an intervention program. Furthermore, it should be stated that the informational value of the diagnosis lies in its usefulness in directing further assessment activities, suggesting risks for associated behavior or learning difficulties, and increasing the probability of choosing effective treatment strategies. Finally, it must be stressed with school team members that ongoing assessment of the child's functioning will be necessary to evaluate the relative efficacy of intervention procedures. When these points are communicated effectively, the focus of the evaluation team can be *balanced* across efforts at multimethod assessment, diagnostic decision making, and the development of a potentially successful treatment protocol. This balance is important, as we see it, as all too often the bulk of professional efforts are aimed at diagnosis, with comparatively small amounts of intervention effort.

Discussions of these issues can help to identify and clarify the expectations held by parents, teachers, and others regarding the utilization and benefits of various assessment procedures. An excellent tool that can prompt and facilitate these types of discussions, as well as discussions of treatment approaches for ADHD, is the Attention Deficit/Hyperactivity Disorder Knowledge and Opinion Survey (AKOS), published by Power and colleagues (2001). The AKOS consists of 43 items answered in either a true/false or Likert-type fashion to determine degree of parent/teacher expectations, knowledge, and opinions about various assessment and intervention strategies pertinent to ADHD. Identifying and clarifying these expectations should result in improved understanding of the need for linkages among assessment, intervention, and education in serving students with ADHD.

EDUCATIONAL TRAINING AND RESPONSIBILITIES

The primary professional responsibilities of education professionals involve the development and delivery of curricula and instruction. As such, educators make decisions and take actions regarding *what* to teach (i.e., selecting curricula and instructional objectives), *how* to teach (i.e., identifying which materials, procedures, and methods to use), *when* to teach (i.e., instructional design and organization), *who* will teach which aspects of a curriculum, and *where* to teach (instructional environment). Decisions surrounding these issues are important for *all students*, including those identified with ADHD, and arguably define the domain of education. Therefore, these issues should be paramount in the decision making of educators responsible for students with ADHD vis-à-vis the child's learning and achievement. In addition, because the diagnosis and treatment of ADHD nearly always involves pediatricians, psychiatrists, clinical psychologists, and other support professionals, collaborative efforts at assessment and treatment will need to be developed and maintained.

The wide range of issues and concerns requiring professional involvement where children diagnosed with ADHD are concerned, clearly warrants interdisciplinary collaboration. Also warranted are frank discussions about appropriate roles and responsibilities for the professionals involved. School psychologists and special educators, in particular, may be faced with challenging demands for service delivery in light of the eligibility for special education services of children identified with ADHD under the "Other Health Impaired" category of the IDEIA 2004 (Public Law 108-446; see Robb et al., 2011; Schnoes, Reid, Wagner, & Marder, 2006). For example, these professionals and their colleagues are likely to need professional development activities to help them obtain knowledge and skills in the DSM psychiatric classification system, developmental psychopathology, psychopharmacology, and the methods and models of clinical psychology and psychiatry.

Additionally, professionals need to be prepared to discuss with parents and others available educational service delivery models and options for students with ADHD. For example, questions will be raised regarding (1) whether a child is eligible for special education services, (2) whether a child should have a "504 accommodation plan," and (3) In what manner is the school system providing appropriate support for this student with ADHD?

Many children with ADHD may be eligible for special education services within their public school systems under the provisions of IDEIA 2004 (Public Law 108-446; see Jacob, Decker, & Hartshorne, 2011, for a review of this legislation). However, children with ADHD do not automatically qualify for services under IDEA by virtue of their ADHD diagnosis. The IDEIA 2004 legislation and its predecessors intend that U.S. students with disabilities should receive a free and appropriate public education, in the least restrictive environment, and have the benefit of an individualized education program. Eligibility for special education services under IDEIA 2004 is contingent on meeting each of two criteria. The first is having a disability as defined in the IDEIA 2004 legislation.

Children with ADHD are most likely to meet this criterion within the categories of "specific learning disability," "other health impaired," and in some cases "emotional disturbance." The second criterion is that a child with an identified disability must have a *demonstrated need for special education services*. This latter criterion often is met through a documented lack of student responsiveness to interventions/supports implemented through general education programs and staff. In many instances parents, and in some instances professionals, are unaware of the second of these criteria, and therefore could benefit from a discussion of the eligibility requirements.

Another legal consideration relative to students with ADHD in the schools is Section 504 of the Rehabilitation Act of 1973 (see Zirkel & Aleman, 2000, for a review of this legislation and its implications for educational practice). In general, this legislation prohibits discrimination on the basis of disability by recipients of federal funds, such as school systems. Section 504 stipulates that students with a mental or physical disability that impairs a major life activity (e.g., education) to a substantial degree are entitled to supports/adjustments to accommodate their participation in either general or special education programs. Efforts will need to be made to help parents and professionals become knowledgeable of the distinctions between IDEIA and Section 504 eligibility and supports.

One further consideration in this arena is that the fields of school psychology, special education, and general education recently have been adopting intervention- and outcomes-oriented models of service delivery and special education eligibility, such as RTI models (Brown-Chidsey & Steege, 2010; Burns & Gibbons, 2008). To date, however, how such models might apply to children with ADHD has received limited professional consideration (see DuPaul, Stoner, & O'Reilly, 2008).

Intervention-oriented service delivery is intended, in part, to prevent an overemphasis on the diagnosis and classification of children, which may preclude school psychologists from taking more active roles and responsibilities in developing and implementing effective interventions. To further illustrate this point, suppose that school professionals are involved with a child who is accurately diagnosed with ADHD. Does this disability necessarily represent a handicapping condition and therefore warrant special services? It has been argued that a recognizable disability, such as ADHD, only becomes a handicap in a nonaccommodating environment (Deno, 2002; Reschly, 2008). That is, if a school is providing instructional and social support such that a student with a recognized disability is not considered to be handicapped (i.e., his or her performance meets or exceeds expectations, and is commensurate with same-age, typical peers), that school should be recognized as providing exemplary services. Of course, given evidence that a student is not meeting the expectations of his or her current environment, reasonable accommodations should be made in attempts to support the student (and teacher) toward meeting those expectations (e.g., matching instructional materials with current academic skills, providing more frequent positive and corrective feedback, enhancing motivation to engage in academic work, increasing opportunities to practice newly acquired skills and knowledge) and achieving academic success. The emphasis here is on encouraging schools to allocate limited resources primarily to procedures that monitor and foster the individual social and academic progress of all students (Reschly, 2008).

These service delivery issues will need to be discussed among all interested parties so that the expectations and responsibilities of each team member may be clarified, and so that parents understand what to expect from the school system personnel with whom they are working. Clarification of team member expectations and responsibilities must be established at a minimum of three points in the evaluation and treatment process. Prior to conducting a multimethod evaluation of ADHD (i.e., Stage II of the assessment process; see Chapter 2), the specific responsibilities of each school-based professional should be delineated clearly. Furthermore, the theoretical and professional "biases" of each team member should be elicited openly and discussed. For example, in some instances teachers and parents may question even the existence of ADHD itself, and a discussion of the International Consensus Statement on ADHD (Barkley, 2002) may be warranted. Although discussion of this type will not necessarily lead to a complete resolution of potential conflicts and disagreements, it will increase the awareness of similarities and differences among the positions of all team members. This is, at least, the first step in promoting greater collaboration in team-based service delivery.

The second point where service delivery issues will need to be discussed is when the intervention plan is designed (Stage IV of the assessment process; see Chapter 2). At this point, decisions must be made not only as to which interventions and supports to recommend but also with respect to who will implement each intervention. There may be initial confusion among some team members as to what ADHD is and the most effective treatments for this disorder. In particular, questions surrounding the use of stimulant medication may arise. It may be helpful to provide written information and/or suggested readings (see Appendix 9.1) about ADHD and its treatment to all interested parties. The appointment of a case manager can facilitate treatment planning as well as enhance the maintenance of consistent service delivery. Given that some treatments for ADHD (e.g., stimulant medication) are provided by community-based professionals, the need for the school to "speak with one voice" is particularly crucial. Potential disagreements among team members should be elicited actively and resolved prior to implementing treatment procedures. It has been our experience that although the latter may delay service delivery, it often prevents more serious and time-consuming conflicts once treatment has begun.

Service delivery expectations and responsibilities should be discussed periodically in the context of ongoing evaluation of the treatment strategies. Several meetings per year should be held for the school-based team, including the parent(s), to discuss the efficacy of each specific intervention and the need for adjustments in programming. This provides the opportunity to make changes in specific responsibilities among team members, if necessary. It is particularly important for those team members (i.e., teachers and parents) who are performing the bulk of the direct intervention to receive reinforcement and support for their efforts. Furthermore, if possible, responsibilities should be rotated among team members to enhance collegiality and prevent the potential "burnout" of a specific individual.

ISSUES SURROUNDING STIMULANT MEDICATION TREATMENT

The most frequent intervention for ADHD is stimulant medication, and this treatment approach therefore influences the lives of a significant number of school-age children. Stimulant medication treatment can be confusing for parents and professionals alike because of the array of forms it takes, dosages, and potential effects and side effects. For example, according to the National Institute of Mental Health (2013):

> Stimulant medications come in different forms, such as a pill, capsule, liquid, or skin patch. Some medications also come in short-acting, long-acting, or extended release varieties. In each of these varieties, the active ingredient is the same, but it is released differently in the body. Long-acting or extended release forms often allow a child to take the medication just once a day before school, so they don't have to make a daily trip to the school nurse for another dose. Parents and doctors should decide together which medication is best for the child and whether the child needs medication only for school hours or for evenings and weekends, too.

And, stimulant medication treatment needs to be undertaken with caution because beneficial effects do not occur for all treated children. Moreover, for those who do benefit, medication response will be dose and behavior specific. Finally, some children will experience adverse effects related to stimulant treatment.

The use of stimulant medication treatment for problems of children's inattention, overactivity, and impulsivity has not been without controversy. Concerns that have arisen around stimulant medication treatment primarily involve discrepancies between defensible professional practices and the personal beliefs of involved parents, educators, and other professionals regarding several key issues including (1) the potential benefits of treatment; (2) the potential harmful effects of treatment; and finally, (3) the values of parents, educators, and other professionals involved in intervention decision making. Communication and discussions of each of these issues will be critical where stimulants and other psychotropic medications are being considered in the treatment of a child with ADHD.

Potential Benefits of Stimulant Medication Treatment

Numerous research investigations conducted since the 1960s have documented positive, short-term benefits of stimulants for *most* children diagnosed with hyperactivity and/or attention problems. These outcomes have been demonstrated in the areas of (1) academic performance; (2) social interactions; and (3) on individually administered, performance assessment tasks. However, it also has been demonstrated that response to stimulants varies from child to child (even those of the same body weight) and across target behaviors for any given child (Rapport & Denney, 2000). As such, the determination of stimulant treatment outcomes for individual children must be made cautiously, and will require the generation and analysis of individual outcome data.

Potential Adverse Effects of Stimulant Medication Treatment

Of concern to parents and professionals considering stimulant treatment for children are potential adverse effects of medication. Children treated with stimulants may experience adverse physical side effects such as appetite suppression, nausea, headaches, irritability, insomnia, growth suppression, and, in rare instances, motor or vocal tics. Furthermore, in a minority of cases, stimulant treatment may result in an "overfocused" child who appears to be overly attentive to specific stimuli and is slow to orient to alternative activities or tasks. Although problems such as these typically have been reported at relatively high doses of medication, the potential for their occurrence is present at low doses as well.

These possibilities and monitoring systems aimed at detecting potential adverse outcomes need to be discussed among professionals and parents.

Values Conflicts or Assumptions on Which Treatment Is Based

From a personal values standpoint, some parents and professionals are resolute in their opposition to using stimulant treatment with children. These values take various forms and are difficult to attribute to any single source or concern. Rather, support for a values position against the use of medication can be found in a variety of professional and popular publications. For example, one researcher (O'Leary, 1980) has argued that identified children need to learn social and self-management skills rather than to be chemically quieted. Similarly, a popular book published in the 1970s (Schrag & Divoky, 1975) asserted that stimulant medication, along with widespread testing, labeling, and "behavior modification" with all children, were all methods of inappropriate institutional control of human rights. More recently, legal suits against prescribing physicians and the picketing of professional conferences have been supported by an organization within the Church of Scientology, the Citizens Commission on Human Rights. This group alleges that the use of stimulants and other psychotropic medications for childhood problems are turning schoolchildren into drug addicts. Nonetheless, these criticisms of stimulant medication are not supported by the empirical literature. Unfortunately, these value-laden critiques are unlikely to be influenced by objective outcome data. However, from an empirical perspective, reliable and valid data regarding meaningful treatment outcomes can and should be critical determinants of parent and professional decision making about the therapeutic usefulness of stimulant medications.

Outcome data have the potential to allow for reasoned judgments to be made regarding the benefits and costs of stimulant medication treatment for any given child. Furthermore, with a focus on a range of carefully measured outcomes (e.g., academic performance, social behavior, adverse physical effects) both the misgivings and the goals of involved parents and professionals may be addressed. Thus, if a child's physician and the school-based evaluation team agree that stimulant medication may be warranted, the student's parents should be provided with accurate and unbiased information regarding the costs and benefits of this treatment as well as how its efficacy will be evaluated. For example, the parents could be provided with a handout, delineating the potential benefits and side effects of stimulants (see Barkley & Murphy, 2006, for a handout on stimulant medication).

Parental decision making about medication treatment should be placed in an appropriate context by support professionals. The initial decision is whether to conduct a *systematically evaluated trial* of stimulants (or other medication), not a decision to permanently and irrevocably place a child on medication. Also, the parents should be made aware of the need for ongoing assessment of medication response to occur on at least an annual basis. Thus, even if the initial trial of medication is successful, professionals are not communicating to the parents that pharmacological treatment is a permanent part of the treatment plan. Nevertheless, given the chronicity of ADHD symptoms, it is realistic to assume that medication may be necessary for at least a year or more.

School Involvement

Management and evaluation of stimulant treatment often involves activities within the school and the classroom. Suggestions for school involvement and collaboration with prescribing physicians have been discussed fully in other places (see Chapter 7; see also Brown & Sawyer, 1998; Gadow, 1993) and include (1) establishing district- or schoolwide policy and communication systems for collaboration with community physicians, (2) establishing a systemwide outcome evaluation system for use with children being treated with stimulant medications, (3) delineating the specific roles of school system personnel in the implementation and monitoring of medication trials, and (4) ensuring that all staff are appropriately trained to fulfill their responsibilities. School psychologists and school nurses should be qualified to facilitate the coordination and implementation of each of these suggestions within their districts.

In addition to discussions of assessment and diagnosis, educational responsibilities, and stimulant medication, involvement with children with ADHD requires education professionals to communicate specific information, requests (e.g., referrals for evaluation), and expectations to parents, other professionals, and children. These person-specific communications are the focus of the remainder of this chapter.

COMMUNICATION BETWEEN EDUCATION PROFESSIONALS AND PARENTS

The following excerpts from the National Association of School Psychologists *Principles for Professional Ethics* outline the ideal approach for school practitioners (National Association of School Psychologists, 2010b):

Standard II.3.10

School psychologists encourage and promote parental participation in designing interventions for their children. When appropriate, this includes linking interventions between the school and the home, tailoring parental involvement to the skills of the family, and helping parents gain the skills needed to help their children.

School psychologists discuss with parents the recommendations and plans for assisting their children. This discussion takes into account the ethnic/cultural values of the family and includes alternatives that may be available. Subsequent recommendations for program changes or additional services are discussed with parents, including any alternatives that may be available.

Parents are informed of sources of support available at school and in the community.

Standard I.1.5

School psychologists respect the wishes of parents who object to school psychological services and attempt to guide parents to alternative resources.

Communication with parents regarding the education of children with ADHD can be conceptualized broadly as intended to involve parents, and support them, in a variety of activities that contribute to educational decision making. The time and effort necessary for these communications and activities will vary widely. For example, compare issues of due-process notification and consent for assessment with completing a behavior rating scale or participating in a structured interview to derive goals for educational planning. Regardless of the time required, our goals should be to communicate as directly and clearly as possible with parents, and to facilitate their involvement and understanding to the fullest extent possible. Particular attention is warranted to issues of due-process notifications, parent involvement in educational decision making, and parent roles in educational program implementation.

Due-Process Notifications

The IDEIA 2004, its predecessors, and related public laws ensure the rights of all children to a free and appropriate education, regardless of disability or handicapping condition. These laws require that parents be notified of and give consent to initial placement of children into special education programs, as well as to assessment activities that might lead to such changes (Jacob et al., 2011). Parental notification also is required as to when a conference will be held for purposes of discussing these decisions. Bersoff and Hofer (1990) note that informed consent involves parental *knowledge* of the action(s) to be taken, *voluntariness* or freedom from coercion, and *capacity* or competence to provide consent. These procedural requirements can best be met via open and informative communication, as can involvement in educational decision making.

Involving Parents in Educational Planning and Decision Making

A number of distinct and related types of educational decisions that can be facilitated by careful assessment have been delineated by Salvia, Ysseldyke, and Bolt (2013). Primary among these are screening, referral, classification or eligibility, instructional program planning, and program evaluation (including student progress evaluation). It is incumbent upon professionals to clarify and discuss with parents the issues and procedures involved in assessment for each these purposes, as well as how they relate to educational decision making. These discussions can help parents to be truly informed and knowledgeable consumers who can better act in the best interest of the child(ren) being served.

As part of these discussions, professionals likely will want to clarify several aspects of their work for parents by providing information along some or all of the following dimensions. For example, what is your model of (or general approach to) professional practice, and, based on the assumptions of that model, what are the implications for service delivery? With respect to assessment, what activities do you and your organization typically engage in when addressing issues of screening, referral, classification, and eligibility for programs? How will you convey to parents the concept that there is no "litmus test" for diagnosing ADHD?

When issues and questions regarding a diagnosis of ADHD are at hand, parents will need to be informed as to the nature and implications of an ADHD diagnosis. For example, how was this diagnosis arrived at? How should parents view this problem? Should they view this as a medical disorder, a developmental disorder, an educational problem, or some combination of the three? What is the prognosis for children diagnosed with ADHD? In our experience, it is helpful to convey to parents of children with ADHD that in a general sense they face two primary problems: first, their child is likely to present with *difficult-to-manage behavior*; and second, their child is likely to be *difficult to teach*. Intervention strategies and options for child management by parents and teachers, as well as by self-management and medication, may be appropriate to discuss at this point. Also, with respect to interventions, the importance of careful planning, implementation, and evaluation of intervention strategies should be conveyed to parents. Finally, professionals should do their best to expose myths regarding ADHD. For example, commonly held beliefs such as ADHD is caused by food allergies or that medication response is a diagnostic indicator of ADHD can be discussed in the course of communications around the appropriate topic (e.g., etiology, assessment, intervention). Discussion of these issues can be facilitated by providing the parents with a brief fact sheet about ADHD and/or a list of suggested readings (see Appendix 9.1).

Parent Involvement in Educational Programming

Professional–parent partnerships, within which collaborative efforts to foster a shared responsibility for student learning, are part of the spirit and the letter of IDEIA 2004 (Public Law 108-446) and related public laws. Furthermore, parent involvement in educational and school-related activities has been documented to enhance student achievement (Christenson & Sheridan, 2001). However, as Epstein (1986) has pointed out, although parents want their children to succeed in school, in general, parents are unclear as to how to assist their children to achieve that success. Christenson and Sheridan (2001) provide an excellent review of literature on those family/parent influences on achievement that have been documented to be both positively correlated with student achievement and are manipulable. Of particular relevance here are parental influences involving school–home communications and the structuring of and participation in learning-related activities at home.

A variety of home–school communication strategies are available for consideration. For example, Christenson and Sheridan (2001) describe and discuss the organization and utility of conferences, informal school visits, telephone calls, log books or notes (see Chapter 5 for a discussion and examples of home–school notes), newsletters, and report cards as viable strategies. In addition, they suggest that school professionals solicit input regarding parent preferences for method and frequency of home–school communication. These strategies can be utilized to foster parental understanding of school programs, as well as to facilitate parental monitoring of student behavior and achievement. In addition, their use can facilitate parental ability to specifically discuss aspects of their children's schooling at home, and to incorporate motivational and feedback strategies around schooling into their routines. Additionally, informed parents can recognize and celebrate student accomplishment(s) on a regular basis, as well as prevent problems and/or manage problems as they arise (see Eddy, Reid, & Curry, 2002, for a discussion of the critical nature of parental monitoring in preventing patterns of antisocial behavior). An important aspect of these activities is their ability to help parents communicate to and teach children that education, learning, and socially appropriate behavior are valued in their homes.

Home-based learning activities also teach children that education and learning are valued. For example, parents can be involved in activities, such as monitoring homework completion and discussing school work, that are linked to children's classroom assignments and responsibilities. Additionally, parents can foster learning by ensuring that books are available at home; that they themselves spend time reading, enjoying, and discussing books and other reading material; and by providing a variety of opportunities for learning. However, it is quite likely that parents will need assistance in organizing and structuring such activities (for useful information and materials, see Christenson & Sheridan, 2001; Power et al., 2001). Also, it should not be assumed that teachers are familiar with strategies to recommend to parents or comfortable with actually making such recommendations. Working together with parents, however, school psychologists, teachers, and administrators can help to promote parent involvement in activities likely to foster learning and achievement.

COMMUNICATION WITH PHYSICIANS AND OTHER PROFESSIONALS

The National Association of School Psychologists (2010b) *Principles for Professional Ethics* provide guidance for inter-professional communication, including the following:

Standard III.3.1

To meet the needs of children and other clients most effectively, school psychologists cooperate with other psychologists and professionals from other disciplines in relationships based on mutual respect. They encourage and support the use of all resources to serve the interests of students. If a child or other client is receiving similar services from another professional, school psychologists promote coordination of services.

And, furthermore, the 2010a National Association of School Psychologists Model for Comprehensive and Integrated School Psychological Services states:

School psychologists promote wellness and resilience by (a) collaborating with other healthcare professionals to provide a basic knowledge of behaviors that lead to good health for children; (b) facilitating environmental changes conducive to good health and adjustment of children; and (c) accessing resources to address a wide variety of behavioral, learning, mental, and physical needs.

In our experience, where ADHD is of concern, educators' communication with and referrals to physicians center around two primary issues: the diagnosis of the disorder and medication treatment. In these instances, families should be involved in the decision-making process (e.g., to make a referral) and should always be treated with dignity and respect. In doing so, the person(s) making the referral should patiently help parents to understand the purpose of the referral. For example, it might be communicated to parents that "I am [we are] concerned about your son, and believe it is reasonable to consider whether or not he can be considered to have attention-deficit/hyperactivity disorder. In many instances where professionals have such concerns, it is helpful to have the input and opinion of physicians. As such, we would like to refer you to your family pediatrician [or other medical professional] for a professional opinion regarding our concerns." If parents are in agreement with a referral, assistance should be offered to them in the form of a letter (or in some cases, a phone contact) to the referee conveying both the specific concerns being raised and what questions the person making the referral would like to have answered (e.g., diagnostic classification, ruling out physical problems). A sample referral letter is included as Appendix 9.2.

For children who already have been diagnosed with ADHD, a referral might be made to inquire about the appropriateness of a medication trial (see Appendix 9.3). Here, the referral might include information about other interventions that have been attempted or that are in place. In addition, school-based professionals might offer to systematically gather information that could be used to evaluate and monitor medication effects (e.g., using side-effects questionnaires, academic performance information, behavior rating scales). In Appendices 9.4 and 9.5, we have included two sample letters discussing the evaluation of a medication trial and its results, respectively. In making professional referrals, it is important to keep in mind that appropriate referrals do not prescribe or dictate to other professionals how to practice. Rather, referrals are requests for professional assistance in producing information to answer particular questions; the manner of producing the information or answering the question remains the professional's prerogative.

Finally, when school-based professionals are responsible for children who are being treated with psychoactive medications, a number of issues and questions should be discussed with parents and physicians. For example, who should be responsible for ensuring that a student takes his or her medication, and what happens if a student refuses to take prescribed medication? Who is responsible for assessing side effects and for monitoring medication effects on a student's social, academic, and physical functioning? Who will be making decisions about changes in the medication regimen? How will these tasks be accomplished? How will changes in the student's physical, social, and academic functioning be measured in valid and reliable ways? (See Brinkman et al., 2009 and Hansen & Hansen, 2006, for some considerations regarding these questions.)

COMMUNICATION WITH STUDENTS

The following excerpt from the NASP Principles for Professional Ethics outlines appropriate communication with students (National Association of School Psychologists, 2010b):

> Standard II.3.11
>
> School psychologists discuss with students the recommendations and plans for assisting them. To the maximum extent appropriate, students are invited to participate in selecting and planning interventions.

As with parents and physicians, students also should be treated with dignity and respect as they are involved in discussions and communications regarding assessment, diagnosis, and interventions, as well as the actual activities. First, in communicating the results and implications to a student diagnosed with ADHD, care should be taken to utilize language the student is likely to understand. Rather than simply telling a child that he or she has a disorder, the focus of the discussion should be on individual strengths and weaknesses. The student should be told what strengths and weaknesses were indicated by the evaluation. It should be pointed out that all of his or her classmates have individual strengths and weaknesses, so that he or she is not unique in this regard. Behaviors and weaknesses related to ADHD should be discussed in terms of problems sustaining attention, inhibiting impulses, and controlling activity level especially in certain situations, such as during independent seatwork. The student might be asked to enumerate specific examples of when, where, and how these problems are experienced on a daily basis. It should be emphasized that many students have weaknesses in these areas and that there are some ways to help with these difficulties. Discussion of various treatment modalities would ensue in language that the child will understand. For example, the use of stimulants would be framed in the context of trying to see whether medication would help the student to pay attention better and get more work done. If positive changes occur, the student is reminded that he or she was responsible for these improvements and that the medication merely helped to make these changes possible.

With older adolescents (e.g., high school students), more specific information about ADHD should be communicated (see Barkley & Murphy, 2006, for useful materials). Depending on the cognitive abilities of the specific student, the handouts and readings recommended for parents and teachers might be provided. Several counseling sessions may be necessary to accurately communicate this information, answer student questions, and provide emotional support. As with younger children, the emphasis of these discussions is not on what the student does wrong but rather that these weaknesses must be addressed in a long-term fashion with the help of teachers and parents.

Other important issues to discuss with adolescents with ADHD will be ones related to current and future academic support (e.g., test accommodations, adjustments to workload), and planning for postsecondary education, employment, and/or other goals. For students participating in special education services, postsecondary school planning is a required part of such services by law. This type of planning is likely to include parents and take the form of family counseling around issues of future planning for the student (see Robin, 1998, for a thorough discussion of working with adolescents with ADHD and their families), as well as issues of self-advocacy, and knowledge and understanding of available and potential educational and vocational options.

Regardless of the individual focus, in an ongoing fashion, time should be taken to involve students in service delivery decisions (e.g., intervention development and choices when possible) as appropriate. As a general rule for educating students diagnosed with ADHD, in every possible way we will want to convey encouragement, reinforce effort, plan for success, and provide constructive feedback and formative evaluation to promote success.

A primary consideration with children diagnosed with ADHD is the attributions that they develop for their behavior, achievement, and academic progress, especially when they are being treated with stimulant (or other) medication. Given that children and adolescents with ADHD tend to view their own competence in an overly positive manner relative to other methods of evaluating their competence (for a review, see Owens, Goldfine, Evangelista, Hoza, & Kaiser, 2007) it is important to consider how evaluations of and attributions for behavior will be influenced by taking prescribed medication. In particular, in practice it is important to evaluate and understand what "messages" children are receiving or sending to others with respect to attributing their behavior to medication or to their own competence. Regardless of whether they are taking medication or not, it is important to help students with ADHD understand that they themselves are responsible for their own behavior.

SUMMARY

Taking the position that child advocacy and student outcomes should drive professional practice has several implications for the services provided by school psychologists to students who are, or may be, diagnosed with ADHD. It requires a focus on the identification and definition of problems and concerns, in addition to diagnoses. Thus, careful communication with parents, physicians, children, and others set the agenda for assessment procedures and intervention activities.

Our comments regarding educational services for children diagnosed with ADHD have focused briefly on the linkages between diagnosis and educational programming, professional responsibilities, stimulant medication use, and communications with parents, physicians, and children. Other perspectives and issues are relevant and certainly will arise to challenge professionals, parents, and children alike. The challenge for those involved will be to balance/divide their attention appropriately between the often competing needs to focus not only on legal or procedural requirements related to diagnosis and classification but on student outcomes. The communication challenge will be to overcome the potential barriers raised by a lack of common vocabulary, training, and perspectives, while building effective interventions through collaboration. However, by initiating and promoting the discussions identified herein, parents, students, and professionals can contribute to improving meaningful student outcomes.

APPENDIX 9.1. Suggested Readings on ADHD and Related Difficulties for Parents and Teachers

Barkley, R. A. (2013). *Taking charge of ADHD: The complete, authoritative guide for parents* (3rd ed.). New York: Guilford Press.

Barkley, R. A., & Robin, A. L., with Benton, C. M. (2014). *Your defiant teen* (2nd ed.): *10 steps to resolve conflict and rebuild your relationship*. New York: Guilford Press.

Christenson, S. L., & Sheridan, S. M. (2001). *Schools and families: Creating essential connections for learning*. New York: Guilford Press.

Dendy, C. A. Z., & Teeter Ellison, P. A. (Eds.). (2006). *CHADD educators manual on attention deficit hyperactivity disorder: An in-depth look from an educational perspective*. Plantation, FL: CHADD.

Forgatch, M. S., & Patterson, G. R. (1989). *Parents and adolescents living together: Part 2. Family problem solving*. Eugene, OR: Castalia.

Patterson, G. R., & Forgatch, M. S. (1989). *Parents and adolescents living together: Part 1. The basics*. Eugene, OR: Castalia.

Power, T. J., Karustis, J. L., & Habboushe, D. F. (2001). *Homework success for children with ADHD: A family–school intervention program*. New York: Guilford Press.

Reif, S. F. (2005) *How to reach and teach children with ADD/ADHD: Practical techniques, strategies and interventions*. San Francisco: Jossey Bass.

Weyandt, L. (2007). *An ADHD primer* (2nd ed.) Mahwah: NJ: Erlbaum.

APPENDIX 9.2. Referral Letter to a Physician

Dr. Janet Williams
755 E. 45th Street
Anywhere, USA 99999

Dear Dr. Williams:

We are writing with a referral question regarding one of your patients, Michael Winston. Michael is a first-grade student with us here at Edgars Elementary, and we have concerns as to whether he might be a child with attention-deficit/hyperactivity disorder. Michael's teacher and our school psychologist have completed systematic observations of Michael's classroom behavior. As compared to his peers, Michael was observed to spend significantly less time engaged in assigned classroom tasks and significantly more time out of his seat and fidgeting while in his seat. At this point, Michael is struggling to keep up with his peers academically, and we are concerned that he frequently does not complete in-class assignments or he completes them quite quickly with little attention to detail. Although, as yet, we have not developed a systematic intervention program for Michael, we are considering developing one. Before doing so, however, we would like your professional opinion as to whether Michael might be diagnosable with ADHD, and, if so, we would appreciate your input as to potential directions for intervention. We would be pleased to provide other information at your request. Thank you for your assistance in this matter.

Sincerely,

School Psychologist   Teacher   School Principal

APPENDIX 9.3. Referral to Physician for Possible Medication Trial

Dr. James Smith
The Anytown Clinic
1162 Willams Street
Anytown USA 99999

RE: Billy Buck

Dear Dr. Smith:

As you are aware, we have been working with the above-named student to address his problems with inattention, impulsivity, and overactivity in the classroom. Previously, you had diagnosed Billy with ADHD. We are writing to provide an update of his progress and to request your input regarding the need for additional intervention (e.g., stimulant medication).

Over the past several months, we have implemented a number of interventions designed to enhance Billy's academic performance and behavior control. These have included a token reinforcement program in the classroom, a home–school communication protocol, and the use of peer tutoring for certain subject areas (e.g., math, spelling). Although these interventions have been helpful, Billy continues to display attentional difficulties throughout the school day and also is very disruptive on the playground and in the lunchroom. We plan to modify and continue these interventions for the remainder of the school year. Nevertheless, we are requesting that you evaluate the need for a stimulant medication trial.

We have discussed the need for this referral with Mr. and Mrs. Buck. They are in agreement with us that further treatment appears necessary. Of course, as with previous cases, we are willing to provide objective data to you regarding Billy's response to stimulant medication.

If you need further information about Billy's school program, please do not hesitate to contact us at any time. We look forward to hearing from you in the near future.

Sincerely,

School Psychologist   Teacher   School Principal

APPENDIX 9.4. Description of Medication Trial to Physician

Dr. James Smith
The Anytown Clinic
1162 Willams Street
Anytown USA 99999

Dear Dr. Smith:

We are pleased to be working with you and your patient, Thomas Jones, in evaluating the effects of stimulant medication on Thomas's academic and social functioning in school. Enclosed you will find a brief description of the project, its purpose, and goals. I am writing to ask your cooperation in prescribing the medication for the trial. Joan Williams, head pharmacist at the Health Center, has agreed to facilitate packaging of medication for the trial. Joan has agreed to label the separate bottles of medication with a code letter and dates (e.g., methylphenidate, dose A, week of April 14). Of the people involved in administering the medication trial, only you and I will be aware of the actual dose on any medication day. Please write four separate prescriptions as follows, and specify that the prescription is to be filled by the Health Center:

> Methylphenidate 5 mg; dispense 6 doses.
> Methylphenidate 10 mg; dispense 6 doses.
> Methylphenidate 15 mg; dispense 6 doses.

Mrs. Jones will pick up the prescriptions from your office when they are ready. The dates and doses (randomly assigned) of Thomas's medication trial will be as follows:

Dates	Dose	
Week of April 7	Baseline	
Week of April 14	Monday thru Saturday	10 mg
Week of April 21	Monday thru Saturday	5 mg
Week of April 28	Monday thru Saturday	15 mg

We will provide you with a summary of the results of this evaluation upon completion of the trial. We look forward to working with you. Please contact us if you have any questions.

Sincerely,

School Psychologist   Teacher   School Principal

APPENDIX 9.5. Report of Results of Medication Trial to Physician

Dr. James Smith
The Anytown Clinic
1162 Willams Street
Anytown USA 99999

Dear Dr. Smith:

We have now completed the methylphenidate evaluation trial for your patient, Thomas Jones. The conditions and dates of the trial were as follows:

Dates	Dose
Week of April 7	Baseline
Week of April 14, Monday thru Saturday	10 mg
Week of April 21, Monday thru Saturday	5 mg
Week of April 28, Monday thru Saturday	15 mg

Ongoing measures consisted of Thomas's reading performance in passages sampled from his curriculum, math performance in basic math skill probes, teacher ratings of classroom behavior and performance, parent ratings of behavior, and side-effects ratings completed by Thomas and his mother. A graph of Thomas's reading data is attached. The overall results of the trial are summarized in the table that follows:

Measure	Optimal dose(s)
Daily curriculum-based reading performance	15 mg
Daily math performance	15 mg
Teacher ratings of classroom behavior	10 mg/15 mg
Parent ratings of behavior	15 mg/5 mg

With respect to side effects, some dizziness, irritability, stomachaches, and difficulty sleeping were reported by both Thomas and his mother at both the 10-mg and 15-mg doses. These problems were reported as minor to moderate in severity, and tended to diminish over the course of each of these weeks.

The results of this evaluation indicate that the 15-mg dose of methylphenidate optimally enhanced Thomas's behavior across social and academic performance measures. Should methylphenidate be prescribed for Thomas at this dose, side effects should be carefully monitored. We hope that you find the results of this evaluation to be useful to you in your work with Thomas and his family. If we can be of further assistance with Thomas or other children, please do not hesitate to contact us.

Sincerely,

School Psychologist   Teacher   School Principal

CHAPTER 10

Conclusions and Future Directions

Meeting the needs of students with ADHD presents significant challenges to educational personnel. The hallmark characteristics of this disorder (i.e., inattention, impulsivity, and overactivity) often lead to disruptions of classroom decorum, academic underachievement, and difficulties making and keeping friends. Each of the characteristics comprising ADHD appears to exist on a continuum (i.e., normal curve) within the population such that the upper 2–5% of children in a given age and gender group could be diagnosed with the disorder. Furthermore, there is an additional 5% of children in a given population who are just out of the range of "clinically diagnosable" ADHD who present with significant, albeit less severe, attention and behavior control problems. Thus, in a general education classroom of 25 children, a teacher would be faced with at least two or three students who have notable difficulties attending to instructional activities and complying with classroom and school rules.

The academic performance of most children with ADHD is deficient due to their poor study habits, lack of work completion, and inconsistent accuracy on seatwork, homework, and tests. In addition, about one-third of these students are significantly below average in academic skills, and therefore are identified as having a learning disability. Federal and state guidelines allow for the provision of special education services to children with ADHD primarily on the basis of this disorder limiting their educational performance. Special education eligibility decisions should be made in the context of a multi-tiered system of support by conducting a reliable and valid assessment of ADHD and related problems, determining the degree to which the child's ADHD impacts his or her academic and social functioning, and evaluating the success of interventions in general education classrooms for ameliorating behaviors related to the disorder.

A major step in addressing the needs of children referred for problems consistent with ADHD is to conduct comprehensive psychological and, if necessary, educational evaluations. The school-based assessment of ADHD is composed of multiple techniques utilized across a variety of settings (e.g., classroom, playground) and sources of information (e.g., parent, teacher, and child). Following a teacher referral for possible ADHD, five stages of assessment are conducted, including initial screening for ADHD symptoms, multimethod assessment, interpretation of results to reach a classification decision, development of a multimodal treatment plan, and ongoing monitoring of progress resulting from intervention(s).

Reaching a diagnosis of ADHD does not signal the end of the evaluation process, nor is it the ultimate goal of an assessment. Rather, the value of the initial assessment lies in the determination of an intervention plan whose success is linked to the information gathered in the evaluation process. The use of behavioral assessment methodologies, including parent and teacher interviews, parent and teacher rating scales, direct observations of school behavior, and collection of academic performance data, is the optimal way to address both goals of the evaluation. Assessment data continue to be collected throughout treatment to determine the efficacy and/or limitations of the various components of an intervention program.

Given that ADHD often begins early in life, typically has a chronic course, and frequently is associated with long-term psychosocial and/or educational impairment, it is important to identify children with the disorder as early as possible so that intervention can begin prior to school entry. We propose a multicomponent model of early intervention that includes family education, consultation with preschool teachers and day-care providers, as well as strategies to promote preacademic skills (i.e., early literacy and numeracy) and safety. A multi-tiered approach is probably warranted such that the breadth and intensity of early intervention services are based on children's demonstrated response to increasingly intensive strategies (DuPaul & Kern, 2011). The objective of early intervention is to reduce the impact of ADHD symptoms on functioning such that conduct problems are delayed or prevented and children's academic functioning is on par with typically developing peers.

The most effective school-based psychosocial interventions are those based on principles of operant conditioning and social learning theory. Typically, these include reactive or consequence-based strategies such as token reinforcement systems, response cost, and self-management interventions. We have articulated a need to develop balanced intervention plans that include both reactive and proactive procedures. The latter include strategies (e.g., choice making and peer tutoring) that involve changes to antecedent conditions in order to prevent disruptive or inappropriate behaviors. Treatment targets include maladaptive behaviors (e.g., inattention to task) to be reduced, as well as competencies (e.g., academic performance, social acceptance) to be enhanced. In fact, when adaptive behaviors are increased, disruptive actions usually are diminished in frequency due to the inherent incompatibilities between these two classes of behavior. Therefore, proactive and positive reinforcement procedures are emphasized, with the realization that mild punishment strategies will be necessary, in some cases, to curtail off-task and/or aggressive actions.

For most children with ADHD, symptoms and associated impairments are chronic through adolescence into adulthood. Thus, school professionals must design, implement, and evaluate intervention strategies that will help secondary school students succeed in the face of possible difficulties with organization, study skills, time management, and related areas of executive functioning. Although empirical studies of school-based intervention for middle and high school students with ADHD are few and far between, we propose several strategies that may be helpful, particularly those that include self-regulation approaches. In addition to ongoing behavioral and educational support, high school students with ADHD will require assistance in making the postsecondary school transition to college or community life. This is particularly critical because approximately 5% of the college student population reports having been diagnosed with ADHD and these students may experience greater academic, psychological, and social difficulties than their peers. College students with ADHD will need a variety of supports including educational accommodations, coaching for time management and self-regulation, academic tutoring, cognitive-behavioral therapy, and/or stimulant medication. Of course, our recommendations for the university population are tempered by the dearth of empirical studies examining treatment strategies for college students with ADHD.

For many children with ADHD the optimal treatment approach may be the combination of behavioral interventions with psychostimulant medication (e.g., MPH). In school settings, stimulant medication can enhance the attention span, task completion and accuracy, and compliance with classroom rules of the majority of treated children. Given that the behavioral effects of stimulants are moderated by dose and individual responsivity, each child's treatment response *must* be assessed in an objective manner across a range of therapeutic doses. School-based professionals should play a major role in helping physicians to evaluate stimulant-induced changes in children's behavior across a variety of

crucial functioning areas (e.g., educational performance, social relationships, and compliance with classroom rules). A subset of the same methods that were used in the initial evaluation of ADHD can be tapped on a
continuous basis over several weeks to objectively determine whether an
individual responds to pharmacotherapy and which dose optimizes the
student's academic and social functioning.

Regardless of the well-established efficacy of stimulant medication
and behavioral interventions, no single treatment approach will be sufficient in ameliorating ADHD-related difficulties. The chronic exhibition
of problem behaviors across settings and with different caretakers likely
will necessitate the implementation of a multimodal treatment approach
over several years or longer. Several intervention strategies can be used
to supplement the use of classroom behavioral interventions and psychotropic medications. These may include both school- (e.g., academic
interventions, peer-relationship support srategies) and home-based (e.g.,
family education) treatments. The focus must be on designing an effective comprehensive program to treat a variety of functional areas while
acknowledging the necessity for long-term treatment. Concurrently, educators and parents, in particular, will need to set their sights on achieving short-term objectives throughout the school year to promote gradual
improvements in the child's overall adjustment.

School-based professionals should carefully evaluate the documented efficacy of proposed treatments for ADHD, as there are a number of therapies that have been touted as "effective" in the treatment
of this disorder (e.g., various diets including restriction of sugar and/
or food dye) that actually have limited or no empirical support. Given
the allure of alternatives to medication or behavioral strategies among
the general public, it is important that someone on the child's treatment team take a cautious, data-based stance toward newly proposed
therapies that are purported to "cure" ADHD. Specifically, the quality
and quantity of empirical support for the treatment should be evaluated
closely. More often than not, it is necessary to point out the limitations
of unsupported treatment modalities in an effort to maintain energy and
resources focused on those interventions more likely to help the child.

Usually, several individuals are involved in the treatment of a child
diagnosed with ADHD. Thus, students and families often interact with
both school- (e.g., teachers, school psychologists, administrators, school
nurse, and guidance counselors) and community-based (e.g., physician,
clinical psychologist) professionals. This necessitates the adoption of a
team approach to treatment wherein the provision of services is coordinated across professionals through ongoing communication. Unfortunately, the latter is more of an ideal than a commonplace circumstance
in the real world. Nevertheless, it is assumed that the more teamwork is
involved in treatment, the better the outcome for the child.

The team approach can be fostered by ensuring that all school professionals are aware of what ADHD is, how to identify students who may potentially require intervention, and how to treat problems related to the disorder. Educators aligned with both general and special education need to understand that ADHD-related behaviors are chronic and rarely fully eliminated, especially in the context of a single academic year. Thus, the focus of professional efforts should be on modifying the classroom and school environment to meet the needs of students with this disorder in order to promote attainment of short-term goals. As short-term improvements in attention, impulse control, and activity level are attained, gradual progress toward long-term amelioration of these problems is achieved. However, in our experience, to maintain the motivation of the student and treatment team members, it is necessary to promote concentration on making "small gains" rather than achieving a permanent "cure" within a short time period.

RECOMMENDATIONS FOR WORKING WITH STUDENTS WITH ADHD: CURRENT AND FUTURE DIRECTIONS

Although there has been substantial progress over the past several decades in the school-based identification and treatment of students with ADHD, significant work remains to be done in a number of key areas. First, the roles and responsibilities of school-based "case managers" continue to require elaboration. Beginning in the preschool and elementary school years, children with ADHD work with a variety of professionals, thus implicating the need for someone to coordinate communication and services across home, school, and community environments. Second, there is continued need to develop instruction in how to address the educational and behavioral challenges of students with ADHD at the preservice level of training (i.e., prior to receiving teacher certification) for both general educators and special education personnel. It continues to be the case that many teachers are not adequately prepared to work effectively with such children even after attending in-service workshops or reading relevant professional literature. Third, there is a significant gap between research and practice such that interventions with established research support are not implemented with integrity in "real-world" school settings. Researchers and practitioners must work together to bridge this gap. Principles of implementation science may be particularly helpful in designing methods to facilitate use of evidence-based interventions in typical classrooms. Finally, researchers and practitioners working with students with ADHD should increase the use of technology to meet the needs of this population. Relatively little empirical attention has been paid to technology-based intervention strategies thus far. Yet there is great potential in using technology to deliver evidence-based interventions to students in classrooms and other school settings. We anticipate that this will be an area of tremendous growth in the coming decades.

School-Based Case Manager to Foster Communication and Integration of Services

The successful treatment of ADHD frequently requires coordination of services among parents, student, teachers, other school professionals, physicians, and community-based service providers (e.g., clinical child psychologists). All too often, service providers associated with a given student's treatment program work independently of one another with little consistent communication occurring among them. This state of affairs increases the potential for redundancy of services or, worse still, the provision of conflicting treatment advice to parents and children. It seems reasonable to assume that effective communication among treatment team members and coordination of services could be enhanced by the efforts of one person serving in the role of a case manager. As children with ADHD spend much of their day in school settings, one cost-effective possibility is for a school-based professional (e.g., school psychologist) to take on case manager responsibilities.

An effective case manager would provide the following services to the child and treatment team:

1. Serve as the liaison between the school and the home by communicating on a regular basis with the student's teachers and parents. In addition, the case manager would have regular contact with all community-based professionals (e.g., physician) working with the student.

2. Coordinate school-based programming among teachers at the elementary, middle, or senior high school level. Either the case manager would meet with each teacher individually or would lead "team" meetings on a regular basis. This process would facilitate consistency in programming across classrooms while preventing potential miscommunication that could lead to ineffective treatment.

3. Coordinate home–school contingency management programming. When home-based contingencies are tied to a child's school performance, consistent communication between the student's parents and teachers is crucial. Also, it is important that all participants in the program are cognizant of their responsibilities and adhere to the tenets of

the intervention. Intervention adherence can be facilitated by the case manager through maintaining contact with parents and teachers, as well as by periodically convening "team" meetings to assess progress and make changes in the format or content of the home–school program.

4. Communicate with physicians regarding medication effects on school behavior and academic performance. The importance of school-based data in determining a child's medication response as well as delineating an individual's optimal dose was discussed in Chapter 7. Having a designated person serve as the link between the physician and the school greatly enhances the probability of effective medication monitoring, and therefore improved outcomes. Thus, the case manager would collate and communicate information regarding changes in the child's school performance to the physician during the initial evaluation of medication response (see Appendices 9.4 and 9.5). In addition, he or she could apprise the physician and/or parents of any unusual changes in the child's behavior that may be occurring as a result of long-term medication administration. Also, the case manager could serve as a go-between when any changes in the child's medication or dosage need to be communicated by the parent or physician to members of the student's school-based team.

5. Serve as a child advocate to facilitate obtaining appropriate school- and community-based services. The case manager should develop an overview of the types of services that a student with ADHD may require versus those currently available. When gaps are found between existing and necessary services, the case manager should advocate for changes in the child's educational and community-based programming with appropriate members of the treatment team (e.g., school administrators, parents). In addition, advocacy for greater professional attention to student outcomes may be warranted.

The above list of case manager responsibilities is not exhaustive: there may well be other roles that the case manager could serve depending upon the child's needs. Furthermore, each of these responsibilities may not be pertinent in some cases. Nevertheless, there is a strong need for a single person to coordinate services on an ongoing basis. In many cases, this should be a school-based professional who can follow a child's education across grade levels (e.g., school psychologist or guidance counselor). School-based professionals have the advantage of daily contact with the child's teachers as well as the opportunity to make contacts with parents and community-based members of the child's treatment team. Ongoing coordination of services and communication among team members is assumed to enhance the overall efficacy of long-term treatment of this disorder.

Preservice Training for Teachers in Working with Students with ADHD

One of the most frequent complaints voiced by parents of children with ADHD is that their children's teachers do not appear to have any background in working with students who have this disorder. Many teachers, particularly those in general education classrooms, readily acknowledge their limitations in working with these students. To address this problem, school systems have endeavored to provide in-service training to their staff in ways to identify, teach, and manage these children in both general and special education settings. Unfortunately, there are no empirical data to indicate that brief didactic training in how to work with children who have ADHD is effective in enhancing the knowledge and skills of educators. In fact, it appears that many teachers are not adequately prepared to work effectively with such children even after attending inservice workshops or reading the relevant professional literature.

Given this state of affairs, instruction in how to meet the educational and behavioral needs of children with ADHD should occur at the preservice level of training (i.e., prior to receiving teacher certification) for all teachers in training, as well as other school personnel. This training would afford the opportunity to provide not only didactic instruction in ADHD but also supervised practice in effective teaching and behavior management strategies. The fact that every educator will typically work with *at least* one student who has ADHD per school year would warrant that this proposal receive serious consideration. Implementation of training models that prepare teachers to be certified in both general and special education are increasing; this combined training focus should prepare teachers to more consistently meet the needs of students with disabilities (including ADHD).

Although it seems reasonable to assume that preservice training in ADHD will enhance educators' skills in working with these children, there are currently no empirical data to support this claim. Thus, the efficacy of preservice training in ADHD should be examined in detail. Specifically, what training activities lead to greater levels of understanding of this disorder and an enhancement of teaching and management skills? Will the combination of didactic instruction, assigned readings, and supervised practice sufficiently prepare teachers to work effectively with this population? Are other training modalities (e.g., practicum placement in school for children with behavior disorders) necessary to teach adequate levels of skills in this area? These are important questions because adequate preservice training for teachers represents a proactive (i.e., preventative) model of service delivery for students with ADHD, and ultimately could reduce the need for more costly and intensive programming at a later date.

Bridging the Gap between Research and Practice

Although various behavioral and cognitive-behavioral interventions for ADHD have been found effective in empirical studies (DuPaul, Eckert, & Vilardo, 2012), there is still a great deal to be learned about how to enhance the school performance of students who have this disorder. In particular, there continues to be a significant gap between research and practice such that interventions established as evidence based may not be used in "real-world" classroom settings.

One reason for this research into practice gap is that investigations may not always provide practitioners with the necessary information to support implementation. For example, behavioral interventions that have been employed for ADHD are quite diverse in scope, content, and intensity. What are the sufficient components of behavioral interventions for ADHD and how much should programming vary as a function of individual (e.g., age, gender, severity of the disorder) and environmental (e.g., general education vs. special education placement, level of teacher stress) factors? Given the chronic course of ADHD, what strategies can be used to promote continued use of effective academic and behavior intervention strategies across school years? Practitioners need to know not only whether an intervention will work but also which treatment will be most effective under a given set of circumstances, and once success is achieved, how to maintain effects over time and across settings.

An additional factor limiting translation of research into practice is that investigators may not directly address the questions that are of greatest interest to school-based professionals. For example, what are the most effective ways to present academic material to students with ADHD? How can we address the needs of students with ADHD within an RTI framework that is implemented in many schools? Will the efficacy of various modes of instruction vary as a function of the behavioral and academic profile of the child? How can we improve children's attention to task directions? Are there ways that we can alter the stimulation level of academic material such that children with ADHD will be more likely to complete their work in a timely and accurate fashion? In particular, greater knowledge of effective ways to modify instruction and other antecedent events would presumably aid in preventing and/ or reducing the severity of many of the behavioral control difficulties associated with this disorder, while enhancing academic skill achievement and performance.

Another challenge to bridging the research into practice gap is the degree to which teachers and other individuals implementing interventions find these strategies acceptable. Despite their effectiveness, teachers frequently find recommended classroom interventions unacceptable due to time constraints, lack of resources, or philosophical differences with the approach to intervening (Witt & Elliott, 1985). Stated differently, many interventions that work well in a research paradigm are not perceived to be very practical, particularly when implemented in general education classrooms. Thus, we need to know how to increase the acceptability of effective interventions. It is not enough to establish that a treatment works; we also must know if it is acceptable to the "consumers" (i.e., teachers, parents, and students) of these interventions. Are there modifications that can be made to currently available interventions that will increase their acceptability and hence their adoption into practice? How can the efficacy of interventions that have greater levels of acceptability, such as self-management strategies, be increased? The true test of whether research in this area contributes to practice will be the degree to which teachers and other school personnel actually implement empirically valid procedures on a consistent basis over lengthy time periods.

Implementation science involves the study of processes that mediate the translation and use of evidence-based practices into community settings like schools (Mendel, Meredith, Schoenbaum, Sherbourne, & Wells, 2008). This relatively new field directly addresses the research into practice gap in attempting to understand factors that hinder implementation while also developing assessment methods and support strategies to enhance use of evidence-based interventions in the community. Although implementation science initially focused on health care settings, this approach has great promise for enhancing "real-world" adoption of research practices in schools. More specifically, an implementation science approach could be very useful in promoting greater use of evidence-based interventions in schools for students with ADHD. Mendel and colleagues (2008) describe a four-stage process for building evidence for implementation that serves as a framework for researchers and practitioners working with the ADHD population. These four stages include (1) developing an understanding of contextual factors and mechanisms by which novel strategies get adopted in schools; (2) identifying how each contextual component can be evaluated in order to explain dissemination of strategies across stakeholder groups (e.g., teachers, principals, parents); (3) developing strategies for adapting, disseminating, and implementing evidence-based interventions using a collaborative, participatory approach with stakeholder groups; and (4) promoting the generalization of findings across different interventions and settings. Collaboration between researchers and practitioners across all phases of the research endeavor, including investigation planning and development of research questions, is a particularly critical component of the implementation science approach.

Using Technology to Deliver Intervention and Support

Although several small-scale studies (e.g., Ota & DuPaul, 2002) have provided initial support for CAI as an academic intervention for students with ADHD, the use of technology has received scant attention in the empirical literature. Perhaps the most prominent technology-based strategy receiving greater attention in recent years is the use of computer-based working memory training for students with ADHD or learning difficulties. Various programs (e.g., CogMed) have been developed to enhance working memory in children, particularly those individuals presumed to have deficits in working memory (e.g., students with ADHD). Typically, these programs involve individual students exposed to visual stimuli on a computer screen and asked to recall those stimuli at various levels of difficulty and complexity. Training sessions typically last anywhere from 15 to 60 minutes. For example, a child may view a series of numbers or letters and then be asked to recall that sequence in either a forward or backward fashion. Although several investigations of working memory training have demonstrated transfer of learning to similar memory tasks, generalization of effects to everyday learning and classroom behavior has been mixed at best (for a review, see Shipstead, Redick, & Engle, 2012). Thus, before widespread adoption of working memory training for students with ADHD can be recommended, additional research is necessary to demonstrate whether such training is effective in reducing ADHD symptomatic behaviors while enhancing academic competence in settings and at times other than when students are engaged in the training activity.

Another potential use for technology is the delivery of clinical health services through telecommunication technology (i.e., telemedicine). In recent years, there has been increased implementation of telemedicine services to populations that may have limited access to health care (e.g., families living in rural and/or remote communities). A telemedicine approach may be particularly valuable for children with ADHD and other behavior disorders who do not have easy access to child psychiatry or clinical child psychology services. Pakyurek, Schweitzer, and Yellowlees (2013) describe several ways a coordinated telemedicine system for students with ADHD can be used to deliver services, including (1) consultation and education for teachers and other school personnel, (2) parent education in behavior management strategies, (3) consultation and training for primary care physicians, and (4) ongoing communication among key stakeholders (e.g., parents, teachers, school nurses, school psychologists). A few studies (e.g., Epstein et al., 2011) provide initial support for some of these components; however, larger-scale studies examining more systemic approaches to the use of telemedicine with the ADHD population are necessary. Telemedicine would seem to have great potential for addressing many of the challenges (e.g., limited access to community-based care, gap between research and practice, lack of teacher and parent training in effective strategies) that negatively impact service delivery for students with ADHD.

CONCLUSIONS

Although our understanding of ADHD has been greatly advanced over the last several decades, children with this disorder continue to encounter significant difficulties succeeding in our schools. To correct this situation, gains must be made in two major areas. First, practitioners in the fields of psychology and education must increase their awareness and understanding of the limitations of students with this disorder. Those professionals possessing expertise in working with such children must educate their colleagues to be similarly proficient. Children with this disorder are encountered in every type of school setting from preschool through college. Therefore, all educators should possess, at the least, minimal competencies in identifying these children and designing effective educational programming to meet their needs and to help them to become successful, productive citizens. Second, the technology of assessing and treating children with ADHD needs improvement. Assessment methodologies must be developed that go beyond the reports of significant others in order to enhance the ecological validity of the evaluation process. Third, treatment modalities that are effective on the one hand, while cost-efficient and acceptable to consumers, are sorely needed. Strategies to promote strong connections between research and practice must be developed and implemented. In particular, the challenge is for research to lead to effective practice such that long-term improvements in school performance are attained for all children with ADHD. Until that goal is reached, however, the many suggestions contained in this book can serve as starting points for guiding current practices to improve educational outcomes for students with ADHD.

References

Abikoff, H. (1985). Efficacy of cognitive training intervention in hyperactive children: A critical review. *Clinical Psychology Review, 5*, 479–512.

Abikoff, H. (2009). ADHD psychosocial treatments: Generalization reconsidered. *Journal of Attention Disorders, 13*(3), 207–210.

Abikoff, H., Gallagher, R., Wells, K. C., Murray, D. W., Huang, L., Lu, F., et al. (2013). Remediating organizational functioning in children with ADHD: Immediate and long-term effects from a randomized controlled trial. *Journal of Consulting and Clinical Psychology, 81*, 113–128.

Abikoff, H., & Gittelman, R. (1985). The normalizing effects of methylphenidate on the classroom behavior of ADDH children. *Journal of Abnormal Child Psychology, 13*, 33–44.

Abikoff, H., Gittelman-Klein, R., & Klein, D. (1977). Validation of a classroom observation code for hyperactive children. *Journal of Consulting and Clinical Psychology, 45*, 772–783.

Abikoff, H., Hechtman, L., Klein, R. G., Gallagher, R., Fleiss, K., Etcovitch, J., et al. (2004). Social functioning in children with ADHD treated with long-term methylphenidate and multimodal psychosocial treatment. *Journal of the American Academy of Child and Adolescent Psychiatry, 43*, 820–829.

Abikoff, H., Hechtman, L., Klein, R. G., Weiss, G., Fleiss, K., Etcovitch, J., et al. (2004). Symptomatic improvement in children with ADHD treated with long-term methylphenidate and multimodal psychosocial treatment. *Journal of the American Academy of Child and Adolescent Psychiatry, 43*, 802–811.

Abramowitz, A. J., Eckstrand, D., O'Leary, S. G., & Dulcan, M. K. (1992). ADHD children's responses to stimulant medication and two intensities of a behavioral intervention. *Behavior Modification, 16*, 193–203.

Abramowitz, A. J., O'Leary, S. G., & Rosen, L. A. (1987). Reducing off-task behavior in the classroom: A comparison of encouragement and reprimands. *Journal of Abnormal Child Psychology, 15*, 153–163.

Achenbach, T. M., & McConaughy, S. H. (1996). Relations between DSM-IV and empirically based assessment. *School Psychology Review, 25*, 329–341.

Achenbach, T. M., & Rescorla, L. A. (2001). *Manual for the ASEBA school-age forms and profiles*. Burlington: University of Vermont, Department of Psychiatry.

Adams, M. J. (1990). *Beginning to read: Thinking and learning about print*. Cambridge, MA: MIT Press.

Adler, L. A., Shaw, D. M., Spencer, T. J., Newcorn, J. H., Hammerness, P., Sitt, D. J., et al. (2012). Preliminary examination of the reliability and concurrent validity of the Attention-Deficit/Hyperactivity Disorder Self-Report Scale v1. 1 Symptom Checklist to rate symptoms of attention-deficit/hyperactivity disorder in adolescents. *Journal of Child and Adolescent Psychopharmacology, 22,* 238–244.

Allsopp, D. H., Minskoff, E. H., & Bolt, L. (2005). Individualized course-specific strategy instruction for college students with learning disabilities and ADHD: Lessons learned from a model demonstration project. *Learning Disabilities Research and Practice, 20,* 103–118.

American Academy of Child and Adolescent Psychiatry. (2007). Practice parameter for the assessment and treatment of children and adolescents with attention-deficit/hyperactivity disorder. *Journal of the American Academy of Child and Adolescent Psychiatry, 46,* 894–921.

American Academy of Pediatrics. (1999). *TIPP—The Injury Prevention Program*. Elk Grove Village, IL: Author.

American Academy of Pediatrics. (2011). ADHD: Clinical practice guideline for the diagnosis, evaluation, and treatment of attention-deficit/hyperactivity disorder in children and adolescents. *Pediatrics, 128,* 1007–1022.

American Psychiatric Association. (1980). *Diagnostic and statistical manual of mental disorders* (3rd ed.). Washington, DC: Author.

American Psychiatric Association. (1987). *Diagnostic and statistical manual of mental disorders* (3rd ed., rev.). Washington, DC: Author.

American Psychiatric Association. (1994). *Diagnostic and statistical manual of mental disorders* (4th ed.). Washington, DC: Author.

American Psychiatric Association. (2000). *Diagnostic and statistical manual of of mental disorders* (4th ed., text rev.). Washington, DC: Author.

American Psychiatric Association. (2013). *Diagnostic and statistical manual of mental disorders* (5th ed.). Arlington, VA: Author.

Anastopoulos, A. D., & Shelton, T. L. (2001). *Assessing attention-deficit/hyperactivity disorder*. New York: Kluwer Academic/Plenum Press.

Anastopoulos, A. D., Smith, J. M., & Wein, E. E. (1998). Counseling and training parents. In R. A. Barkley, *Attention-deficit hyperactivity disorder: A handbook for diagnosis and treatment* (2nd ed., pp. 373–393). New York: Guilford Press.

Anastopoulos, A. D., Spisto, M. A., & Maher, M. (1994). The WISC-III Freedom from Distractibility factor: Its utility in identifying children with attention deficit hyperactivity disorder. *Psychological Assessment, 6,* 368–371.

Anderson, R. C., Hiebert, E. H., Scott, J. A., & Wilkinson, I. A. G. (1985). *Becoming a nation of readers: The report of the commission on reading*. Washington, DC: National Institute of Education, U.S. Department of

Education. Available from the Center for the Study of Reading, University of Illinois, Champaign.

Anesko, K. M., Schoiock, G., Ramirez, R., & Levine, F. M. (1987). The Homework Problem Checklist: Assessing children's homework difficulties. *Behavioral Assessment, 9,* 179–185.

Ang, R. P., & Hughes, J. N. (2002). Differential benefits of skills training with antisocial youth based on group composition: A meta-analytic investigation. *School Psychology Review, 31,* 164–185.

Archer, A., & Gleason, M. (2002). *Skills for school success (grades 3–7+).* North Billerica, MA: Curriculum Associates.

Archer, A. L., & Hughes, C. A. (2011). *Explicit instruction: Effective and efficient teaching strategies.* New York: Guilford Press.

Arnold, L. E., Hurt, E. A., Mayes, T., & Lofthouse, N. (2011). Ingestible alternative and complementary treatments for attention deficit hyperactivity disorder. In S. W. Evans & B. Hoza (Eds.), *Treating attention deficit hyperactivity disorder: Assessment and intervention in developmental context* (pp. 14-1–14-40). Kingston, NJ: Civic Research Institute.

Atkins, M. S., Pelham, W. E., & Licht, M. H. (1985). A comparison of objective classroom measures and teacher ratings of attention deficit disorder. *Journal of Abnormal Child Psychology, 13,* 155–167.

Axelrod, M. I., Zhe, E. J., Haugen, K. A., & Klein, J. A. (2009). Self-management of on-task homework behavior: A promising strategy for adolescents with attention and behavior problems. *School Psychology Review, 38,* 325–333.

Baker, S., Gersten, R., & Grossen, B. (2002). Interventions for students with reading comprehension problems. In M. R. Shinn, H. M. Walker, & G. Stoner (Eds.), *Interventions for academic and behavior problems, II: Preventive and remedial approaches* (pp. 731–754). Bethesda, MD: National Association of School Psychologists.

Bambara, L. M., & Kern, L. (2005). *Individualized supports for students with problem behaviors: Designing positive behavior plans.* New York: Guilford Press.

Bambara, L. M., & Knoster, T. P. (1995). *Guidelines: Effective behavioral support.* Harrisburg: Pennsylvania Department of Education, Bureau of Special Education.

Banaschewski, T., Becker, K., Scherag, S., Franke, B., & Coghill, D. (2010). Molecular genetics of attention-deficit/hyperactivity disorder: An overview. *European Child and Adolescent Psychiatry, 19,* 237–257.

Barbaresi, W. J., Katusic, S. K., Colligan, R. C., Weaver, A. L., & Jacobsen, S. J. (2007). Modifiers of long term school outcomes for children with attention-deficit/hyperactivity disorder: Does treatment with stimulant medication make a difference? Results from a population-based study. *Journal of Developmental and Behavioral Pediatrics, 28,* 274–287.

Barkley, R. A. (1979). Using stimulant drugs in the classroom. *School Psychology Digest, 8,* 412–425.

Barkley, R. A. (1988). The effects of methylphenidate on the interactions of preschool ADHD children with their mothers. *Journal of the American Academy of Child and Adolescent Psychiatry, 27,* 336–341.

Barkley, R. A. (1989). Attention-deficit hyperactivity disorder. In E. J. Mash & R. A. Barkley (Eds.), *Treatment of childhood disorders* (pp. 39–72). New York: Guilford Press.

Barkley, R. A. (1990). *Attention-deficit hyperactivity disorder: A handbook for diagnosis and treatment.* New York: Guilford Press.

Barkley, R. A. (1991). The ecological validity of laboratory and analogue assessment methods of ADHD symptoms. *Journal of Abnormal Child Psychology, 19,* 149–178.

Barkley, R. A. (1997a). *ADHD and the nature of self-control.* New York: Guilford Press.

Barkley, R. A. (1997b). *Defiant children: A clinician's manual for assessment and parent training* (2nd ed.). New York: Guilford Press.

Barkley, R. A. (1998). *Attention-deficit hyperactivity disorder: A handbook for diagnosis and treatment* (2nd ed.). New York: Guilford Press.

Barkley, R. A. (2001). Accidents and ADHD. *Economics of Neuroscience, 3,* 64–68.

Barkley, R. A. (2002). International consensus statement on ADHD. *Clinical Child and Family Psychology Review, 5,* 89–111.

Barkley, R. A. (2004). Driving impairments in teens and adults with attention-deficit/hyperactivity disorder. *Psychiatric Clinics of North America, 27,* 233–260.

Barkley, R. A. (2006). *Attention-deficit/hyperactivity disorder: A handbook for diagnosis and treatment* (3rd ed.). New York: Guilford Press.

Barkley, R. A. (2013a). *Defiant children: A clinician's manual for assessment and parent training* (3rd ed.). New York: Guilford Press.

Barkley, R. A. (2013b). *Taking charge of ADHD: The complete, authoritative guide for parents* (3rd ed.). New York: Guilford Press.

Barkley, R. A. (in press). *Attention-deficit/hyperactivity disorder: A handbook for diagnosis and treatment* (4th ed.). New York: Guilford Press.

Barkley, R. A., Anastopoulos, A. D., Guevremont, D. C., & Fletcher, K. E. (1991). Adolescents with attention deficit hyperactivity disorder: Patterns of behavioral adjustment, academic functioning, and treatment utilization. *Journal of the American Academy of Child and Adolescent Psychiatry, 30,* 752–861.

Barkley, R. A., Copeland, A., & Sivage, C. (1980). A self-control classroom for hyperactive children. *Journal of Autism and Developmental Disorders, 10,* 75–89.

Barkley, R. A., DuPaul, G. J., & McMurray, M. B. (1990). A comprehensive evaluation of attention deficit disorder with and without hyperactivity as defined by research criteria. *Journal of Consulting and Clinical Psychology, 58,* 775–789.

Barkley, R. A., DuPaul, G. J., & McMurray, M. B. (1991). Attention deficit disorder with and without hyperactivity: Clinical response to three dose levels of methylphenidate. *Pediatrics, 87,* 519–531.

Barkley, R. A., Edwards, G., Laneri, M., Fletcher, K., & Metevia, L. (2001). The efficacy of problem-solving communication training alone, behavior management training alone, and their combination for parent–adolescent conflict in teenagers with ADHD and ODD. *Journal of Consulting and Clinical Psychology, 69,* 926–941.

Barkley, R. A., Edwards, G. H., & Robin, A. L. (1999). *Defiant teens: A clinician's guide for assessment and family intervention.* New York: Guilford Press.

Barkley, R. A., Fischer, M., Edelbrock, C. S., & Smallish, L. (1990). The adolescent outcome of hyperactive children diagnosed by research criteria: I. An 8–year prospective follow-up study. *Journal of the American Academy of Child and Adolescent Psychiatry, 29,* 546–557.

Barkley, R. A., Fischer, M., Newby, R., & Breen, M. (1988). Development of a multi-method clinical protocol for assessing stimulant drug responses in ADHD children. *Journal of Clinical Child Psychology, 17,* 14–24.

Barkley, R. A., Fischer, M., Smallish, L., & Fletcher, K. (2002). The persistence of attention-deficit/hyperactivity disorder into young adulthood as a function of reporting source and definition of disorder. *Journal of Abnormal Psychology, 111,* 279–289.

Barkley, R. A., Fischer, M., Smallish, L., & Fletcher, K. (2006). Young adult outcome of hyperactive children: Adaptive functioning in major life activities. *Journal of the American Academy of Child and Adolescent Psychiatry, 45*(2), 192–202.

Barkley, R. A., Guevremont, D. C., Anastopoulos, A. D., DuPaul, G. J., & Shelton, T. L. (1993). Driving-related risks and outcomes of attention-deficit hyperactivity disorder in adolescents and young adults: A 3–5 year follow-up survey. *Pediatrics, 92,* 212–218.

Barkley, R. A., Guevremont, D. C., Anastopoulos, A. D., & Fletcher, K. E. (1992). A comparison of three family therapy programs for treating family conflicts in adolescents with attention-deficit hyperactivity disorder. *Journal of Consulting and Clinical Psychology, 60,* 450–462.

Barkley, R. A., Karlsson, J., Strzelecki, E., & Murphy, J. (1984). Effects of age and Ritalin dosage on the mother–child interactions of hyperactive children. *Journal of Consulting and Clinical Psychology, 52,* 750–758.

Barkley, R. A., McMurray, M. B., Edelbrock, C. S., & Robbins, K. (1989). The response of aggressive and non-aggressive ADHD children to two doses of methylphenidate. *Journal of the American Academy of Child and Adolescent Psychiatry, 28,* 873–881.

Barkley, R. A., McMurray, M. B., Edelbrock, C. S., & Robbins, K. (1990). The side effects of Ritalin in ADHD children: A systematic placebo-controlled evaluation of two doses. *Pediatrics, 86,* 184–192.

Barkley, R. A., Murphy, K., DuPaul, G. J., & Bush, T. (2002). Driving knowledge, performance, and adverse outcomes in teens and young adults with attention deficit hyperactivity disorder. *Journal of the International Neuropsychological Society, 8,* 655–672.

Barkley, R. A., & Murphy, K. R. (2006). *Attention-deficit hyperactivity disorder: A clinical workbook* (3rd ed.). New York: Guilford Press.

Barkley, R. A., Murphy, K. R., & Fischer, M. (2008). *ADHD in adults: What the science says.* New York: Guilford Press.

Barkley, R. A., & Robin, A. L. (2014). *Defiant teens: A clinician's manual for assessment and family intervention* (2nd ed.). New York: Guilford Press.

Barkley, R. A., Shelton, T. L., Crosswait, C., Moorehouse, M., Fletcher, K., Barrett, S., et al. (2000). Multi-method psycho-educational intervention for preschool children with disruptive behavior: Preliminary results at post-treatment. *Journal of Child Psychology and Psychiatry, 41,* 319–332.

Barkley, R. A., Smith, K. M., Fischer, M., & Navia, B. (2006). An examination of the behavioral and neuropsychological correlates of three ADHD candidate gene polymorphisms (DRD4 7+, DBH TaqI A2, and DAT1 40 bp VNTR) in hyperactive and normal children followed to adulthood. *American Journal of Medical Genetics Part B (Neuropsychiatric Genetics), 141B,* 487–498.

Barlow, D. H. (Ed.). (1981). *Behavioral assessment of adult disorders.* New York: Guilford Press.

Barrios, B., & Hartmann, D. P. (1986). The contributions of traditional assessment: Concepts, issues, and methodologies. In R. O. Nelson & S. C. Hayes (Eds.), *Conceptual foundations of behavioral assessment* (pp. 81–110). New York: Guilford Press.

Bauermeister, J. J., Barkley, R. A., Bauermeister, J. A., Martinez, J. V., & McBurnett, K. (2012). Validity of the sluggish cognitive tempo, inattention, and hyperactivity dimensions: Neuropsychological and psychosocial correlates. *Journal of Abnormal Child Psychology, 50,* 683–697.

Beck, I. L., Perfetti, C. A., & McKeown, M. E. (1982). The effects of long-term vocabulary instruction on lexical access and reading comprehension. *Journal of Educational Psychology, 74,* 506–521.

Bergan, J. R., & Kratochwill, T. R. (1990). *Behavioral consultation and therapy.* New York: Plenum Press.

Bersoff, D. N., & Hofer, P. T. (1990). The legal regulation of school psychology. In T. B. Gutkin & C. R. Reynolds (Eds.), *The handbook of school psychology* (2nd ed., pp. 939–961). New York: Wiley.

Biederman, J., Faraone, S. V., Milberger, S., Curtis, S., Chen, L., Marrs, A., et al. (1996). Predictors of persistence and remission of ADHD into adolescence: Results from a four-year prospective follow-up study. *Journal of the American Academy of Child and Adolescent Psychiatry, 35,* 343–351.

Biederman, J., Melmed, R. D., Patel, A., McBurnett, K., Konow, J., Lyne, A., et al. (2008). A randomized, double-blind, placebo-controlled study of guanfacine extended release in children and adolescents with attention-deficit/hyperactivity disorder. *Pediatrics, 121,* e73–e84.

Biederman, J., Monuteaux, M. C., Spencer, T., Wilens, T. E., MacPherson, H. A., & Faraone, S. V. (2008). Stimulant therapy and risk for subsequent substance use disorders in male adults with ADHD: A naturalistic controlled 10–year follow-up study. *American Journal of Psychiatry, 165,* 597–603.

Biederman, J., Wilens, T., Mick, E., Faraone, S. V., Weber, W., Curtis, S., et al. (1997). Is ADHD a risk factor for psychoactive substance use disorders?: Findings from a four-year prospective follow-up study. *Journal of the American Academy of Child and Adolescent Psychiatry, 36,* 21–29.

Blackman, G. L., Ostrander, R., & Herman, K. C. (2005). Children with ADHD and depression: A multisource, multimethod assessment of clinical, social, and academic functioning. *Journal of Attention Disorders, 8*(4), 195–207.

Blackman, J. A., Westervelt, V. D., Stevenson, R., & Welch, A. (1991). Management of preschool children with attention deficit-hyperactivity disorder. *Topics in Early Childhood Special Education, 11*, 91–104.

Booster, G. D., DuPaul, G. J., Power, T. J., & Eiraldi, R. (2012). Functional impairments in children with ADHD: Unique effects of age and comorbid status. *Journal of Attention Disorders, 16*, 179–189.

Boyajian, A. E., DuPaul, G. J., Wartel Handler, M., Eckert, T. L., & McGoey, K. E. (2001). The use of classroom-based brief functional analyses with preschoolers at-risk for attention deficit hyperactivity disorder. *School Psychology Review, 30*, 278–293.

Bracken, B. A. (1998). *Examiner's manual for the Bracken Basic Concept Scale–Revised*. San Antonio, TX: The Psychological Corporation, Harcourt Brace.

Bremness, A. B., & Sverd, J. (1979). Methylphenidate-induced Tourette syndrome: Case report. *American Journal of Psychiatry, 136*, 1334–1335.

Brinkman, W. B., Sherman, S. N., Zmitrovich, A. R., Visscher, M. O., Crosby, L. E., Phelan, K. J., et al. (2009). Parental angst making and revisiting decisions about treatment of attention-deficit hyperactivity disorder. *Pediatrics, 124*(2), 580–589.

Brown, R. T., & Sawyer, M. G. (1998). *Medications for school-age children: Effects on learning and behavior*. New York: Guilford Press.

Brown, R. T., & Sleator, E. K. (1979). Methylphenidate in hyperkinetic children: Differences in dose effects on impulsive behavior. *Pediatrics, 64*, 408–411.

Brown-Chidsey, R., & Steege, M. W. (2010). *Response to intevention: Principles and strategies for effective practice* (2nd ed.). New York: Guilford Press.

Buhrmester, D., Whalen, C. K., Henker, B., MacDonald, V., & Hinshaw, S. P. (1992). Prosocial behavior in hyperactive boys: Effects of stimulant medication and comparison with normal boys. *Journal of Abnormal Child Psychology, 20*, 103–122.

Burns, M. K., Deno, S. L., & Jimerson, S. R. (2007). Toward a unified response-to-intervention model. In S. R. Jimerson, M. K. Burns, & A. M. VanDer-Heyden (Eds.), *Handbook of response to intervention* (pp. 428–440). New York: Springer.

Burns, M. K., & Gibbons, K. A. (2008). *Implementing response-to-intervention in elementary and secondary schools*. New York: Routledge.

Burns, M. K., & Wagner, D. (2008). Determining an effective intervention within a brief experimental analysis for reading: A meta-analytic review. *School Psychology Review, 37*, 126–136.

Bussing, R., Mason, D. M., Bell, L., Porter, P., & Garvan, C. (2010). Adolescent outcomes of childhood attention-deficit/hyperactivity disorder in a diverse community sample. *Journal of the American Academy of Child and Adolescent Psychiatry, 49*, 595–605.

Campbell, S. B., Endman, M. W., & Bernfield, G. (1977). A three-year follow-up of hyperactive preschoolers into elementary school. *Journal of Child Psychology and Psychiatry, 18*, 239–249.

Campbell, S. B., & Ewing, L. J. (1990). Follow-up of hard to manage preschoolers: Adjustment at age 9 and predictors of continuing symptoms. *Journal of Child Psychology and Psychiatry, 31*, 871–889.

Campbell, S. B., Schleifer, M., & Weiss, G. (1978). Continuities in maternal reports and child behaviors over time in hyperactive and comparison groups. *Journal of Abnormal Child Psychology, 6*, 33–45.

Cantwell, D. P. (1986). Attention deficit disorder in adolescents. *Clinical Psychology Review, 6*, 237–247.

Cantwell, D. P., & Baker, L. (1991). Association between attention-deficit hyperactivity disorder and learning disorders. *Journal of Learning Disabilities, 24*, 88–95.

Cantwell, D. P., & Satterfield, J. H. (1978). The prevalence of academic underachievement in hyperactive children. *Journal of Pediatric Psychology, 3*, 168–171.

Carlson, C. L., & Mann, M. (2000). Attention-deficit/hyperactivity disorder predominantly inattentive subtype. *Child and Adolescent Psychiatric Clinics of North America, 9*, 499–510.

Carlson, C. L., & Mann, M. (2002). Sluggish cognitive tempo predicts a different pattern of impairment in the attention deficit hyperactivity disorder, predominantly inattentive type. *Journal of Clinical Child and Adolescent Psychology, 31*, 123–129.

Carnine, D., Kame'enui, E., & Silbert, J. (1990). *Direct instruction reading.* Columbus, OH: Merrill.

Carnine, D., & Kinder, D. (1985). Teaching low-performing students to apply generative and schema strategies to narrative and expository material. *Remedial and Special Education, 6*, 20–30.

Carroll County Public Schools. (1997). *ADHD procedural guidelines.* Westminster, MD: Author.

Castellanos, F. X., Giedd, J. N., Elia, J., Marsh, W. L., Ritcline, G. F., Hamburger, S. P., et al. (1997). Controlled stimulant treatment of ADHD and comorbid Tourette's syndrome: Effects of stimulant and dose. *Journal of the American Academy of Child and Adolescent Psychiatry, 36*, 589–596.

Centers for Disease Control and Prevention. (2010). Increasing prevalence of parent-reported attention-deficit/hyperactivity disorder among children—United States, 2003 and 2007. *Morbidity and Mortality Weekly Report, 59*(44), 1439–1443.

Centers for Disease Control and Prevention (2013, May 17). Mental health surveillance among children—United States, 2005–2011. *Morbidity and Mortality Weekly Report, 62*(Suppl. 2), 1–35.

Chacko, A., Wymbs, B. T., Chimiklis, A., Wymbs, F. A., & Pelham, W. E. (2012). Evaluating a comprehensive strategy to improve engagement to group-based behavioral parent training for high-risk families of children with ADHD. *Journal of Abnormal Child Psychology, 40*, 1351–1362.

Chacko, A., Wymbs, B. T., Flammer-Rivera, L. M., Pelham, W. E., Walker, K. S., Arnold, F. W., et al. (2008). A pilot study of the feasibility and efficacy of the Strategies to Enhance Positive Parenting (STEPP) program for single mothers of children with ADHD. *Journal of Attention Disorders, 12,* 270–280.

Chafouleas, S., Riley-Tillman, T. C., & Sugai, G. (2007). *School-based behavioral assessment: Informing intervention and instruction.* New York: Guilford Press.

Chan, E., Zhan, C., & Homer, C. J. (2002). Health care use and costs for children with attention-deficit/hyperactivity disorder. *Archives of Pediatric and Adolescent Medicine, 156,* 504–511.

Charach A., Dashti B., Carson P., Booker L., Lim C. G., Lillie E., et al. (2010). *Attention deficit hyperactivity disorder: Effectiveness of treatment in at-risk preschoolers; long-term effectiveness in all ages; and variability in prevalence, diagnosis, and treatment. Comparative Effectiveness Review No. 44* (prepared by the McMaster University Evidence-Based Practice Center under Contract No. MME2202 290-02-0020; AHRQ Publication No. 12-EHC003-EF). Rockville, MD: Agency for Healthcare Research and Quality. Available at *www.effectivehealthcare.ahrq.gov/reports/final.cfm.*

Charach, A., Yeung, E., Climans, T., & Lillie, E. (2011). Childhood attention-deficit/hyperactivity disorder and future substance use disorders: Comparative meta-analyses. *Journal of the American Academy of Child and Adolescent Psychiatry, 50,* 9–21.

Christenson, S. L., & Sheridan, S. M. (2001). *Schools and families: Creating essential connections for learning.* New York: Guilford Press.

Chronis, A. M., Chacko, A., Fabiano, G. A., Wymbs, B. T., & Pelham, W. E. (2004). Enhancements to the behavioral parent training paradigm for families of children with ADHD: Review and future directions. *Clinical Child and Family Psychology Review, 7,* 1–27.

Chronis-Tuscano, A., Molina, B. S. G., Pelham, W. E., Applegate, B., Dahlke, A., Overmyer, A. M., et al. (2010). Very early predictors of adolescent depression and suicide attempts in children with attention-deficit/hyperactivity disorder. *Archives of General Psychiatry, 67,* 1044–1051.

Cipani, E., & Schock, K. M. (2011). *Functional behavioral assessment, diagnosis, and treatment: A complete system for education and mental health settings.* New York: Springer.

Clarfield, J., & Stoner, G. (2005). The effects of computerized reading instruction on the academic performance of students identified with ADHD. *School Psychology Review, 34*(2), 246–254.

Coghill, D., & Sonuga-Barke, E. J. S. (2012). Annual research review: Categories versus dimensions in the classification and conceptualisation of child and adolescent mental disorders-implications of recent empirical study. *Journal of Child Psychology and Psychiatry, 53,* 469–489.

Coles, E. K., Pelham, W. E., Gnagy, E. M., Burrows-Maclean, L., Fabiano, G. A., Chacko, A., et al. (2005). A controlled evaluation of behavioral treatment with children with ADHD attending a summer treatment program. *Journal of Emotional and Behavioral Disorders, 13*(2), 99–112.

Columbia University DISC Development Group. (2000). *C-DISC 4 Young Child Version.* New York: Author.

Cone, J. D. (1986). Idiographic, nomothetic, and related perspectives in behavioral assessment. In R. O. Nelson & S. C. Hayes (Eds.), *Conceptual foundations of behavioral assessment* (pp. 111–128). New York: Guilford Press.

Conners, C. K. (2000). *Conners Continuous Performance Test*. North Tonawanda NY: Multi-Health Systems.

Conners, C. K. (2008). *Conners 3rd edition*. Toronto: Multi-Health Systems.

Conners, C. K., Epstein, J. N., March, J. S., Angold, A., Wells, K. C., Klaric, J., et al. (2001). Multimodal treatment of ADHD in the MTA: An alternative outcome analysis. *Journal of the American Academy of Child and Adolescent Psychiatry, 40*, 159–167.

Connor, D. F. (2006a). Other medications. In R. A. Barkley, *Attention-deficit/hyperactivity disorder: A handbook for diagnosis and treatment (3rd ed.)* (pp. 658–677). New York: Guilford Press.

Connor, D. F. (2006b). Stimulants. In R. A. Barkley, *Attention-deficit/hyperactivity disorder: A handbook for diagnosis and treatment* (3rd ed., pp. 608–647). New York: Guilford Press.

Connor, D. F., Barkley, R. A., & Davis, H. T. (2000). A pilot study of methylphenidate, clonidine, or the combination in ADHD comorbid with aggressive oppositional defiant or conduct disorder. *Clinical Pediatrics, 39*, 15–25.

Connor, D. F., & Doerfler, L. A. (2008). ADHD with comorbid oppositional defiant disorder or conduct disorder: Discrete or nondistinct behavior disorders? *Journal of Attention Disorders, 12*(2), 126–134.

Connor, D. F., Fletcher, K. E., & Swanson, J. M. (1999). A meta-analysis of clonidine for symptoms of attention-deficit/hyperactivity disorder. *Journal of the American Academy of Child and Adolescent Psychiatry, 38*, 1551–1559.

Connor, D. F., Glatt, S. J., Lopez, I. D., Jackson, D., & Melloni, R. H. (2002). Psychopharmacology and aggression, I: A meta-analysis of stimulant effects on overt/covert aggression-related behaviors in ADHD. *Journal of the American Academy of Child and Adolescent Psychiatry, 41*, 253–261.

Connors, L. L., Connolly, J., & Toplak, M. E. (2012). Self-reported inattention in early adolescence in a community sample. *Journal of Attention Disorders, 16*, 60–70.

Cooper, H., Robinson, J. C., & Patall, E. A. (2006). Does homework improve academic achievement?: A synthesis of research 1987–2003. *Review of Educational Research, 76*, 1–62.

Crawford, S. G., Kaplan, B. J., & Dewey, D. (2006). Effects of coexisting disorders on cognition and behavior in children with ADHD. *Journal of Attention Disorders, 10*(2), 192–199.

Crenshaw, T. M., Kavale, K. A., Forness, S. R., & Reeve, R. E. (1999). Attention deficit hyperactivity disorder and the efficacy of stimulant medication: A meta-analysis. In T. Scruggs & M. Mastropieri (Eds.), *Advances in learning and behavioral disabilities* (Vol. 13, pp. 135–165). Stamford, CT: JAI Press.

Cunningham, C. E. (2006). COPE: Large-group, community-based, family-centered parent training. In R. A. Barkley, *Attention-deficit/hyperactivity disorder: A handbook for diagnosis and treatment* (3rd ed., pp. 480–498). New York: Guilford Press.

Cunningham, C. E., & Barkley, R. A. (1979). The interactions of hyperactive and normal children with their mothers during free play and structured task. *Child Development, 50,* 217–224.

Cunningham, C. E., Bremner, R., & Secord, M. (1998). *The Community Parent Education Program: A school-based family systems oriented workshop for parents of children with disruptive behavior disorders.* Hamilton, Ontario, Canada: Hamilton Health Sciences Corporation.

Cunningham, C. E., & Cunningham, L. J. (2006). Student-mediated conflict resolution programs. In R. A. Barkley, *Attention-deficit/hyperactivity disorder: A handbook for diagnosis and treatment* (3rd ed., pp. 590–607). New York: Guilford Press.

Cunningham, C. E., Siegel, L. S., & Offord, D. R. (1985). A developmental dose response analysis of the effects of methylphenidate on the peer interactions of attention deficit disordered boys. *Journal of Child Psychology and Psychiatry, 26,* 955–971.

Dang, M. T., Warrington, D., Tung, T., Baker, D., & Pan, R. J. (2007). A school-based approach to early identification and management of students with ADHD. *Journal of School Nursing, 23,* 2–12.

Dawson, P., & Guare, R. (1998). *Coaching the ADHD student.* North Tonowanda, NY: Multi-Health Systems.

Dawson, P., & Guare, R. (2012). *Coaching students with executive skills deficits.* New York: Guilford Press.

Demaray, M. K., & Elliott, S. N. (2001). Perceived social support by children with characteristics of attention-deficit/hyperactivity disorder. *School Psychology Quarterly, 16,* 68–90.

Demaray, M. K., Schaefer, K., & DeLong, L. K. (2003). Attention-deficit/hyperactivity disorder (ADHD): A national survey of training and current assessment practices in the schools. *Psychology in the Schools, 40,* 583–597.

Deno, S. L. (2002). Problem solving as "best practice." In A. Thomas & J. Grimes (Eds.), *Best practices in school psychology IV* (pp. 37–55). Bethesda, MD: National Association of School Psychologists.

Denton, C. A., & Vaughn, S. (2010). Preventing and remediating reading difficulties: Perspectives from research. In M. R. Shinn & H. M. Walker (Eds.), *Interventions for achievement and behavior problems in a three-tier model including RTI* (pp. 469–500). Bethesda, MD: National Association of School Psychologists.

DeRisi, W. J., & Butz, G. (1975). *Writing behavioral contracts: A case simulation practice manual.* Champaign, IL: Research Press.

Dinkmeyer, D., McKay, G. D., Dinkmeyer, J. S., Dinkmeyer, D., & McKay, J. L. (1997). *Early Childhood Systematic Training for Effective Parenting (STEP).* Circle Pines, MN: American Guidance Services.

DiPerna, J. C., & Elliott, S. N. (2000). *Academic Competence Evaluation Scale.* San Antonio, TX: Psychological Corporation.

Dishion, T. J., & Patterson, G. R. (1997). The timing and severity of antisocial behavior: Three hypotheses within an ecological framework. In D. M. Stoff, J. Breiling, & J. D. Maser (Eds.), *Handbook of antisocial behavior* (pp. 205–217). New York: Wiley.

Dishion, T. J., Patterson, G. R., & Kavanagh, K. A. (1992). An experimental test of the coercion model: Linking theory, measurement, and intervention. In J. McCord & R. E. Tremblay (Eds.), *Preventing antisocial behavior: Interventions from birth through adolescence* (pp. 253–282). New York: Guilford Press.

Dittmann, R. W., Schacht, A., Helsberg, K., Scheider-Fresenius, C., Lehmann, M., Lehmkuhl, G., et al. (2011). Atomoxetine versus placebo in children and adolescents with attention-deficit/hyperactivity disorder and comorbid oppositional defiant disorder: A double-blind, randomized, multicenter trial in Germany. *Journal of Child and Adolescent Psychopharmacology, 21,* 97–110.

Donnelly, C., Bangs, M., Trzepacz, P., Jin, L., Zhang, S., Witte, M. M., et al. (2009). Safety and tolerability of atomoxetine over 3 to 4 years in children and adolescents with ADHD. *Journal of the American Academy of Child and Adolescent Psychiatry, 48,* 176–185.

Donnelly, M., & Rapoport, J. L. (1985). Attention deficit disorders. In J. M. Wiener (Ed.), *Diagnosis and psychopharmacology of childhood and adolescent disorders* (pp. 179–197). New York: Wiley.

Doshi, J. A., Hodgkins, P., Kahle, J., Sikirica, V., Cangelosi, M. J., Setyawan, J., et al. (2012). Economic impact of childhood and adult attention-deficit/hyperactivity disorder in the United States. *Journal of the American Academy of Child and Adolescent Psychiatry, 51,* 990–1002.

Douglas, V. I. (1980). Higher mental processes in hyperactive children: Implications for training. In R. Knights & D. Bakker (Eds.), *Treatment of hyperactive and learning disordered children* (pp. 65–92). Baltimore: University Park Press.

Douglas, V. I., Barr, R. G., O'Neill, M. E., & Britton, B. G. (1986). Short term effects of methylphenidate on the cognitive, learning and academic performance of children with attention deficit disorder in the laboratory and the classroom. *Journal of Child Psychology and Psychiatry, 27,* 191–211.

Dunlap, G., de Perczel, M., Clarke, S., Wilson, D., Wright, S., White, R., & Gomez, A. (1994). Choice making to promote adaptive behavior for students with emotional and behavioral challenges. *Journal of Applied Behavior Analysis, 27,* 505–518.

DuPaul, G. J. (1992). How to assess attention-deficit hyperactivity disorder within school settings. *School Psychology Quarterly, 7,* 45–58.

DuPaul, G. J., Anastopoulos, A. D., Kwasnik, D., Barkley, R. A., & McMurray, M. B. (1996). Methylphenidate effects on children with attention deficit hyperactivity disorder: Self-report of symptoms, side-effects, and self-esteem. *Journal of Attention Disorders, 1,* 3–15.

DuPaul, G. J., Anastopoulos, A. D., Shelton, T. L., Guevremont, D. C., & Metevia, L. (1992). Multimethod assessment of attention-deficit hyperactivity disorder: The diagnostic utility of clinic-based tests. *Journal of Clinical Child Psychology, 21,* 394–402.

DuPaul, G. J., & Barkley, R. A. (1992). Situational variability of attention problems: Psychometric properties of the revised Home and School Situations Questionnaires. *Journal of Clinical Child Psychology, 21*, 178–188.

DuPaul, G. J., Barkley, R. A., & Connor, D. F. (1998). Stimulants. In R. A. Barkley, *Attention-deficit hyperactivity disorder: A handbook for diagnosis and treatment* (2nd ed., pp. 510–551). New York: Guilford Press.

DuPaul, G. J., Barkley, R. A., & McMurray, M. B. (1994). Response of children with ADHD to methylphenidate: Interaction with internalizing symptoms. *Journal of the American Academy of Child and Adolescent Psychiatry, 33*, 894–903.

DuPaul, G. J., & Eckert, T. L. (1994). The effects of social skills curricula: Now you see them, now you don't. *School Psychology Quarterly, 9*, 113–132.

DuPaul, G. J., & Eckert, T. L. (1997). School-based interventions for children with attention-deficit/hyperactivity disorder: A meta-analysis. *School Psychology Review, 26*, 5–27.

DuPaul, G. J., Eckert, T. L., & McGoey, K. E. (1997). Interventions for students with attention-deficit/hyperactivity disorder: One size does not fit all. *School Psychology Review, 26*, 369–381.

DuPaul, G. J., Eckert, T. L., & Vilardo, B. (2012). The effects of school-based interventions for attention deficit hyperactivity disorder: A meta-analysis 1996–2010. *School Psychology Review, 41*, 387–412.

DuPaul, G. J., & Ervin, R. A. (1996). Functional assessment of behaviors related to attention-deficit/hyperactivity disorder: Linking assessment to intervention design. *Behavior Therapy, 27*, 601–622.

DuPaul, G. J., Ervin, R. A., Hook, C. L., & McGoey, K. E. (1998). Peer tutoring for children with attention deficit hyperactivity disorder: Effects on classroom behavior and academic performance. *Journal of Applied Behavior Analysis, 31*, 579–592.

DuPaul, G. J., Gormley, M. J., & Laracy, S. D. (2013). Comorbidity of LD and ADHD: Implications of DSM-5 for assessment and treatment. *Journal of Learning Disabilities, 46*, 43–51.

DuPaul, G. J., Guevremont, D. C., & Barkley, R. A. (1991). Attention-deficit hyperactivity disorder in adolescence: Critical assessment parameters. *Clinical Psychology Review, 11*, 231–245.

DuPaul, G. J., Guevremont, D. C., & Barkley, R. A. (1992). Behavioral treatment of attention-deficit hyperactivity disorder in the classroom: The use of the Attention Training System. *Behavior Modification, 16*, 204–225.

DuPaul, G. J., & Henningson, P. N. (1993). Peer tutoring effects on the classroom performance of children with attention deficit hyperactivity disorder. *School Psychology Review, 22*, 134–143.

DuPaul, G. J., Jitendra, A. K., Volpe, R. J., Tresco, K. E., Lutz, J. G., Vile Junod, R. E., et al. (2006). Consultation-based academic interventions for children with ADHD: Effects on reading and mathematics achievement. *Journal of Abnormal Child Psychology, 34*, 635–648.

DuPaul, G. J., & Kern, L. (2011). *Young children with ADHD: Early identification and intervention.* Washington, DC: American Psychological Association.

DuPaul, G. J., Kern, L., Volpe, R. J., Caskie, G. I. L., Sokol, N., Arbolino, L., et al. (2013). Comparison of parent education and functional assessment-based intervention across 24 months for young children with ADHD. *School Psychology Review, 42,* 56–75.

DuPaul, G. J., McGoey, K. E., Eckert, T. L., & VanBrakle, J. (2001). Preschool children with attention-deficit/hyperactivity disorder: Impairments in behavioral, social, and school functioning. *Journal of the American Academy of Child and Adolescent Psychiatry, 40,* 508–515.

DuPaul, G. J., & Power, T. J. (2000). Educational interventions for students with attention-deficit disorders. In T. E. Brown (Ed.), *Attention-deficit disorders and comorbidities in children, adolescents, and adults* (pp. 607–635). Washington, DC: American Psychiatric Press.

DuPaul, G. J., Power, T. J., Anastopoulos, A. D., & Reid, R. (1998). *ADHD Rating Scale–IV (for Children and Adolescents): Checklists, norms, and clinical interpretation.* New York: Guilford Press.

DuPaul, G. J., & Rapport, M. D. (1993). Does methylphenidate normalize the classroom performance of children with attention deficit disorder? *Journal of the American Academy of Child and Adolescent Psychiatry, 32,* 190–198.

DuPaul, G. J., Rapport, M. D., & Perriello, L. M. (1991). Teacher ratings of academic skills: The development of the Academic Performance Rating Scale. *School Psychology Review, 20,* 284–300.

DuPaul, G. J., & Stoner, G. (2010). Interventions for attention-deficit hyperactivity disorder. In H. M. Walker & M. R. Shinn (Eds.), *Interventions for achievement and behavior in a three-tier model including RTI* (3rd ed., pp. 825–848). Bethesda, MD: National Association of School Psychologists.

DuPaul, G. J., Stoner, G., & O'Reilly, M. J. (2008). Best practices in classroom interventions for attention problems. In A. Thomas & J. Grimes (Eds.), *Best practices in school psychology* (5th ed., pp. 1421–1437). Bethesda, MD: National Association of School Psychologists.

DuPaul, G. J., Weyandt, L. L., O'Dell, S. M., & Varejao, M. (2009). College students with ADHD: Current status and future directions. *Journal of Attention Disorders, 13,* 234–250.

DuPaul, G. J., Weyandt, L. L., Rossi, J. S., Vilardo, B. A., O'Dell, S. M., Carson, K. M., et al. (2012). Double-blind, placebo-controlled, crossover study of the efficacy and safety of lisdexamfetamine dimesylate in college students with ADHD. *Journal of Attention Disorders, 16*(3), 202–220.

Dyer, K., Dunlap, G., & Winterling, V. (1990). Effects of choice making on the serious problem behaviors of students with severe handicaps. *Journal of Applied Behavior Analysis, 23,* 515–524.

Eckert, T. L., DuPaul, G. J., McGoey, K. E., & Volpe, R. J. (2002). *Young children at-risk for attention-deficit/hyperactivity disorder: A needs assessment of parents, community service providers, and experts.* Unpublished manuscript, Lehigh University, Bethlehem, PA.

Eddy, J. M., Reid, J. B., & Curry, V. (2002). The etiology of youth antisocial behavior, delinquency, and violence and a public health approach to prevention. In M. R. Shinn, H. M. Walker, & G. Stoner (Eds.), *Interventions for academic and behavior problems, II: Preventive and remedial approaches* (pp. 27–51). Bethesda, MD: National Association of School Psychologists.

Edwards, G., Barkley, R. A., Laneri, M., Fletcher, K., & Metevia, L. (2001). Parent–adolescent conflict in teenagers with ADHD and ODD. *Journal of Abnormal Child Psychology, 29,* 557–572.

Egger, H. L., Kondo, D., & Angold, A. (2006). The epidemiology and diagnostic issues in preschool attention-deficit/hyperactivity disorder: A review. *Infants and Young Children, 19,* 109–122.

Elia, J., & Rapoport, J. L. (1991). Ritalin versus dextroamphetamine in ADHD: Both should be tried. In L. L. Greenhill & B. B. Osman (Eds.), *Ritalin: Theory and patient management* (pp. 69–74). New York: Liebert.

Epstein, J. L. (1986). Parents' reactions to teacher practices of parent involvement. *Elementary School Journal, 86,* 277–294.

Epstein, J. N., Erkanli, A., Conners, C. K., Klaric, J., Costello, J. E., & Angold, A. (2003). Relations between continuous performance test performance measures and ADHD behaviors. *Journal of Abnormal Child Psychology, 31,* 543–544.

Epstein, J. N., Langberg, J. M., Lichtenstein, P. K., Kolb, R., Altaye, M., & Simon, J. O. (2011). Use of an Internet portal to improve community-based pediatric ADHD care: A cluster randomized trial. *Pediatrics, 128,* e1201–e1208.

Ervin, R. A., DuPaul, G. J., Kern, L., & Friman, P. C. (1998). Classroom-based functional and adjunctive assessments: Proactive approaches to intervention selection for adolescents with attention deficit hyperactivity disorder. *Journal of Applied Behavior Analysis, 31,* 65–78.

Ervin, R. A., Ehrhardt, K. E., & Poling, A. (2001). Functional assessment: Old wine in new bottles. *School Psychology Review, 30,* 173–179.

Escobar, R., Montoya, A., Polavieja, P., Cardo, E., Artigas, J., Hervas, A., et al. (2009). Evaluation of patients' and parents' quality of life in a randomized placebo-controlled atomoxetine study in attention-deficit/hyperactivity disorder. *Journal of Child and Adolescent Psychopharmacology, 19,* 253–263.

Evans, R. W., Gualtieri, C. T., & Amara, I. (1986). Methylphenidate and memory: Dissociated effects in hyperactive children. *Psychopharmacology, 90,* 211–216.

Evans, S. W., Allen, J., Moore, S., & Strauss, V. (2005). Measuring symptoms and functioning of youth with ADHD in middle schools. *Journal of Abnormal Child Psychology, 33,* 695–706.

Evans, S. W. Axelrod, J. L., & Langberg, J. (2004). Efficacy of a school-based treatment program for middle school youth with ADHD: Pilot data. *Behavior Modification, 28,* 528–547.

Evans, S. W., Owens, J. S., & Bunford, N. (in press). Evidence-based psychosocial treatments for children and adolescents with attention-deficit/hyperactivity disorder. *Journal of Clinical Child and Adolescent Psychology.*

Evans, S. W., Owens, J. S., Mautone, J. A., DuPaul, G. J., & Power, T. J. (2014). Toward a comprehensive, life course model of care for youth with ADHD. In M. Weist, N. Lever, C. Bradshaw, & J. S. Owens (Eds.), *Handbook of school mental health* (2nd ed., pp. 413–426). New York: Springer.

Evans, S. W., & Pelham, W. E. (1991). Psychostimulant effects on academic and behavioral measures for ADHD junior high school students in a lecture format classroom. *Journal of Abnormal Child Psychology, 19,* 537–552.

Evans, S. W., Pelham, W. E., Smith, B. H., Bukstein, O., Gnagy, E. M., Greiner, A. R., et al. (2001). Dose–response effects of methylphenidate on ecologically valid measures of academic performance and classroom behavior in adolescents with ADHD. *Experimental and Clinical Psychopharmacology, 9,* 163–175.

Evans, S., Schultz, B., DeMars, C., & Davis, H. (2011). Effectiveness of the Challenging Horizons after-school program for young adolescents with ADHD. *Behavior Therapy, 42,* 462–474.

Evans, S. W., Schultz, B. K., Casey White, L., Brady, C., Sibley, M. H., & Van Eck, K. (2009). A school-based organization intervention for young adolescents with attention deficit/hyperactivity disorder. *School Mental Health, 1*(2), 78–88.

Evans, S. W., Serpell, Z. N., Schultz, B. K., & Pastor, D. A. (2007). Cumulative benefits of secondary school-based treatment of students with attention deficit hyperactivity disorder. *School Psychology Review, 36,* 256–273.

Eyberg, S. M., Funderburk, B. W., Hembree-Kigin, T. L., McNeil, C. B., Querido, J. G., & Hood, K. K. (2001). Parent–child interaction therapy with behavior problem children: One and two year maintenance of treatment effects in the family. *Child and Family Behavior Therapy, 23,* 1–20.

Eyberg, S. M., Nelson, M. M., & Boggs, S. R. (2008). Evidence-based psychosocial treatments for children and adolescents with disruptive behavior. *Journal of Clinical Child and Adolescent Psychology, 37,* 215–237.

Fabiano, G. A., Pelham, W. E. Jr., Coles, E. K., Gnagy, E. M., Chronis-Tuscano, A., & O'Connor, B. C. (2009). A meta-analysis of behavioral treatments for attention-deficit/hyperactivity disorder. *Clinical Psychology Review, 29,* 29–140.

Fabiano, G. A., Pelham, W. E., Gnagy, E. M., Kipp, H., Lahey, B. B., Burrows-MacLean, L., et al. (1999, November). *The reliability and validity of the Children's Impairment Rating Scale: A practical measure of impairment in children with ADHD.* Poster presented at the annual meeting of the Association for the Advancement of Behavior Therapy, Toronto, Ontario, Canada.

Fabiano, G. A., Pelham, W. E., Jr., Gnagy, E. M., Burrows-MacLean, L., Coles, E. K., Chacko, A., et al. (2007). The single and combined effects of multiple intensities of behavior modification and methylphenidate for children with attention deficit hyperactivity disorder. *School Psychology Review, 36,* 195–216.

Fabiano, G. A., Pelham, W. E., Jr., Manos, M. J., Gnagy, E. M., Chronis, A. M., Onyango, A. N., et al. (2004). An evaluation of three time-out procedures for children with attention deficit/hyperactivity disorder. *Behavior Therapy, 35,* 449–469.

Fabiano, G. A., Pelham, W. E., Jr., Waschbusch, D. A., Gnagy, E. M., Lahey, B. B., Chronis, A. M., et al. (2006). A practical measure of impairment: Psychometric properties of the Impairment Rating Scale in samples of children with attention deficit hyperactivity disorder and two school-based samples. *Journal of Clinical Child and Adolescent Psychology, 35,* 369–385.

Faraone, S. V., Biederman, J., Krifcher, B., Lehmann, B., Keenan, K., Norman, D., et al. (1993). Evidence for the independent familial transmission of attention deficit hyperactivity disorder and learning disabilities: Results from a family genetic study. *American Journal of Psychiatry, 150,* 891–895.

Faraone, S. V., Biederman, J., Weber, W., & Russell, R. L. (1998). Psychiatric, neuropsychological, and psychosocial features of DSM-IV subtypes of attention-deficit/hyperactivity disorder: Results from a clinically referred sample. *Journal of the American Academy of Child and Adolescent Psychiatry, 37,* 185–193.

Faraone, S. V., & Buitelaar, J. (2010). Comparing the efficacy of stimulants for ADHD in children and adolescents using meta-analysis. *European Child and Adolescent Psychiatry, 19,* 353–364.

Faraone, S. V., & Glatt, S. J. (2010). Effects of extended-release guanfacine on ADHD symptoms and sedation-related adverse events in children with ADHD. *Journal of Attention Disorders, 13,* 532–538.

Feil, E. G., Walker, H. M., & Severson, H. H. (1995). Young children with behavior problems: Research and development of the Early Screening Project. *Journal of Emotional and Behavioral Disorders, 3,* 194–202.

Feingold, B. F. (1975). Hyperkinesis and learning disabilities linked to artificial food flavors and colors. *American Journal of Nursing, 75,* 797–803.

Fergusson, D. M., & Horwood, L. J. (1995). Early disruptive behavior, IQ, and later school achievement and delinquent behavior. *Journal of Abnormal Child Psychology, 23,* 183–199.

Fergusson, D. M., Horwood, L. J., & Lynskey, M. T. (1993). The effects of conduct disorder and attention deficit in middle childhood on offending and scholastic ability at age 13. *Journal of Child Psychology and Psychiatry, 34,* 899–916.

Fergusson, D. M., Lynskey, M. T., & Horwood, L. J. (1997). Attentional difficulties in middle childhood and psychosocial outcomes in young adulthood. *Journal of Child Psychology and Psychiatry, 38,* 633–644.

Fielding, L. T., Murphy, R. J., Reagan, M. W., & Peterson, T. L. (1980). An assessment program to reduce drug use with the mentally retarded. *Hospital and Community Psychiatry, 31,* 771–773.

Finn, C. A., & Sladeczek, I. E. (2001). Assessing the social validity of behavioral interventions: A review of treatment acceptability measures. *School Psychology Quarterly, 16,* 176–206.

Fischer, M. (1990). Parenting stress and the child with attention deficit hyperactivity disorder. *Journal of Clinical Child Psychology, 19,* 337–346.

Flood, W. A., & Wilder, D. A. (2002). Antecedent assessment and assessment-based treatment of off-task behavior in a child diagnosed with attention deficit hyperactivity disorder (ADHD). *Education and Treatment of Children, 25,* 331–338.

Floyd, R. G., Hojnoski, R. L., & Key, J. M. (2006). Preliminary evidence of technical adequacy of the Preschool Numeracy Indicators. *School Psychology Review, 35,* 627–644.

Forness, S. R., & Kavale, K. A. (2001). ADHD and a return to the medical model of special education. *Education and Treatment of Children, 24*, 224–247.

Forness, S. R., Kavale, K. A., Sweeney, D. P., & Crenshaw, T. M. (1999). The future of research and practice in behavioral disorders: Psychopharmacology and its school treatment implications. *Behavioral Disorders, 24*, 305–318.

Frazier, T. W., Demaree, H. A., & Youngstrom, E. A. (2004). Meta-analysis of intellectual and neuropsychological test performance in attention-deficit/hyperactivity disorder. *Neuropsychology, 18*, 543–555.

Frazier, T. W., Youngstrom, E. A., Glutting, J. J., & Watkins, M. (2007). ADHD and achievement: Meta-analysis of the child, adolescent, and young adult literatures and a concomitant study with college students. *Journal of Learning Disabilities, 40*, 49–65.

Frick, P. J., Kamphaus, R. W., Lahey, B. B., Loeber, R., Christ, M. A. G., Hart, E. L., et al. (1991). Academic underachievement and the disruptive behavior disorders. *Journal of Consulting and Clinical Psychology, 59*, 289–294.

Froehlich, T. E., Lamphear, B. P., Epstein, J. N., Barbaresi, W. J., Katusic, S. K., & Kahn, R. S. (2007). Prevalence, recognition, and treatment of attention-deficit/hyperactivity disorder in a national sample of U.S. children. *Archives of Pediatric and Adolescent Medicine, 161*, 857–864.

Gadow, K. D. (1993). A school-based medication evaluation program. In J. L. Matson (Ed.), *Handbook of hyperactivity in children* (pp. 186–219). Boston: Allyn & Bacon.

Gadow, K. D., Nolan, E. E., Paolicelli, L. M., & Sprafkin, J. (1991). A procedure for assessing the effects of methylphenidate on hyperactive children in public school settings. *Journal of Clinical Child Psychology, 20*, 268–276.

Gadow, K. D., Nolan, E. E., Sverd, J., Sprafkin, J., & Paolicelli, L. (1990). Methylphenidate in aggressive-hyperactive boys: I. Effects on peer aggression in public school settings. *Journal of the American Academy of Child and Adolescent Psychiatry, 29*, 710–718.

Gadow, K. D., & Sprafkin, J. (2010). *Early Childhood Inventory–4R: Norms manual.* Stony Brook, NY: Checkmate Plus.

Gadow, K. D., Sprafkin, J., Carlson, C. A., Schneider, J., Nolan, E. E., Mattison, R. E., et al. (2002). A DSM-IV-referenced, adolescent self-report rating scale. *Journal of the American Academy of Child and Adolescent Psychiatry, 41*, 671–679.

Gadow, K. D., Sprafkin, J., & Nolan, E. E. (1996). *ADHD School Observation Code.* Stony Brook, NY: Checkmate Plus.

Gadow, K. D., Sverd, J., Nolan, E. E., Sprafkin, J., & Schneider, J. (2007). Immediate-release methylphenidate for ADHD in children with comorbid chronic multiple tic disorder. *Journal of the American Academy of Child and Adolescent Psychiatry, 46*, 840–848.

Galéra, C., Melchior, M., Chastang, J. F., Bouvard, M. P., & Fombonne, E. (2009). Childhood and adolescent hyperactivity–inattention symptoms and academic achievement 8 years later: The GAZEL Youth Study. *Psychological Medicine, 39*, 1895–1906.

Galéra, C., Messiah, A., Melchior, M., Chastang, J., Encrenaz, G., Lagarde, E., et al. (2010). Disruptive behaviors and early sexual intercourse: The GAZEL Youth Study. *Psychiatry Research, 177,* 361–363.

Garmezy, N. (1978). DSM-III. Never mind the psychologists: Is it good for the children? *Clinical Psychologist, 31,* 1–6.

Gaub, M., & Carlson, C. L. (1997). Gender differences in ADHD: A meta-analysis and critical review. *Journal of the American Academy of Child and Adolescent Psychiatry, 36,* 1036–1045.

Gersten, R., Fuchs, L. S., Williams, J. P., & Baker, S. (2001). Teaching reading comprehension strategies to students with learning disabilities: A review of research. *Review of Educational Research, 71*(2), 279–320.

Gersten, R., Jordan, N. C., & Flojo, J. R. (2005). Early identification and interventions for students with mathematics difficulties. *Journal of Learning Disabilities, 38,* 293–304.

Ghuman, J. K., Arnold, L. E., & Anthony, B. J. (2008). Psychopharmacological and other treatments in preschool children with attention-deficit/hyperactivity disorder: Current evidence and practice. *Journal of Child and Adolescent Psychopharmacology, 18,* 413–447.

Ginsburg-Block, M. D., Rohrbeck, C. A., & Fantuzzo, J. W. (2006). A meta-analytic review of the social, self-concept, and behavioral conduct outcomes of peer assisted learning. *Journal of Educational Psychology, 98,* 732–749.

Gioia, G. A., Isquith, P. K., Guy, S. C., & Kenworthy, L. (2000). *Behavioral Rating Inventory of Executive Function.* Lutz, FL: Psychological Assessment Resources.

Gittelman, R., Mannuzza, S., Shenker, R., & Bonagura, N. (1985). Hyperactive boys almost grown up. *Archives of General Psychiatry, 42,* 937–947.

Gleason, M. M., Archer, A. L., & Colvin, G. (2010). Study skills: Making the invisible visible. In M. R. Shinn & H. M. Walker (Eds.), *Interventions for achievement and behavior problems in a three-tier model including RTI* (pp. 571–607). Bethesda, MD: National Association of School Psychologists.

Golden, S. M. (2009). Does childhood use of stimulant medication as a treatment for ADHD affect the likelihood of future drug abuse and dependence?: A literature review. *Journal of Child and Adolescent Substance Abuse, 18,* 343–358.

Goldstein, S., & Goldstein, M. (1998). *Managing attention deficit hyperactivity disorder in children: A guide for practitioners* (2nd ed.). New York: Wiley.

Gordon, M. (1983). *The Gordon diagnostic system.* DeWitt, NY: Gordon Systems.

Gordon, M. (1986). How is a computerized attention test used in the diagnosis of attention deficit disorder? *Journal of Children in Contemporary Society, 19,* 53–64.

Graham, S., MacArthur, C. A., & Fitzgerald, J. (2013). *Best practices in writing instruction* (2nd ed.). New York: Guilford Press.

Graham-Day, K. J., Gardner, R., III, & Hsin, Y. W. (2010). Increasing on-task behaviors of high school students with attention deficit hyperactivity disorder: Is it enough? *Education and Treatment of Children, 33,* 205–221.

Grauvogel-MacAleese, A. N., & Wallace, M. D. (2010). Use of peer-mediated intervention in children with attention deficit hyperactivity disorder. *Journal of Applied Behavior Analysis, 43*, 547–551.

Greene, R. W., Beszterczey, S. K., Katzenstein, T., Park, K., & Goring, J. (2002). Are students with ADHD more stressful to teach?: Patterns of teacher stress in an elementary school sample. *Journal of Emotional and Behavioral Disorders, 10*, 79–89.

Greene, R. W., Biederman, J., Faraone, S. V., Ouellette, C. A., Penn, C., & Griffin, S. (1996). Toward a new psychometric definition of social disability in children with attention-deficit hyperactivity disorder. *Journal of the American Academy of Child and Adolescent Psychiatry, 35*, 571–578.

Greenhill, L., Kollins, S., Abikoff, H., McCracken, J., Riddle, M., Swanson, J., et al. (2006). Efficacy and safety of immediate-release methylphenidate treatment for preschoolers with ADHD. *Journal of the American Academy of Child and Adolescent Psychiatry, 45*, 1284–1293.

Greenhill, L. L. (1984). Stimulant related growth inhibition in children: A review. In L. Greenhill & B. Shopsin (Eds.), *The psychobiology of childhood* (pp. 135–157). New York: Spectrum.

Greenwood, C. R., Delquadri, J., & Carta, J. J. (1988). *Classwide peer tutoring.* Seattle, WA: Educational Achievement Systems.

Greenwood, C. R., Maheady, L., & Delquadri, J. (2002). Classwide peer tutoring programs. In M. R. Shinn, H. M. Walker, & G. Stoner (Eds.), *Interventions for academic and behavior problems, II: Preventive and remedial approaches* (pp. 611–649). Bethesda, MD: National Association of School Psychologists.

Greenwood, C. R., Seals, K., & Kamps, D. (2010). Peer teaching interventions for multiple levels of support. In M. R. Shinn & H. M. Walker (Eds.), *Interventions for achievement and behavior problems in a three-tier model including RTI* (pp. 633–675). Bethesda, MD: National Association of School Psychologists.

Gregory, R. J. (1996). *Psychological testing: History, principles, and applications* (2nd ed). Boston: Allyn & Bacon.

Gresham, F. M. (1989). Assessment of treatment integrity in school consultation and prereferral intervention. *School Psychology Review, 18*, 37–50.

Gresham, F. M. (1991). Conceptualizing behavior disorders in terms of resistance to intervention. *School Psychology Review, 20*, 23–36.

Gresham, F. M. (2009). Evolution of the treatment integrity concept: Current status and future directions. *School Psychology Review, 38*(4), 533–540.

Gresham, F. M., & Elliott, S. N. (2008). *Social Skills Improvement System.* Minneapolis, MN: Pearson Assessments.

Gresham, F. M., & Gansle, K. A. (1992). Misguided assumptions of DSM-III-R: Implications for school psychological practice. *School Psychology Quarterly, 7*, 79–95.

Gresham, F. M., Gansle, K. A., Noell, G. H., Cohen, S., & Rosenblum, S. (1993). Treatment integrity of school-based behavioral intervention studies: 1980–1990. *School Psychology Review, 22*, 254–272.

Gresham, F. M., Watson, T. S., & Skinner, C. H. (2001). Functional behavioral assessment: Principles, procedures, and future directions. *School Psychology Review, 30,* 156–172.

Griffin, S. A., Case, R., & Siegler, R. S. (1994). Rightstart: Providing the central conceptual prerequisites for first formal learning of arithmetic to students at risk for school failure. In K. McGilly (Ed.), *Classroom lessons: Integrating cognitive theory and classroom practice* (pp. 25–49). Cambridge, MA: MIT Press.

Grossen, B., & Carnine, D. (1991). Strategies for maximizing reading success in the regular classroom. In G. Stoner, M. R. Shinn, & H. M. Walker (Eds.), *Interventions for achievement and behavior problems* (pp. 333–355). Silver Spring, MD: National Association of School Psychologists.

Guevara, J., Lozano, P., Wickizer, T., Mell, L., & Gephart, H. (2001). Utilization and cost of health care services for children with attention-deficit/hyperactivity disorder. *Pediatrics, 108,* 71–78.

Gureasko-Moore, D. P., DuPaul, G. J., & Power, T. J. (2005). Stimulant treatment for attention-deficit/hyperactivity disorder: Medication monitoring practices of school psychologists. *School Psychology Review, 34,* 232–245.

Gureasko-Moore, S., DuPaul, G., & White, G. (2007). Self-management of classroom preparedness and homework: Effects on school functioning of adolescents with attention-deficit hyperactivity disorder. *School Psychology Review, 36,* 647–664.

Gureasko-Moore, S., DuPaul, G. J., & White, G. P. (2006). The effects of self-management in general education classrooms on the organizational skills of adolescents with ADHD. *Behavior Modification, 30,* 159–183.

Hakola, S. (1992). Legal rights of students with attention deficit disorder. *School Psychology Quarterly, 7,* 285–297.

Handler, M. W., & DuPaul, G. J. (2002). Diagnosis of childhood ADHD: Differences across psychology specialty areas. *ADHD Report, 10*(3), 7–9.

Hansen, D. L., & Hansen, E. H. (2006). Caught in a balancing act: Parents' dilemmas regarding their ADHD child's treatment with stimulant medication. *Qualitative Health Research, 16,* 1267–1285.

Harris, K. R., & Graham, S. (1996). *Making the writing process work: Strategies for composition and self-regulation.* Cambridge MA: Brookline Books.

Harrison, J. R., Bunford, N., Evans, S. W., & Owens, J. S. (2013). Educational accommodations for students with behavioral challenges: A systematic review of the literature. *Review of Educational Research, 83,* 551–597.

Harrison, J. R., Vannest, K., Davis, J., & Reynolds, C. (2012). Common problem behaviors of children and adolescents in general education classrooms in the United States. *Journal of Emotional and Behavioral Disorders, 20,* 55–64.

Harrison, J. R., Vannest, K. J., & Reynolds, C. R. (2011). Behaviors that discriminate ADHD in children and adolescents: Primary symptoms, symptoms of comorbid conditions, or indicators of functional impairment? *Journal of Attention Disorders, 15*(2), 147–160.

Hart, B., & Risley, T. R. (1995). *Meaningful differences in the everyday experience of young American children.* Baltimore: Brookes.

Harty, S. C., Ivanov, I., Newcorn, J. H., & Halperin, J. M. (2011). The impact of conduct disorder and stimulant medication on later substance use in an ethnically diverse sample of individuals with attention-deficit/hyperactivity disorder in childhood. *Journal of Child and Adolescent Psychopharmacology, 21,* 331–339.

Harty, S. C., Miller, C. J., Newcorn, J. H., & Halperin, J. M. (2009). Adolescents with childhood ADHD and comorbid disruptive behavior disorders: Aggression, anger, and hostility. *Child Psychiatry Human Development, 40,* 85–97.

Haynes, S. N. (1986). The design of intervention programs. In R. O. Nelson & S. C. Hayes (Eds.), *Conceptual foundations of behavioral assessment* (pp. 386–429). New York: Guilford Press.

Haynes, S. N., Mumma, G. H., & Pinson, C. (2009). Idiographic assessment: Conceptual and psychometric foundations of individualized behavioral assessment. *Clinical Psychology Review, 29,* 179–191.

Hazell, P. L., Kohn, M. R., Dickson, R., Walton, R. J., Granger, R. E., & van Wyk, G. W. (2011). Core ADHD symptom improvement with atomoxetine versus methylphenidate: A direct comparison meta-analysis. *Journal of Attention Disorders, 15,* 674–683.

Healey, D. M., Miller, C. J., Castelli, K. L., Marks, D. J., & Halperin, J. M. (2008). The impact of impairment criteria on rates of ADHD diagnoses in preschoolers. *Journal of Abnormal Child Psychology, 36,* 771–778.

Heaton, R. K., Chelune, G. J., Talley, J. L., Kay, G. G., & Curtiss, G. (1993). *Wisconsin Card Sorting Test manual.* Odessa, FL: Psychological Assessment Resources.

Heiligenstein, E., & Keeling, R. P. (1995). Presentation of unrecognized attention deficit hyperactivity disorder in college students. *Journal of American College Health, 43*(5), 226–228.

Hinshaw, S. P. (1991). Stimulant medication and the treatment of aggression in children with attentional deficits. *Journal of Clinical Child Psychology, 20,* 301–312.

Hinshaw, S. P. (1992). Academic underachievement, attention deficits, and aggression: Comorbidity and implications for intervention. *Journal of Consulting and Clinical Psychology, 60,* 893–903.

Hinshaw, S. P., Henker, B., & Whalen, C. K. (1984). Self-control in hyperactive boys in anger-inducing situations: Effects of cognitive-behavioral training and of methylphenidate. *Journal of Abnormal Child Psychology, 12,* 55–77.

Hinshaw, S. P., Henker, B., Whalen, C. K., Erhardt, D., & Dunnington, R. E., Jr. (1989). Aggressive, prosocial, and nonsocial behavior in hyperactive boys: Dose effects of methylphenidate in naturalistic settings. *Journal of Consulting and Clinical Psychology, 57,* 636–643.

Hinshaw, S. P., & Melnick, S. (1992). Self-management therapies and attention-deficit hyperactivity disorder: Reinforced self-evaluation and anger control interventions. *Behavior Modification, 16,* 253–273.

Hinshaw, S. P., Owens, E. B., Sami, N., & Fargeon, S. (2006). Prospective follow-up of girls with attention-deficit/hyperactivity disorder into adolescence: Evidence for continuing cross-domain impairment. *Journal of Consulting and Clinical Psychology, 74*(3), 489–499.

Hinshaw, S. P., Owens, E. B., Zalecki, C., Huggins, S. P., Montenegro-Nevado, A. J., Schrodek, E., et al. (2012). Prospective follow-up of girls with attention-deficit/hyperactivity disorder into early adulthood: Continuing impairment includes elevated risk for suicide attempts and self-injury. *Journal of Consulting and Clinical Psychology, 80,* 1041–1051.

Hinshaw, S. P., Zupan, B. A., Simmel, C., Nigg, J. T., & Melnick, S. (1997). Peer status in boys with and without attention-deficit hyperactivity disorder: Predictions from overt and covert antisocial behavior, social isolation, and authoritative parenting beliefs. *Child Development, 68,* 880–896.

Hodgens, J. B., Cole, J., & Boldizar, J. (2000). Peer-based differences among boys with ADHD. *Journal of Clinical Child Psychology, 29,* 443–452.

Hoff, K., & DuPaul, G. J. (1998). Reducing disruptive behavior in general education classrooms: The use of self-management strategies. *School Psychology Review, 27,* 290–303.

Hojnoski, R. L., Silberglitt, B., & Floyd, R. G. (2009). Sensitivity to growth over time of the Preschool Numeracy Indicators with a sample of preschoolers in Head Start. *School Psychology Review, 38,* 402–418.

Hook, C. L., & DuPaul, G. J. (1999). Parent tutoring for students with attention deficit hyperactivity disorder: Effects on reading at home and school. *School Psychology Review, 28,* 60–75.

Horner, R. H., Salentine, S., & Albin, R. W. (2003). Self-assessment of contextual fit in school (rating scale). Retrieved from *www.pbis.org.*

Houghton, S., Alsalmi, N., Tan, C., Taylor, M., & Durkin, K. (in press). Treating comorbid anxiety in adolescents with ADHD using a cognitive behavior therapy program. *Journal of Attention Disorders.*

Hoza, B., Pelham, W. E., Dobbs, J., Owens, J. S., & Pillow, D. R. (2002). Do boys with attention-deficit/hyperactivity disorder have positive illusory self-concepts? *Journal of Abnormal Psychology, 111,* 268–278.

Hoza, B., Pelham, W. E., Sams, S. E., & Carlson, C. (1992). An examination of the "dosage" effects of both behavior therapy and methylphenidate on the classroom performance of two ADHD children. *Behavior Modification, 16,* 164–192.

Huff, K. E., & Robinson, S. L. (2002). Best practices in peer-mediated interventions. In A. Thomas & J. Grimes (Eds.), *Best practices in school psychology IV* (pp. 1555–1567). Bethesda, MD: National Association of School Psychologists.

Hunt, R. D., Mindera, R. B., & Cohen, D. J. (1985). Clonidine benefits children with attention deficit disorder and hyperactivity: Report of a double-blind placebo-crossover therapeutic trial. *Journal of the American Academy of Child and Adolescent Psychiatry, 24,* 617–629.

Imeraj, L., Antrop, I., Sonuga-Barke, E., Deboutte, D., Deschepper, E., Bal, S., et al. (2013). The impact of instructional context on classroom on-task behavior: A matched comparison of children with ADHD and non-ADHD classmates. *Journal of School Psychology, 51,* 487–498.

Individuals with Disabilities Education Improvement Act. (2004). Public Law 108-446.

Ingersoll, B., & Goldstein, S. (1993). *Attention deficit disorder and learning disabilities: Realities, myths, and controversial treatments.* New York: Doubleday.

Invernizzi, M., Sullivan, A., & Meier, J. (2001). *Phonological Awareness Literacy Screening for Preschool.* Charlottesville, VA: University Press.

Jacob, R. G., O'Leary, K. D., & Rosenblad, C. (1978). Formal and informal classroom settings: Effects on hyperactivity. *Journal of Abnormal Child Psychology, 6,* 47–59.

Jacob, S., Decker, D. M., & Hartshorne, T. S. (2011). *Ethics and law for school psychologists* (6th ed.). Hoboken, NJ: Wiley.

Jacobsen, N. S., & Truax, P. (1991). Clinical significance: A statistical approach to defining meaningful change in psychotherapy research. *Journal of Consulting and Clinical Psychology, 59,* 12–19.

Jacobson, L. T., & Reid, R. (2010). Improving the persuasive essay writing of high school students with ADHD. *Exceptional Children, 76,* 157–174.

James, R. S., Sharp, W. S., Bastain, T. M., Lee, P. P., Walter, J. M., Czarnolewski, M., et al. (2001). Double-blind, placebo-controlled study of single-dose amphetamine formulations in ADHD. *Journal of the American Academy of Child and Adolescent Psychiatry, 40,* 1268–1276.

Jarrett, M. A., & Ollendick, T. H. (2008). A conceptual review of the comorbidity of attention-deficit/hyperactivity disorder and anxiety: Implications for future research and practice. *Clinical Psychology Review, 28,* 1266–1280.

Jarrett, M. A., & Ollendick, T. H. (2012). Treatment of comorbid attention-deficit/hyperactivity disorder and anxiety in children: A multiple baseline design analysis. *Journal of Consulting and Clinical Psychology, 80(2),* 239–244.

Jensen, P. S., Arnold, L. E., Swanson, J. M., Vitiello, B., Abikoff, H. B., Greenhill, L. L., et al. (2007). 3-year follow-up of the NIMH MTA study. *Journal of the American Academy of Child and Adolescent Psychiatry, 46,* 989–1002.

Jensen, P. S., Martin, D., & Cantwell, D. P. (1997). Comorbidity in ADHD: Implications for research, practice, and DSM-V. *Journal of the American Academy of Child and Adolescent Psychiatry, 36,* 1065–1079.

Jimerson, S. R., Burns, M. K., & VanDerHeyden, A. M. (Eds.). (2007). *Handbook of response to intervention: The science and practice of assessment and intervention.* New York: Springer.

Jitendra, A. K., DuPaul, G. J., Someki, F., & Tresco, K. E. (2008). Enhancing academic achievement for chidren with attention deficit hyperactivity disorder: Evidence from school-based intervention research. *Developmental Disabilities Research Reviews, 14,* 325–330.

Johnson, J. W., Reid, R., & Mason, L. H. (2012). Improving the reading recall of high school students with ADHD. *Remedial and Special Education, 33,* 258–268.

Johnson, R. C., & Rosén, L. A. (2000). Sports behavior of ADHD children. *Journal of Attention Disorders, 4,* 150–160.

Johnston, C., & Mash, E. J. (2001). Families of children with attention-deficit/ hyperactivity disorder: Review and recommendations for future research. *Clinical Child and Family Psychology Review, 4,* 183–207.

Johnston, C., Pelham, W. E., Hoza, J., & Sturges, J. (1987). Psychostimulant rebound in attention deficit disordered boys. *Journal of the American Academy of Child and Adolescent Psychiatry, 27*, 806–810.

Kaiser Permanente Center for Health Research. (2013). *Adolescents coping with depression course.* Retrieved from *www.kpchr.org/research/public/acwd/acwd.html.*

Kaminski, R. A., & Good, R. H. (1996). Toward a technology for assessing basic early literacy skills. *School Psychology Review, 25*, 215–227.

Karustis, J. L., Power, T. J., Rescorla, L. A., Eiraldi, R. B., & Gallagher, P. R. (2000). Anxiety and depression in children with ADHD: Unique associations with academic and social functioning. *Journal of Attention Disorders, 4*, 133–149.

Kavale, K. A., & Mattson, P. D. (1983). One jumped off the balance beam: Meta-analysis of perceptual-motor training. *Journal of Learning Disabilities, 16*, 165–173.

Kazdin, A. E. (1992). *Research design in clinical psychology* (2nd ed.). Boston: Allyn & Bacon.

Kazdin, A. E. (2000). *Psychotherapy for children and adolescents: Directions for research and practice.* London: Oxford University Press.

Kazdin, A. E. (2011). *Single-case research designs: Methods for clinical and applied settings* (2nd ed.). New York: Oxford University Press.

Keenan, K., Shaw, D. S., Walsh, B., Deliquadri, E., & Giovanelli, J. (1997). DSM-III-R disorders in preschool children from low-income families. *Journal of the American Academy of Child and Adolescent Psychiatry, 36*, 620–627.

Kelley, M. L. (1990). *School–home notes: Promoting children's classroom success.* New York: Guilford Press.

Kelly, K. (2001). *An assessment of the peer relationships of elementary school children diagnosed with attention deficit hyperactivity disorder.* Unpublished doctoral dissertation, Lehigh University, Bethlehem, PA.

Kelsey, D. K., Sumner, C. R., Casat, C. D., Coury, D. L., Quintana, H., Saylor, K. E., et al. (2004). Once-daily atomoxetine treatment for children with attention-deficit/hyperactivity disorder, including an assessment of evening and morning behavior: A double-blind, placebo-controlled trial. *Pediatrics, 114*, e1–e8.

Kendall, P. C., & Hedtke, K. A. (2006). *Coping Cat workbook* (2nd ed.). Ardmore, PA: Workbook.

Kent, K. M., Pelham, W. E., Jr., Molina, B. S. G., Sibley, M. H., Waschbusch, D. A., Yu, J., et al. (2011). The academic experience of male high school students with ADHD. *Journal of Abnormal Child Psychology, 39*, 451–462.

Keown, L. J., & Woodward, L. J. (2002). Early parent–child relations and family functioning of preschool boys with pervasive hyperactivity. *Journal of Abnormal Child Psychology, 30*, 541–553.

Kern, L., Childs, K. E., Dunlap, G., Clarke, S., & Falk, G. D. (1994). Using assessment-based curricular intervention to improve the classroom behavior of a student with emotional and behavioral challenges. *Journal of Applied Behavior Analysis, 27*, 7–19.

Kern, L., DuPaul, G. J., Volpe, R. J., Sokol, N. G., Lutz, J. G., Arbolino, L. A., et al. (2007). Multisetting assessment-based intervention for young children at risk for attention deficit hyperactivity disorder: Initial effects on academic and behavioral functioning. *School Psychology Review, 36*, 237–255.

Kessler, R. C., Avenevoli, S., Costello, J., Georgiades, K., Green, J. G., Gruber, M. J., et al. (2012). Prevalence, persistence, and sociodemographic correlates of DSM-IV disorders in the National Comorbidity Survey Replication Adolescent Supplement. *Archives of General Psychiatry, 69*, 372–380.

King, S., Waschbusch, D. A., Pelham, W. E., Jr., Frankland, B. W., Andrade, B. F., Jacques, S., et al. (2009). Social information processing in elementary-school aged children with ADHD: Medication effects and comparisons with typical children. *Journal of Abnormal Child Psychology, 37*, 579–589.

Klorman, R., Brumaghim, J. T., Salzman, L. F., Strauss, J., Borgsted, A. D., McBride, M. C., et al. (1988). Effects of methylphenidate on attention-deficit hyperactivity disorder with and without aggressive/noncompliant features. *Journal of Abnormal Psychology, 97*, 413–422.

Knowledge Adventure, Inc. (producer). (2013). *Math Blaster.* Retrieved from *www.knowledgeadventure.com/school/mathblaster/Default.aspx.*

Koegel, R. L., Dyer, K., & Bell, L. K. (1987). The influence of child-preferred activities on autistic children's social behavior. *Journal of Applied Behavior Analysis, 20*, 243–252.

Kofler, M. J., Rapport, M. D., & Alderson, R. M. (2008). Quantifying ADHD classroom inattentiveness, its moderators, and variability: A meta-analytic review. *Journal of Child Psychology and Psychiatry, 49*, 59–69.

Kollins, S., Greenhill, L., Swanson, J., Wigal, S., Abikoff, H., McCracken, J., et al. (2006). Rationale, design, and methods of the Preschool ADHD Treatment Study (PATS). *Journal of the American Academy of Child and Adolescent Psychiatry, 45*, 1275–1283.

Kratochwill, T. R., & Levin, J. R. (Eds.). (1992). *Single-case research design and analysis: New directions for psychology and education.* Hillsdale, NJ: Erlbaum.

Kwon, K., Kim, E. M., & Sheridan, S. M. (2012). A contextual approach to social skills assessment in the peer group: Who is the best judge? *School Psychology Quarterly, 27*, 121–133.

Lahey, B. B., & Carlson, C. (1992). Validity of the diagnostic category of attention deficit disorder without hyperactivity: A review of the literature. In S. E. Shaywitz & B. A. Shaywitz (Eds.), *Attention deficit disorder comes of age: Toward the twenty-first century* (pp. 119–144). Austin, TX: Pro-Ed.

Lahey, B. B., Pelham, W. E., Loney, J., Kipp, H., Ehrhardt, A., Lee, S. S., et al. (2004). Three-year predictive validity of DSM-IV attention deficit hyperactivity disorder in children diagnosed at 4–6 years of age. *American Journal of Psychiatry, 161*, 2014–2020.

Lahey, B. B., Pelham, W. E., Loney, J., Lee, S. S., & Willcutt, W. (2005). Instability of the DSM-IV subtypes of ADHD from preschool through elementary school. *Archives of General Psychiatry, 62*, 896–902.

Lahey, B. B., Pelham, W. E., Stein, M. A., Loney, J., Trapani, C., Nugent, K., et al. (1998). Validity of DSM-IV attention-deficit/hyperactivity disorder for younger children. *Journal of the American Academy of Child and Adolescent Psychiatry, 37,* 695–702.

Lahey, B. B., & Willcutt, E. G. (2010). Predictive validity of a continuous alternative to nominal subtypes of attention-deficit/hyperactivity disorder for DSM-V. *Journal of Clinical Child and Adolescent Psychology, 39,* 761–765.

Lam, A. L., Cole, C. L., Shapiro, E. S., & Bambara, L. M. (1994). Relative effects of self-monitoring on-task behavior, academic accuracy, and disruptive behavior in students with behavior disorders. *School Psychology Review, 23,* 44–58.

Lambek, R., Tannock, R., Dalsgaard, S., Trillingsgaard, A., Damm, D., & Thomsen, P. H. (2011). Executive dysfunction in school-aged children with ADHD. *Journal of Attention Disorders, 15,* 646–655.

Lambert, N. (2005). The contribution of childhood ADHD, conduct problems, and stimulant treatment to adolescent and adult tobacco and psychoactive substance abuse. *Ethical Human Psychology and Psychiatry, 7,* 197–221.

Landau, S., Milich, R., & Widiger, T. A. (1991). Conditional probability of child interview symptoms in the diagnosis of attention deficit disorder. *Journal of Child Psychology and Psychiatry, 32,* 501–513.

Langberg, J., Epstein, J., Urbanowicz, C., Simon, J., & Graham, A. (2008). Efficacy of an organization skills intervention to improve the academic functioning of students with ADHD. *School Psychology Quarterly, 23,* 407–417.

Langberg, J., Molina, B., Arnold, L., Epstein, J., Altaye, M., Hinshaw, S., et al. (2011). Patterns and predictors of adolescent academic achievement and performance in a sample of children with attention-deficit/hyperactivity disorder (ADHD). *Journal of Clinical Child and Adolescent Psychology, 40,* 519–531.

Langberg, J. M. (2011). *Homework, Organization, and Planning Skills (HOPS) interventions.* Bethesda, MD: National Association of School Psychologists.

Langberg, J. M., Epstein, J. N., Becker, S. P., Girio-Herrera, E., & Vaughn, A. J. (2012). Evaluation of the Homework, Organization, and Planning Skills (HOPS) intervention for middle school students with attention deficit hyperactivity disorder as implemented by school mental health providers. *School Psychology Review, 41,* 342–364.

Langley, K., Fowler, T., Ford, T., Thapar, A. K., van den Bree, M., Harold, G., et al. (2010). Adolescent clinical outcomes for young people with attention-deficit hyperactivity disorder. *British Journal of Psychiatry, 196*(3), 235–240.

Lavigne, J. V., LeBailly, S. A., Hopkins, J., Gouze, K. R., & Binns, H. J. (2009). The prevalence of ADHD, ODD, depression, and anxiety in a community sample of 4–year-olds. *Journal of Clinical Child and Adolescent Psychology, 38,* 315–328.

Lee, L., Harrington, R. A., Chang, J. J., & Connors, S. L. (2008). Increased risk of injury in children with developmental disabilities. *Research in Developmental Disabilities, 29,* 247–255.

Lee, S. S., Humphreys, K. L., Flory, K., Liu, R., & Glass, K. (2011). Prospective association of childhood attention-deficit/hyperactivity disorder (ADHD) and substance use and abuse/dependence: A meta-analytic review. *Clinical Psychology Review, 31,* 328–341.

Lee, S. S., Lahey, B. B., Owens, E. B., & Hinshaw, S. P. (2008). Few preschool boys and girls with ADHD are well-adjusted during adolescence. *Journal of Abnormal Child Psychology, 36,* 373–383.

Lenz, B. K., Ehren, B. J., & Deshler, D. D. (2005). The Content Literacy Continuum: A school-reform framework for improving adolescent literacy for all students. *Teaching Exceptional Children, 37*(6), 60–63.

Levin, J. R., Ferron, J. M., & Kratochwill, T. R. (2012). Nonparametric statistical tests for single-case systematic and randomized ABAB . . . AB and alternating treatment intervention designs: New developments, new directions. *Journal of School Psychology, 50,* 599–624.

Levy, F., Hay, D. A., McStephen, M., Wood, C., & Waldman, I. (1997). Attention-deficit hyperactivity disorder: A category or a continuum? Genetic analysis of a large-scale twin study. *Journal of the American Academy of Child and Adolescent Psychiatry, 36,* 737–744.

Lillie, D. L., Hannun, W. H., & Stuck, G. B. (1989). *Computers and effective instruction.* New York: Longman.

Lindsley, O. R. (1991). From technical jargon to plain English for application. *Journal of Applied Behavior Analysis, 24,* 449–458.

Loney, J., Weissenburger, F. E., Woolson, R. F., & Lichty, E. C. (1979). Comparing psychological and pharmacological treatments for hyperkinetic boys and their classmates. *Journal of Abnormal Child Psychology, 7,* 133–143.

Lord, C., Rutter, M., & Le Couteur, A. (1994). Autism Diagnostic Interview–Revised: A revised version of a diagnostic interview for caregivers of individuals with possible pervasive developmental disorders. *Journal of Autism and Developmental Disabilities, 24,* 659–685.

Mahone, M. E., Crocetti, D., Ranta, M. E., Gaddis, A., Cataldo, M., Silfer, K. J., et al. (2011). A preliminary neuroimaging study of preschool children with ADHD. *The Clinical Neuropsychologist, 25,* 1009–1028.

Mangus, R. S., Bergman, D., Zieger, M., & Coleman, J. J. (2004). Burn injuries in children with attention-deficit/hyperactivity disorder. *Burns, 30,* 148–150.

Mannuzza, S., & Klein, R. G. (2000). Long-term prognosis in attention-deficit/hyperactivity disorder. *Child and Adolescent Psychiatric Clinics of North America, 9*(3), 711–726.

Mannuzza, S., Klein, R. G., Truong, N. L., Moulton, J. L., III, Roizen, E. R., Howell, K. H., et al. (2008). Age of methylphenidate treatment initiation in children with ADHD and later substance abuse: Prospective follow-up into adulthood. *American Journal of Psychiatry, 165,* 604–609.

Marks, D. J., Mlodnicka, A., Bernstein, M., Chacko, A., Rose, S., & Halperin, J. M. (2009). Profiles of service utilization and the resultant economic impact in preschoolers with attention deficit/hyperactivity disorder. *Journal of Pediatric Psychology, 34,* 681–689.

Martel, M. M., Nikolas, M., Jernigan, K., Friderici, K., Waldman, I., & Nigg, J. (2011). The dopamine receptor D4 gene (DRD4) moderates family environmental effects on ADHD. *Journal of Abnormal Child Psychology,* *39*, 1–10.

Mautone, J. A., DuPaul, J. A., & Jitendra, A. K. (2005). The effects of computer-assisted instruction on the mathematics performance and classroom behavior of children with ADHD. *Journal of Attention Disorders, 9,* 301–312.

Mayer, G. R., Sulzer-Azaroff, B., & Wallace, M. (2014). *Behavior analysis for lasting change* (3rd ed.). Cornwall-on-Hudson, NY: Sloan.

Mayes, R., Bagwell, C., & Erkulwater, J. (2008). ADHD and the rise of stimulant use among children. *Harvard Review of Psychiatry, 16,* 151–166.

McBurnett, K., Pfiffner, L. J., & Frick, P. (2001). Symptom properties as a function of ADHD type: An argument for continued study of sluggish cognitive tempo. *Journal of Abnormal Child Psychology, 29,* 207–213.

McConaughy, S. H., Achenbach, T. M., & Gent, C. L. (1988). Multiaxial empirically based assessment: Parent, teacher, observational, cognitive, and personality correlates of child behavior profile types for 6– to 11–year-old boys. *Journal of Abnormal Child Psychology, 16,* 485–509.

McConaughy, S. H., Volpe, R. J., Antshel, K. M., Gordon, M., & Eiraldi, R. B. (2011). Academic and social impairments of elementary school children with attention deficit hyperactivity disorder. *School Psychology Review, 40,* 200–225.

McDermott, P. A., Leigh, N. M., & Perry, M. A. (2002). Development and validation of the Preschool Learning Behaviors Scale. *Psychology in the Schools, 39,* 353–365.

McGee, R., & Share, D. L. (1988). Attention deficit disorder-hyperactivity and academic failure: Which comes first and what should be treated? *Journal of the American Academy of Child and Adolescent Psychiatry, 27,* 318–325.

McGee, R. A., Clark, S. E., & Symons, D. K. (2000). Does the Conners' Continuous Performance Test aid in ADHD diagnosis? *Journal of Abnormal Child Psychology, 28,* 415–424.

McGoey, K. E., & DuPaul, G. J. (2000). Token reinforcement and response cost procedures: Reducing the disruptive behavior of preschool children with ADHD. *School Psychology Quarterly, 15,* 330–343.

McGoey, K. E., DuPaul, G. J., Haley, E., & Shelton, T. L. (2007). Parent and teacher ratings of attention-deficit/hyperactivity disorder in preschool: The ADHD Rating Scale–IV Preschool Version. *Journal of Psychopathology and Behavioral Assessment, 29,* 269–276.

McGoey, K. E., Eckert, T. L., & DuPaul, G. J. (2002). Early intervention for preschool-age children with ADHD: A literature review. *Journal of Emotional and Behavioral Disorders, 10,* 14–28.

McKinley, L. A., & Stormont, M. A. (2008). The School Supports Checklist: Identifying support needs and barriers for children with ADHD. *Teaching Exceptional Children, 41*(2), 14–19.

Mendel, P., Meredith, L. S., Schoenbaum, M., Sherbourne, C. D., & Wells, K. B. (2008). Interventions in organizational and community context: A framework for building evidence on dissemination and implementation in health services research. *Administration and Policy in Mental Health and Mental Health Services, 35,* 21–37.

Merikangas, K. R., He, J., Burstein, M., Swendsen, J., Avenevoli, S., Case, B., et al. (2011). Service utilization for lifetime mental disorders in U. S. adolescents: Results of the National Comorbidity Survey–Adolescent Supplement (NCS-A). *Journal of the American Academy of Child and Adolescent Psychiatry, 50,* 32–45.

Merrell, K. (2003). *Preschool and Kindergarten Behavior Scales* (2nd ed.). Longmont, CO: Sopris-West.

Merrell, K. W. (1994). *Preschool and Kindergarten Behavior Scales.* Brandon, VT: Clinical Psychology.

Merrell, K. W., Ervin, R. A., & Gimpel Peacock, G. (2012). *School psychology for the 21st Century: Foundations and practices* (2nd ed.). New York: Guilford Press.

Meyer, L. H., & Evans, I. M. (1989). *Nonaversive interventions for behavior problems: A manual for home and community.* Baltimore: Brookes.

Meyer, K., & Kelley, M. L. (2007). Improving homework in adolescents with attention-deficit/hyperactivity disorder: Self vs. parent monitoring of homework behavior and study skills. *Child and Family Behavior Therapy, 29,* 25–42.

Mick, E., Biederman, J., Faraone, S. V., Sayer, J., & Kleinman, S. (2002). Case–control study of attention-deficit hyperactivity disorder and maternal smoking, alcohol use, and drug use during pregnancy. *Journal of the American Academy of Child and Adolescent Psychiatry, 41,* 378–385.

Mick, E., Biederman, J., Prince, J., Fischer, M. J., & Faraone, S. V. (2002). Impact of low birth weight on attention-deficit hyperactivity disorder. *Journal of Developmental and Behavioral Pediatrics, 23,* 16–22.

Mikami, A. Y., Griggs, M. S., Lerner, M. D., Emeh, C. C., Reuland, M. M., Jack, A., et al. (2013). A randomized trial of a classroom intervention to increase peers' social inclusion of children with attention-deficit/hyperactivity disorder. *Journal of Consulting and Clinical Psychology, 81,* 100–112.

Mikami, A. Y., Lerner, M. D., Griggs, M. S., McGrath, A., & Calhoun, C. D. (2010). Parental influence on children with attention-deficit/hyperactivity disorder: II. Results of a pilot intervention training parents as friendship coaches for children. *Journal of Abnormal Child Psychology, 38,* 737–749.

Milberger, S., Biederman, J., Faraone, S. V., Chen, L., & Jones, J. (1996). Is maternal smoking during pregnancy a risk factor for attention deficit hyperactivity disorder in children? *American Journal of Psychiatry, 153,* 1138–1142.

Milich, R., Balentine, A. C., & Lynam, D. R. (2001). ADHD combined type and ADHD predominately inattentive type are distinct and unrelated disorders. *Clinical Psychology: Science and Practice, 8,* 463–488.

Milich, R., Carlson, C. L., Pelham, W. E., Jr., & Licht, B. G. (1991). Effects of methylphenidate on the persistence of ADHD boys following failure experiences. *Journal of Abnormal Child Psychology, 19,* 519–536.

Milich, R., Landau, S., Kilby, G., & Whitten, P. (1982). Preschool peer perceptions of the behavior of hyperactive and aggressive children. *Journal of Abnormal Child Psychology, 10,* 497–510.

Miller, M., Nevado-Montenegro, A. J., & Hinshaw, S. P. (2012). Childhood executive function continues to predict outcomes in young adult females with and without childhood-diagnosed ADHD. *Journal of Abnormal Child Psychology, 40,* 657–668.

Miller, T. W., Nigg, J. T., & Miller, R. L. (2009). Attention deficit hyperactivity disorder in African American children: What can be concluded from the past ten years? *Clinical Psychology Review, 29,* 77–86.

Minuchin, S. (1974). *Families and family therapy.* Cambridge, MA: Harvard University Press.

Molina, B. S. G., Hinshaw, S. P., Arnold, L. E., Swanson, J. M., Pelham, W. E., Hechtman, L., et al. (2013). Adolescent substance use in the Multimodal Treatment Study of Attention-Deficit/Hyperactivity Disorder (ADHD MTA) as a function of childhood ADHD, random assignment to childhood treatments, and subsequent medication. *Journal of the American Academy of Child and Adolescent Psychiatry, 52,* 250–263.

Molina, B. S. G., Hinshaw, S. P., Swanson, J. M., Arnold, L. E., Vitiello, B., Jensen, P. S., et al. (2009). MTA at 8 years: Prospective follow-up of children treated for combined-type ADHD in a multisite study. *Journal of the American Academy of Child and Adolescent Psychiatry, 48,* 484–500.

Molina, B. S. G., Pelham, W. E., Jr., Cheong, J., Marshal, M. P., Gnagy, E. M., & Curran, P. J. (2012). Childhood attention-deficit/hyperactivity disorder and growth in adolescent alcohol use: The roles of functional impairments, ADHD symptom persistence, and parental knowledge. *Journal of Abnormal Psychology.*

Morgan, P. L., Staff, J., Hillemeier, M. M., Farkas, G., & Maczuga, S. (2013). Racial and ethnic disparities in ADHD diagnosis from kindergarten to eighth grade. *Pediatrics, 132,* 85–93.

Mrug, S., Molina, B. S. G., Hoza, B., Gerdes, A. C., Hinshaw, S. P., Hechtman, L., et al. (2012). Peer rejection and friendships in children with attention-deficit/hyperactivity disorder: Contributions to long-term outcomes. *Journal of Abnormal Child Psychology, 40,* 1013–1026.

MTA Cooperative Group. (1999). A 14-month randomized clinical trial of treatment strategies for attention-deficit/hyperactivity disorder. *Archives of General Psychiatry, 56,* 1073–1086.

Murray, H. A. (1943). *Thematic Apperception Test.* Cambridge, MA: Harvard University Press.

Murray, L. K., & Kollins, S. H. (2000). Effects of methylphenidate on sensitivity to reinforcement in children diagnosed with attention deficit hyperactivity disorder: An application of the matching law. *Journal of Applied Behavior Analysis, 33,* 573–591.

National Association of School Psychologists. (2010a). *National Association of School Psychologists model for comprehensive and integrated school psychological services.* Bethesda, MD: Author.

National Association of School Psychologists. (2010b). *National Association of School Psychologists principles for professional ethics.* Bethesda, MD: Author.

National Association of School Psychologists. (2011). *Students with attention deficit hyperactivity disorder* (Position statement). Bethesda, MD: Author.

NationalInstituteofMentalHealth.(2013).*ADHD*.RetrievedAugust1,2013,from *www.nimh.nih.gov/health/publications/attention-deficit-hyperactivity-disorder/index.shtml.*

National Reading Panel. (2000). *Teaching children to read: An evidence-based assessment of the scientific research literature on reading and its implications for reading instruction.* Available at *www.nichd.nih.gov/publications/ nrp/smallbook.htm.*

National Research Council. (1998). *Preventing reading difficulties in young children.* Washington, DC: National Academy Press.

Nigg, J. T. (2006). *What causes ADHD?: Understanding what goes wrong and why.* New York: Guilford Press.

Nigg, J. T., Goldsmith, H. H., & Sachek, J. (2004). Temperament and attention deficit hyperactivity disorder: The development of a multiple pathway model. *Journal of Clinical Child and Adolescent Psychology, 33,* 42–53.

Nixon, R. D. (2002). Treatment of behavior problems in preschoolers: A review of parent training programs. *Clinical Psychology Review, 22,* 525–546.

Noell, G. H., Witt, J. C., Slider, N. J., Connell, J. E., Gatti, S. L., & Wi, K. L. (2005). Treatment implementation following behavioral consultation in schools: A comparison of three follow-up strategies. *School Psychology Review, 34,* 87–106.

Northup, J., Fusilier, I., Swanson, V., Huete, J., Bruce, T., Freeland, J., et al. (1999). Further analysis of the separate and interactive effects of methylphenidate and common classroom contingencies. *Journal of Applied Behavior Analysis, 32,* 35–50.

Northup, J., & Gulley, V. (2001). Some contributions of functional analysis to the assessment of behaviors associated with attention deficit hyperactivity disorder and the effects of stimulant medication. *School Psychology Review, 30,* 227–238.

Northup, J., Jones, K., Broussard, C., DiGiovanni, G., Herring, M., Fusilier, I., et al. (1997). A preliminary analysis of interactive effects between common classroom contingencies and methylphenidate. *Journal of Applied Behavior Analysis, 30,* 121–125.

Northup, J., Wacker, D., Sasso, G., Steege, M., Cigrand, K., Cook, J., et al. (1991). A brief functional analysis of aggressive and alternative behavior in an outclinic setting. *Journal of Applied Behavior Analysis, 24,* 509–522.

Notari-Syverson, A., O'Connor, R. E., & Vadasy, P. F. (1998). *Ladders to literacy: A preschool activity book.* Baltimore: Brookes.

Ohan, J. L., & Johnston, C. (2011). Positive illusions of social competence in girls with and without ADHD. *Journal of Abnormal Child Psychology, 39,* 527–539.

Olazagasti, M. A. R., Klein, R. G., Mannuzza, S., Belsky, E. R., Hutchison, J. A., Lashua-Shriftman, E. C., et al. (2013). Does childhood attention-deficit/ hyperactivity disorder predict risk-taking and medical illnesses in adulthood? *Journal of the American Academy of Child and Adolescent Psychiatry, 52,* 153–162.

O'Leary, K. D. (1980). Pills or skills for hyperactive children. *Journal of Applied Behavior Analysis, 13,* 191–204.

Olfson, M., Marcus, S. C., Weissman, M. M., & Jensen, P. S. (2002). National trends in the use of psychotropic medications by children. *Journal of the American Academy of Child and Adolescent Psychiatry, 41*, 514–521.

Olympia, D. E., Jenson, W. R., & Hepworth-Neville, M. (1996). *Sanity savers for parents: Tips for tackling homework.* Longmont, CO: Sopris-West.

O'Reilly, M. J. (2002). *The early literacy skill development of kindergartners and first graders at-risk for externalizing behavior disorders.* Unpublished manuscript, University of Massachusetts, Amherst.

O'Shea, L. J., Sindelar, P. T., & O'Shea, D. J. (1987). The effects of repeated readings and attentional cues on the reading fluency and comprehension of learning disabled readers. *Learning Disabilities Research, 2*, 103–109.

Ostrander, R., & Herman, K. C. (2006). Potential cognitive, parenting, and developmental mediators of the relationship between ADHD and depression. *Journal of Consulting and Clinical Psychology, 74* (1), 89–98.

Ota, K. R., & DuPaul, G. J. (2002). Task engagement and mathematics performance in children with attention deficit hyperactivity disorder: Effects of supplemental computer instruction. *School Psychology Quarterly, 17*, 242–257.

Owens, J. S., Goldfine, M. E., Evangelista, N. M., Hoza, B., & Kaiser, N. M. (2007). A critical review of self-perceptions and the positive illusory bias in children with ADHD. *Clinical Child and Family Psychology Review, 10*, 335–351.

Owens, J. S., Holdaway, A. S., Zoromski, A. K., Evans, S. W., Himawan, L. K., Girio-Herrera, E., et al. (2012). Incremental benefits of a daily report card intervention over time for youth with disruptive behavior. *Behavior Therapy, 43*, 848–861.

Owens, J. S., Johannes, L. M., & Karpenko, V. (2009). The relation between change in symptoms and functioning in children with ADHD receiving school-based mental health services. *School Mental Health, 1*, 183–195.

Pakyurek, M., Schweitzer, J., & Yellowlees, P. (2013, February). Telepsychiatry and ADHD. *The ADHD Report, 21*(1), 1–5, 11.

Paniagua, F. A. (1992). Verbal–nonverbal correspondence training with ADHD children. *Behavior Modification, 16*, 226–252.

Pany, D., Jenkins, J. R., & Schreck, J. (1982). Vocabulary instruction: Effects on word knowledge and reading comprehension. *Learning Disability Quarterly, 5*, 202–214.

Parker, J. G., & Asher, S. R. (1987). Peer relations and later personal adjustment: Are low-accepted children at risk? *Psychological Bulletin, 102*, 357–389.

Pastor, P. N., & Reuben, C. A. (2002). Attention deficit disorder and learning disability: United States, 1997–98. In *National Center for Health Statistics: Vital Health Statistics* (DHHS Publication No. PHS 2002-1534). Hyattsville, MD: Department of Health and Human Services.

Pastor, P. N., & Reuben, C. A. (2008). Diagnosed attention deficit disorder and learning disability: United States, 2004–2006. National Center for Health Statistic. *Vital and Health Statistics, 10*(237). Retrieved from *www.cdc.gov/nchs/products/series/series10.htm.*

Patterson, G. R., & Chamberlain, P. (1994). A functional analysis of resistance during parent-training therapy. *Clinical Psychology: Science and Practice, 1,* 53–70.

Patterson, G. R., Reid, J. B., & Dishion, T. J. (1992). *Antisocial boys.* Eugene, OR: Castalia.

Pelham, W. E. (1989). Behavior therapy, behavioral assessment, and psycho-stimulant medication in treatment of attention deficit disorders: An interactive approach. In J. Swanson & L. Bloomingdale (Eds.), *Attention deficit disorders: IV. Current concepts and emerging trends in attentional and behavior disorders of childhood* (pp. 169–195). London: Pergamon Press.

Pelham, W. E., Bender, M. E., Caddell, J., Booth, S., & Moorer, S. H. (1985). Methylphenidate and children with attention deficit disorder. *Archives of General Psychiatry, 42,* 948–952.

Pelham, W. E., Carlson, C., Sams, S. E., Vallano, G., Dixon, M. J., & Hoza, B. (1993). Separate and combined effects of methylphenidate and behavior modification on boys with attention deficit-hyperactivity disorder in classroom. *Journal of Consulting and Clinical Psychology, 61,* 506–515.

Pelham, W. E., Foster, E. M., & Robb, J. A. (2007). The economic impact of attention-deficit/hyperactivity disorder in children and adolescents. *Journal of Pediatric Psychology, 32,* 711–727.

Pelham, W. E., McBurnett, K., Harper, G. W., Milich, R., Murphy, D. A., Clinton, J., et al. (1990). Methylphenidate and baseball playing in ADHD children: Who's on first? *Journal of Consulting and Clinical Psychology, 58,* 130–133.

Pelham, W. E., & Milich, R. (1991). Individual differences in response to Ritalin in classwork and social behavior. In L. L. Greenhill & B. B. Osman (Eds.), *Ritalin: Theory and patient management* (pp. 203–221). New York: Liebert.

Pelham, W. E., & Murphy, H. A. (1986). Attention deficit and conduct disorders. In M. Hersen (Ed.), *Pharmacological and behavioral treatment: An integrative approach* (pp. 108–148). New York: Wiley.

Pelham, W. E., Vodde-Hamilton, M., Murphy, D. A., Greenstein, J. L., & Vallano, G. (1991). The effects of methylphenidate on ADHD adolescents in recreational, peer group, and classroom settings. *Journal of Clinical Child Psychology, 20,* 293–300.

Pelham, W. E., Jr., & Fabiano, G. A. (2008). Evidence-based psychosocial treatments for attention-deficit/hyperactivity disorder. *Journal of Clinical Child and Adolescent Psychology, 37,* 184–214.

Pelham, W. E., Jr., Fabiano, G. A., & Massetti, G. M. (2005). Evidence-based assessment of attention deficit hyperactivity disorder in children and adolescents. *Journal of Clinical Child & Adolescent Psychology, 34,* 449–476.

Perepletchikova, F., Treat, T. A., & Kazdin, A. E. (2007). Treatment integrity in psychotherapy research: Analysis of the studies and examination of the associated factors. *Journal of Consulting and Clinical Psychology, 75,* 829–841.

Pfiffner, L. J., Barkley, R. A., & DuPaul, G. J. (2006). Treatment of ADHD in school settings. In R. A. Barkley, *Attention-deficit hyperactivity disorder: A handbook for diagnosis and treatment* (3rd ed., pp. 547–589). New York: Guilford Press.

Pfiffner, L. J., & DuPaul, G. J. (in press). Treatment of ADHD in school settings. In R. A. Barkley, *Attention-deficit hyperactivity disorder: A handbook for diagnosis and treatment* (4th ed.). New York: Guilford Press.

Pfiffner, L. J., & McBurnett, K. (1997). Social skills training with parent generalization: Treatment effects for children with attention deficit disorder. *Journal of Consulting and Clinical Psychology, 65,* 749–757.

Pfiffner, L. J., & O'Leary, S. G. (1987). The efficacy of all-positive management as a function of the prior use of negative consequences. *Journal of Applied Behavior Analysis, 20,* 265–271.

Pfiffner, L. J., & O'Leary, S. G. (1993). School-based psychological treatments. In J. L. Matson (Ed.), *Handbook of hyperactivity in children* (pp. 234–255). Boston: Allyn & Bacon.

Pfiffner, L. J., O'Leary, S. G., Rosen, L. A., & Sanderson, W. C., Jr. (1985). A comparison of the effects of continuous and intermittent response cost and reprimands in the classroom. *Journal of Clinical Child Psychology, 14,* 348–352.

Pfiffner, L. J., Villodas, M., Kaiser, N., Rooney, M., & McBurnett, K. (2013). Educational outcomes of a collaborative school–home behavioral intervention for ADHD. *School Psychology Quarterly, 28,* 25–36.

Phillips, P. L., Greenson, J. N., Collett, B. R., & Gimpel, G. A. (2002). Assessing ADHD symptoms in preschool children: Use of the ADHD Symptoms Rating Scale. *Early Education and Development, 13,* 283–299.

Pierce, E. W., Ewing, L. J., & Campbell, S. B. (1999). Diagnostic status and symptomatic behavior of hard-to-manage preschool children in middle childhood and early adolescence. *Journal of Clinical Child Psychology, 28,* 44–57.

Pingault, J. B., Tremblay, R. E., Vitaro, F., Carbonneau, R., Genolini, C., Falissard, B., et al. (2011). Childhood trajectories of inattention and hyperactivity and prediction of educational attainment in early adulthood: A 16–year longitudinal population-based study. *American Journal of Psychiatry, 168,* 1164–1170.

Platzman, K. A., Stoy, M. R., Brown, R. T., Coles, C. D., Smith, I. E., & Falek, A. (1992). Review of observational methods in attention deficit hyperactivity disorder (ADHD): Implications for diagnosis. *School Psychology Quarterly, 7,* 155–177.

Pliszka, S. R. (2011). *Treating ADHD and comorbid disorders: Psychosocial and psychopharmacological interventions.* New York: Guilford Press.

Pliszka, S. R., Carlson, C. L., & Swanson, J. M. (1999). *ADHD with comorbid disorders: Clinical assessment and management.* New York: Guilford Press.

Plotts, C. A., & Lasser, J. (2013). *School psychologist as counselor.* Bethesda, MD: National Association of School Psychologists.

Plumer, P. J., & Stoner, G. (2005). The relative effects of classwide peer tutoring and peer coaching on the positive social behaviors of children with attention deficit hyperactivity disorder. *Journal of Attention Disorders, 9*(1), 290–300.

Pope, D., Whiteley, H., Smith, C., Lever, R., Wakelin, D., Dudiak, H., et al. (2007). Relationships between ADHD and dyslexia screening scores and academic performance in undergraduate psychology students: Implications for teaching, learning, and assessment. *Psychology Learning and Teaching, 6*(2), 114–120.

Powell, S. G., Thomsen, P. H., Frydenberg, M., & Rasmussen, H. (2011). Long-term treatment of ADHD with stimulants: A large observational study of real-life patients. *Journal of Attention Disorders, 15*, 439–451.

Power, T. J. (2002). Preparing school psychologists as interventionists and preventionists. In M. R. Shinn, H. M. Walker, & G. Stoner (Eds.), *Interventions for academic and behavior problems: II. Preventive and remedial approaches* (pp. 1047–1065). Bethesda, MD: National Association of School Psychologists.

Power, T. J., DuPaul, G. J., Shapiro, E. S., & Kazak, A. E. (2003). *Promoting children's health: Integrating school, family, and community.* New York: Guilford Press.

Power, T. J., Karustis, J. L., & Habboushe, D. F. (2001). *Homework success for children with ADHD: A family–school intervention program.* New York: Guilford Press.

Power, T. J., Mautone, J. A., & Ginsburg-Block, M. (2010). Training school psychologists for prevention and intervention in a three-tier model. In M. R. Shinn & H. M. Walker (Eds.), *Interventions for achievement and behavior problems in a three-tier model including RTI* (pp. 151–173). Bethesda, MD: National Association of School Psychologists.

Power, T. J., Mautone, J. A., Soffer, S. L., Clarke, A. T., Marshall, S. A., Sharman, J., et al. (2012). Family–school intervention for children with ADHD: Results of a randomized clinical trial. *Journal of Consulting and Clinical Psychology, 80*, 611–623.

Power, T. J., Werba, B. E., Watkins, M. W., Angelucci, J. G., & Eiraldi, R. B. (2006). Patterns for parent-reported homework problems among ADHD-referred and non-referred children. *School Psychology Quarterly, 21*, 13–33.

Powers, R. L., Marks, D. J., Miller, C. J., Newcorn, J. H., & Halperin, J. M. (2008). Stimulant treatment in children with attention-deficit/hyperactivity disorder moderates adolescent academic outcome. *Journal of Child and Adolescent Psychopharmacology, 18*, 449–459.

Pryor, J. H., DeAngelo, L., Palucki Blake, L., Hurtado, S., & Tran, S. (2010). *The American freshman: National norms fall 2010.* Los Angeles: Higher Education Research Institute, University of California, Los Angeles.

Purpura, D. J., & Lonigan, C. J. (2009). Conners' Teacher Rating Scale for preschool children: A revised, brief, age-specific measure. *Journal of Clinical Child and Adolescent Psychology, 38*, 263–272.

Ramsay, J. R., & Rostain, A. L. (2006). Cognitive behavior therapy for college students with attention-deficit/hyperactivity disorder. *Journal of College Student Psychotherapy, 21*(1), 3–20.

Rapoport, J., Buchsbaum, M., Weingartner, H., Zahn, T., Ludlow, C., Bartko, J., et al. (1980). Dextroamphetamine: Cognitive and behavioral effects in normal and hyperactive boys and normal adult males. *Archives of General Psychiatry, 37*, 933–946.

Rapport, M. D. (1987a). Attention deficit disorder with hyperactivity. In M.

Hersen & V. B. Van Hasselt (Eds.), *Behavior therapy with children and adolescents* (pp. 325–361). New York: Wiley.

Rapport, M. D. (1987b). *The attention training system: User's manual.* DeWitt, NY: Gordon Systems.

Rapport, M. D., Chung, K. M., Shore, G., Denney, C. B., & Isaacs, P. (2000). Upgrading the science and technology of assessment and diagnosis: Laboratory and clinic-based assessment of children with ADHD. *Journal of Clinical Child Psychology, 29,* 555–568.

Rapport, M. D., & Denney, C. B. (1997). Titrating methylphenidate in children with attention-deficit/hyperactivity disorder: Is body mass predictive of clinical response? *Journal of the American Academy of Child and Adolescent Psychiatry, 36,* 523–530.

Rapport, M. D., & Denney, C. B. (2000). Attention deficit hyperactivity disorder and methylphenidate: Assessment and prediction of clinical response. In L. L. Greenhill & B. B. Osman (Eds.), *Ritalin: Theory and practice* (2nd ed., pp. 45–70). Larchmont, NY: Liebert.

Rapport, M. D., Denney, C. B., DuPaul, G. J., & Gardner, M. J. (1994). Attention deficit disorder and methylphenidate: Normalization rates, clinical effectiveness, and response prediction in 76 children. *Journal of the American Academy of Child and Adolesecent Psychiatry, 33,* 882–893.

Rapport, M. D., DuPaul, G. J., & Kelly, K. L. (1989). Attention-deficit hyperactivity disorder and methylphenidate: The relationship between gross body weight and drug response in children. *Psychopharmacology Bulletin, 25,* 285–290.

Rapport, M. D., DuPaul, G. J., & Smith, N. F. (1985). Rate-dependency and hyperactivity: Methylphenidate effects upon operant performance. *Pharmacology, Biochemistry, and Behavior, 23,* 77–83.

Rapport, M. D., DuPaul, G. J., Stoner, G., & Jones, J. T. (1986). Comparing classroom and clinic measures of attention deficit disorder: Differential, idiosyncratic, and dose–response effects of methylphenidate. *Journal of Consulting and Clinical Psychology, 54,* 334–341.

Rapport, M. D., Jones, J. T., DuPaul, G. J., Kelly, K. L., Gardner, M. J., Tucker, S. B., et al. (1987). Attention deficit disorder and methylphenidate: Group and single-subject analyses of dose effects on attention in clinic and classroom settings. *Journal of Clinical Child Psychology, 16,* 329–338.

Rapport, M. D., & Kelly, K. L. (1991). Psychostimulant effects on learning and cognitive function: Findings and implications for children with attention-deficit hyperactivity disorder. *Clinical Psychology Review, 11,* 61–92.

Rapport, M. D., Kofler, M. J., Coiro, M. M., Raiker, J. S., Sarver, D. E., & Alderson, R. M. (2008). Unexpected effects of methylphenidate in attention-deficit/hyperactivity disorder reflect decreases in core/secondary symptoms and physical complaints common to all children. *Journal of Child and Adolescent Psychopharmacology, 18,* 237–247.

Rapport, M. D., & Moffitt, C. (2002). Attention deficit/hyperactivity disorder and methylphenidate: A review of height/weight, cardiovascular, and somatic complaint side effects. *Clinical Psychology Review, 22,* 1107–1131.

Rapport, M. D., Murphy, A., & Bailey, J. S. (1980). The effects of a response cost treatment tactic on hyperactive children. *Journal of School Psychology, 18*, 98–111.

Rapport, M. D., Murphy, A., & Bailey, J. S. (1982). Ritalin vs. response cost in the control of hyperactive children: A within-subject comparison. *Journal of Applied Behavior Analysis, 15*, 205–216.

Rapport, M. D., Scanlan, S. W., & Denney, C. B. (1999). Attention-deficit/ hyperactivity disorder and scholastic achievement: A model of dual developmental pathways. *Journal of Child Psychology and Psychiatry, 40*, 1169–1183.

Rapport, M. D., Stoner, G., DuPaul, G. J., Kelly, K. L., Tucker, S. B., & Schoeler, T. (1988). Attention deficit disorder and methylphenidate: A multilevel analysis of dose–response effects on children's impulsivity across settings. *Journal of the American Academy of Child and Adolescent Psychiatry, 27*, 60–69.

Rapport, M. D., Tucker, S. B., DuPaul, G. J., Merlo, M., & Stoner, G. (1986). Hyperactivity and frustration: The influence of size and control over rewards in delaying gratification. *Journal of Abnormal Child Psychology, 14*, 191–204.

Reeve, E., & Garfinkel, B. (1991). Neuroendocrine and growth regulation: The role of sympathomimetic medication. In L. L. Greenhill & B. B. Osman (Eds.), *Ritalin: Theory and patient management* (pp. 289–300). New York: Liebert.

Reich, W. (2000). *Diagnostic Interview for Children and Adolescents: Preschool Version*. St. Louis, MO: Washington University.

Reid, J. B., & Eddy, J. M. (1997). The prevention of antisocial behavior: Some considerations in the search for effective interventions. In D. M. Stoff, J. Breiling, & J. D. Maser (Eds.), *Handbook of antisocial behavior* (pp. 343–356). New York: Wiley.

Reid, R., DuPaul, G. J., Power, T. J., Anastopoulos, A. D., & Riccio, C. (1998). Assessing culturally different students for attention deficit hyperactivity disorder using behavior rating scales. *Journal of Abnormal Child Psychology, 26*, 187–198.

Reschly, D. J. (2008). School psychology paradigm shift and beyond. In A. Thomas & J. Grimes (Eds.), *Best practices in school psychology V* (pp. 3–15). Bethesda, MD: National Association of School Psychologists.

Resnick, A., & Reitman, D. (2011). The use of homework success for a child with attention-deficit/hyperactivity disorder, predominantly inattentive type. *Clinical Case Studies, 10*, 23–36.

Reynolds, C. R., & Kamphaus, R. W. (2004). *BASC-2: Behavior Assessment System for Children, second edition manual*. Circle Pines, MN: American Guidance Service.

Reynolds, W. M. (2002). *Reynolds Adolescent Depression Scale—Second Edition: Professional manual*. Odessa FL: Psychological Assessment Resources.

Rhode, G., Morgan, D. P., & Young, K. R. (1983). Generalization and maintenance of treatment gains of behaviorally handicapped students from resource rooms to regular classrooms using self-evaluation procedures. *Journal of Applied Behavior Analysis, 16*, 171–188.

Richard, M. (1992). Considering student support services in college selection. *CH.A.D.D.ER,* 5(6), 1, 6, 7.

Riddle, M. A., Yershova, K., Lazzaretto, D., Paykina, N., Yenokyan, G., Greenhill, L., et al. (2013). The Preschool Attention-Deficit/Hyperactivity Disorder Treatment Study (PATS) 6–year follow-up. *Journal of the American Academy of Child and Adolescent Psychiatry, 52,* 264–278.

Riley-Tillman, T. C., & Burns, M. K. (2009). *Evaluating educational interventions: Single-case design for measuring response to intervention.* New York: Guilford Press.

Risley, T. R., & Hart, B. (1968). Developing correspondence between the nonverbal and verbal behavior of preschool children. *Journal of Applied Behavior Analysis, 1,* 267–281.

Robb, J. A., Sibley, M. H., Pelham, W. E., Jr., Foster, E. M., Molina, B. S. G., Gnagy, E. M., et al. (2011). The estimated annual cost of ADHD to the U.S. education system. *School Mental Health, 3,* 169–177.

Roberts, M. L., & Landau, S. (1995). Using curriculum-based data for assessing children with attention deficits. *Journal of Psychoeducational Assessment, ADHD Special Edition,* 75–88.

Robin, A. L. (1998). *ADHD in adolescents: Diagnosis and treatment.* New York: Guilford Press.

Robin, A. L., & Foster, S. L. (1989). *Negotiating parent–adolescent conflict: A behavioral–family systems approach.* New York: Guilford Press.

Rose, T. L., & Sherry, L. (1984). Relative effects of two previewing procedures on LD adolescents' oral reading performance. *Learning Disability Quarterly, 7,* 39–44.

Rosen, L. A., O'Leary, S. G., Joyce, S. A., Conway, G., & Pfiffner, L. J. (1984). The importance of prudent negative consequences for maintaining the appropriate behavior of hyperactive students. *Journal of Abnormal Child Psychology, 12,* 581–604.

Rosvold, H. E., Mirsky, A. F., Sarason, I., Bransome, E. D., & Beck, L. H. (1956). A continuous performance test of brain damage. *Journal of Consulting Psychology, 20,* 343–350.

Rourke, B. P. (1988). Socioemotional disturbances of learning disabled children. *Journal of Consulting and Clinical Psychology, 56,* 801–810.

Rowe, K. J., & Rowe, K. S. (1992). The relationship between inattentiveness in the classroom and reading achievement, part B: An explanatory study. *Journal of the American Academy of Child and Adolescent Psychiatry, 31,* 357–368.

Safer, D. J., & Zito, J. M. (2000). Pharmacoepidemiology of methylphenidate and other stimulants for the treatment of attention deficit hyperactivity disorder. In L. L. Greenhill & B. B. Osman (Eds.), *Ritalin: Theory and practice* (2nd ed., pp. 7–26). Larchmont, NY: Liebert.

Sallee, F. R., Lyne, A., Wigal, T., & McGough, J. J. (2009). Long-term safety and efficacy of guanfacine extended release in children and adolescents with attention-deficit/hyperactivity disorder. *Journal of Child and Adolescent Psychopharmcology, 19,* 215–226.

Sallee, F. R., McGough, J., Wigal, T., Donahue, J., Lyne, A., & Biederman,

J. (2009). Guanfacine extended release in children and adolescents with attention-deficit/hyperactivity disorder: A placebo-controlled trial. *Journal of the American Academy of Child and Adolescent Psychiatry, 48,* 155–165.

Salvia, J., & Ysseldyke, J. (1998). *Assessment in special and remedial education* (7th ed.). Boston: Houghton Mifflin.

Salvia, J., Ysseldyke, J. E., & Bolt, S. (2013). *Assessment for special and inclusive education* (12th ed.). Belmont, CA: Wadsworth, Cengage Learning.

Samuels, S. J. (1979). The method of repeated readings. *The Reading Teacher, 32,* 403–408.

Schacht, T., & Nathan, P. E. (1977). But is it good for the psychologists?: Appraisal and status of DSM-III. *American Psychologist, 32,* 1017–1025.

Schatz, D. B., & Rostain, A. L. (2006). ADHD with comorbid anxiety: A review of current literature. *Journal of Attention Disorders, 10*(2), 141–149.

Scheffler, R. M., Brown, T. T., Fulton, B. D., Hinshaw, S. P., Levine, P., & Stone, S. (2009). Positive association between attention-deficit/hyperactivity disorder medication use and academic achievement during elementary school. *Pediatrics, 123,* 1273–1279.

Schnoes, C., Reid, R., Wagner, M., & Marder, C. (2006). ADHD among students receiving special education services: A national survey. *Exceptional Children, 72*(4), 483–496.

Schopler, E., Reichler, R. J., & Renner, B. R. (1988). *The Childhood Autism Rating Scale (CARS).* Los Angeles: Western Psychological Services.

Schrag, P., & Divoky, D. (1975). *The myth of the hyperactive child.* New York: Pantheon.

Schumaker, J. B., Denton, P. H., & Deshler, D. D. (1984). *The paraphrasing strategy.* Lawrence: University of Kansas Press.

Schumaker, J. B., & Deshler, D. D. (2010). Using a tiered intervention model in secondary schools to improve academic outcomes in subject-area courses. In M. R. Shinn & H. M. Walker (Eds.), *Interventions for achievement and behavior problems in a three-tier model including RTI* (pp. 609–632). Bethesda, MD: National Association of School Psychologists.

Schwartz, I. S., & Baer, D. M. (1991). Social validity assessments: Is current practice state of the art? *Journal of Applied Behavior Analysis, 24,* 189–204.

Schwebel, D. C., Speltz, M. L., Jones, K., & Bardina, P. (2002). Unintentional injury in preschool boys with and without early onset of disruptive behavior. *Journal of Pediatric Psychology, 27,* 727–737.

Schwiebert, V. L., Sealander, K. A., & Bradshaw, M. L. (1998). Preparing students with attention deficit disorders for entry into the workplace and post-secondary education. *Professional School Counseling, 2,* 26–33.

Semrud-Clikeman, M., Biederman, J., Sprich-Buckminster, S., Lehman, B. K., Faraone, S. V., & Norman, D. (1992). Comorbidity between ADDH and learning disability: A review and report in a clinically referred sample. *Journal of the American Academy of Child and Adolescent Psychiatry, 31,* 439–448.

Shapiro, E. S. (1996). *Academic skills problems: Direct assessment and intervention* (2nd ed.). New York: Guilford Press.

Shapiro, E. S. (2011a). *Academic skills problems: Direct assessment and intervention* (4th ed.). New York: Guilford Press.

Shapiro, E. S. (2011b). *Academic skills problems fourth edition workbook.* New York: Guilford Press.

Shapiro, E. S., & Cole, C. L. (1994). *Behavior change in the classroom: Self-management interventions.* New York: Guilford Press.

Shapiro, E. S., DuPaul, G. J., & Bradley, K. L. (1998). Self-management as a strategy to improve the classroom behavior of adolescents with ADHD. *Journal of Learning Disablities, 31,* 545–555.

Shapiro, E. S., & Kratochwill, T. R. (Eds.). (2000). *Behavioral assessment in schools: Theory, research, and clinical foundations* (2nd ed.). New York: Guilford Press.

Shaw-Zirt, B., Popali-Lehane, L., Chaplin, W., & Bergman, A. (2005). Adjustment, social skills, and self-esteem in college students with symptoms of ADHD. *Journal of Attention Disorders, 8*(3), 109–120.

Shaywitz, B. A., Fletcher, J. M., & Shaywitz, S. E. (1995). Defining and classifying learning disabilities and attention-deficit/hyperactivity disorder. *Journal of Child Neurology, 10,* 50–57.

Shaywitz, B. A., & Shaywitz, S. E. (1991). Comorbidity: A critical issue in attention deficit disorder. *Journal of Child Neurology, 6,* 13–22.

Shelton, T. L., Barkley, R. A., Crosswait, C., Moorehouse, M., Fletcher, K., Barrett, S., et al. (2000). Multimethod psychoeducational intervention for preschool children with disruptive behavior: Two-year post-treatment follow-up. *Journal of Abnormal Child Psychology, 28,* 253–266.

Shelton, T. L., Woods, J. E., Williford, A. P., Dobbins, T. R., & Neal, J. M. (2002). *Project Mastery: Early intervention with Head Start preschoolers at risk for AD/HD.* Unpublished manuscript, University of North Carolina at Greensboro.

Sheridan, S. M. (1995). *The tough kid social skills book.* Longmont, CO: Sopris-West.

Sheridan, S. M., Dee, C. C., Morgan, J. C., McCormick, M. E., & Walker, D. (1996). A multimethod intervention for social skills deficits in children with ADHD and their parents. *School Psychology Review, 25,* 57–76.

Sheridan, S. M., & Kratochwill, T. R. (2008). *Conjoint behavioral consultation: Promoting family-school connections and interventions* (2nd ed.). New York: Springer-Verlag.

Sheridan, S. M., Kratochwill, T. R., & Bergan, J. (1996). *Conjoint behavioral consultation: A procedural manual.* New York: Plenum Press.

Shimabukuro, S. M., Prater, M. A., Jenkins, A., & Edelin-Smith, P. (1999). The effects of self-monitoring of academic performance on students with learning disabilities and ADD/ADHD. *Education and Treatment of Children, 22*(4), 397–414.

Shinn, M. R. (Ed.). (1989). *Curriculum-based measurement: Assessing special children.* New York: Guilford Press.

Shinn, M. R. (Ed.). (1998). *Advanced applications of curriculum-based measurement.* New York: Guilford Press.

Shinn, M. R. (2010). Building a scientifically based data system for progress monitoring and universal screening across three tiers, including RTI using curriculum-based measurement. In M. R. Shinn & H. M. Walker (Eds.), *Interventions for achievement and behavior problems in a three-tier model including RTI* (pp. 259–292). Bethesda, MD: National Association of School Psychologists.

Shinn, M. R., & Walker, H. M. (Eds.). (2010). *Interventions for achievement and behavior problems in a three-tier model including RTI*. Bethesda, MD: National Association of School Psychologists.

Shipstead, Z., Redick, T. S., & Engle, R. W. (2012). Is working memory training effective? *Psychological Bulletin, 138*, 628–654.

Sibley, M. H., Evans, S. W., & Serpell, Z. N. (2010). Social cognition and interpersonal impairment in young adolescents with ADHD. *Journal of Psychopathology and Behavioral Assessment, 32*, 193–202.

Sibley, M. H., Pelham, W. E., Evans, S. W., Gnagy, E. M., Ross, J. M., & Greiner, A. R. (2011). An evaluation of a summer treatment program for adolescents with ADHD. *Cognitive and Behavioral Practice, 18*, 530–544.

Sibley, M. H., Pelham, W. E., Jr., Molina, B. S. G., Gnagy, E. M., Waschbusch, D. A., Garefino, A. C., et al. (2012). Diagnosing ADHD in adolescence. *Journal of Consulting and Clinical Psychology, 80*, 139–150.

Sibley, M. H., Smith, B. H., Evans, S. W., Pelham, W. E., & Gnagy, E. M. (2012). Treatment response to an intensive summer treatment program for adolescents with ADHD. *Journal of Attention Disorders, 16*(6), 443–448.

Sihvoia, E., Rose, R. J., Dick, D. M., Korhonen, T., Puikkinen, L., Raevuori, A., et al. (2011). Prospective relationships of ADHD symptoms with developing substance use in a population-derived sample. *Psychological Medicine, 41*, 2615–2623.

Silver, L. B. (1990). Attention deficit-hyperactivity disorder: Is it a learning disability or a related disorder? *Journal of Learning Disabilities, 23*, 394–397.

Simmons, D. C., Kame'enui, E. J., Good, R. H., III, Harn, B. A., Cole, C., & Braun. D. (2002). Building, implementing, and sustaining a beginning reading improvement model: Lessons learned school by school. In M. R. Shinn, H. M. Walker, & G. Stoner (Eds.), *Interventions for academic and behavior problems, II: Preventive and remedial approaches* (pp. 537–569). Bethesda, MD: National Association of School Psychologists.

Simonsen, B., MacSuga-Gage, A. S., Briere, D. E., III, Freeman, J., Myers, D., Scott, T. M., et al. (in press). Multitiered support framework for teachers' classroom-management practices: Overview and case study of building the triangle for teachers. *Journal of Positive Behavior Interventions*.

Sindelar, P. T., Lane, H. B., Pullen, P. C., & Hudson, R. F. (2002). Remedial interventions for students with reading decoding problems. In M. R. Shinn, H. M. Walker, & G. Stoner (Eds.), *Interventions for academic and behavior problems: II. Preventive and remedial approaches* (pp. 703–729). Bethesda, MD: National Association of School Psychologists.

Sindelar, P. T., & Stoddard, K. (1991). Teaching reading to mildly disabled students in regular classes. In G. Stoner, M. R. Shinn, & H. M. Walker (Eds.),

Interventions for achievement and behavior problems (pp. 357–378). Silver Spring, MD: National Association of School Psychologists.

Sinkovits, H. S., Kelly, M., & Ernst, M. (2003). Medication administration in day care centers for children. *Journal of the American Pharmacists Association, 43,* 379–382.

Skiba, R., & Peterson, R. (2003): Teaching the social curriculum: School discipline as instruction. *Preventing School Failure: Alternative Education for Children and Youth, 47*(2), 66–73.

Skinner, C. H., Johnson, C. W., Larkin, M. J., Lessley, D. J., & Glowacki, M. L. (1995). The influence of rate of presentation during taped-words interventions on reading performance. *Journal of Emotional and Behavior Disorders, 4,* 214–223.

Smith, B. H., Pelham, W. E., Jr., Evans, S., Gnagy, E., Molina, B., Bukstein, O., et al. (1998). Dosage effects of methylphenidate on the social behavior of adolescents diagnosed with attention-deficit hyperactivity disorder. *Experimental and Clinical Psychopharmacology, 6,* 187–204.

Smith, B. H., Pelham, W. E., Jr., Gnagy, E., Molina, B., & Evans, S. (2000). The reliability, validity, and unique contributions of self-report by adolescents receiving treatment for attention-deficit/hyperactivity disorder. *Journal of Consulting and Clinical Psychology, 68,* 489–499.

Smith, D. J., Young, K. R., Nelson, J. R., & West, R. P. (1992). The effect of a self- management procedure on the classroom academic behavior of students with mild handicaps. *School Psychology Review, 21,* 59–72.

Snow, C. E., Burns, M. S., & Griffin, P. (Eds.). (1998). *Preventing reading difficulties in young children.* Washington, DC: National Academies Press.

Sokol, N. G. (2002). *Early Numeracy Screening Assessment.* Unpublished test, Department of Education and Human Services, Lehigh University, Bethlehem, PA.

Solanto, M. V. (1984). Neuropharmacological basis of stimulant drug action in attention deficit disorder with hyperactivity: A review and synthesis. *Psychological Bulletin, 95,* 387–409.

Solanto, M. V. (2000). Dose–response effects of Ritalin on cognitive self-regulation, learning and memory, and academic performance. In L. L. Greenhill & B. B. Osman (Eds.), *Ritalin: Theory and practice* (2nd ed., pp. 219–236). Larchmont, NY: Liebert.

Solanto, M. V., & Wender, E. H. (1989). Does methylphenidate constrict cognitive functioning? *Journal of the American Academy of Child and Adolescent Psychiatry, 28,* 897–902.

Sonuga-Barke, E. J., Daley, D., Thompson, M., Laver-Bradbury, C., & Weeks, A. (2001). Parent-based therapies for preschool attention-deficit/hyperactivity disorder: A randomized controlled trial with a community sample. *Journal of the American Academy of Child and Adolescent Psychiatry, 40,* 402–408.

Speer, D. C. (1992). Clinically significant change: Jacobson and Truax (1991) revisited. *Journal of Consulting and Clinical Psychology, 60,* 402–408.

Spencer, T. J., Biederman, J., & Mick, E. (2007). Attention-deficit/hyperactivity disorder: Diagnosis, lifespan, comorbidities, and neurobiology. *Journal of Pediatric Psychology, 32*(6), 631–642.

Spira, E. G., & Fischel, J. E. (2005). The impact of preschool inattention, hyperactivity, and impulsivity on social and academic development: A review. *Journal of Child Psychology and Psychiatry, 46,* 755–773.

Sprague, R. K., & Sleator, E. K. (1977). Methylphenidate in hyperkinetic children: Differences in dose effects on learning and social behavior. *Science, 198,* 1274–1276.

Stahr, B., Cushing, D., Lane, K., & Fox, J. (2006). Efficacy of a function-based intervention in decreasing off-task behavior exhibited by a student with ADHD. *Journal of Positive Behavior Interventions, 8,* 201–211.

Stein, M. A., & Pao, M. (2000). Attention deficit hyperactivity disorder and Ritalin side effects: Is sleep delayed, disrupted, or disturbed? In L. L. Greenhill & B. B. Osman (Eds.), *Ritalin: Theory and practice* (2nd ed., pp. 287–300). Larchmont, NY: Liebert.

Sterba, S., Egger, H. L., & Angold, A. (2007). Diagnostic specificity and nonspecificity in the dimensions of preschool psychopathology. *Journal of Child Psychology and Psychiatry, 48,* 1005–1013.

Stoner, G., Carey, S. P., Ikeda, M. J., & Shinn, M. R. (1994). The utility of curriculum-based measurement for evaluating the effects of methylphenidate on academic performance. *Journal of Applied Behavior Analysis, 27,* 101–114.

Stormont, M. (2001). Social outcomes of children with AD/HD: Contributing factors and implications for practice. *Psychology in the Schools, 38,* 521–531.

Stormont, M., & Stebbins, M. S. (2001). Teachers' comfort and importance ratings for interventions for preschoolers with AD/HD. *Psychology in the Schools, 38,* 259–267.

Strayhorn, J. M., & Weidman, C. S. (1989). Reduction of attention deficit and internalizing symptoms through parent–child interaction training. *Journal of the American Academy of Child and Adolescent Psychiatry, 28,* 888–896.

Strayhorn, J. M., & Weidman, C. S. (1991). Follow-up one year after parent–child interaction training: Effects on behavior of preschool children. *Journal of the American Academy of Child and Adolescent Psychiatry, 30,* 138–143.

Strickland, J., Keller, J., Lavigne, J. V., Gouze, K., Hopkins, J., & LeBailly, S. (2011). The structure of psychopathology in a community sample of preschoolers. *Journal of Abnormal Child Psychology, 39,* 601–610.

Sugai, G., & Horner, R. H. (2006). A promising approach for expanding and sustaining school-wide positive behavior support. *School Psychology Review, 35,* 245–259.

Sugai, G., Horner, R. H., Dunlap, G., Hieneman, M., Lewis, T. J., Nelson, C. M., et al. (2000). Applying positive behavioral support and functional behavioral assessment in schools. *Journal of Positive Behavioral Interventions, 2,* 131–143.

Swanson, J., Greenhill, L., Wigal, T., Kollins, S., Stehli, A., Davies, M., et al. (2006). Stimulant-related reductions of growth rates in the PATS. *Journal of the American Academy of Child and Adolescent Psychiatry, 45,* 1304–1313.

Swanson, J., & Kinsbourne, M. (1975). Stimulant-related state-dependent learning in hyperactive children. *Science, 192,* 1354–1357.

Swanson, J. M., Kraemer, H. C., Hinshaw, S. P., Arnold, L. E., Conners, C. K., Abikoff, H. B., et al. (2001). Clinical relevance of the preliminary findings of the MTA: Success rates based on severity of ADHD and ODD symptoms at the end of treatment. *Journal of the American Academy of Child and Adolescent Psychiatry, 40,* 168–179.

Swartz, S. L., Prevatt, F., & Proctor, B. E. (2005). A coaching intervention for college students with attention deficit/hyperactivity disorder. *Psychology in the Schools, 42*(6), 647–656.

Szasz, T. S. (1960). The myth of mental illness. *American Psychologist, 15,* 113–118.

Szatmari, P., Offord, D. R., & Boyle, M. H. (1989). Ontario Child Health Study: Prevalence of attention deficit disorder with hyperactivity. *Journal of Child Psychology and Psychiatry, 30,* 219–230.

Telzrow, C. F., & Tankersley, M. (2000). *IDEA amendments of 1997: Practice guidelines for school-based teams.* Bethesda, MD: National Association of School Psychologists.

Theule, J., Wiener, J., Tannock, R., & Jenkins, J. M. (2013). Parenting stress in families of children with ADHD: A meta-analysis. *Journal of Emotional and Behavioral Disorders, 21,* 3–17.

Timmermanis, V., & Wiener, J. (2011). Social correlates of bullying in adolescents with attention-deficit/hyperactivity disorder. *Canadian Journal of School Psychology, 26,* 301–318.

Todd, R. D., Sitdhirakso, N., Reich, W., Ji, T. H., Joyner, C. A., Heath, A. C., et al. (2002). Discrimination of DSM-IV and latent class attention-deficit/ hyperactivity disorder subtypes by educational and cognitive performance in a population-base sample of child and adolescent twins. *Journal of the American Academy of Child and Adolescent Psychiatry, 41,* 820–828.

Torgesen, J. K., & Young, K. A. (1983). Priorities for the use of microcomputers with learning disabled children. *Journal of Learning Disabilities, 16,* 234–237.

Touchette, P. E., MacDonald, R. F., & Langer, S. N. (1985). A scatter plot for identifying stimulus control of problem behavior. *Journal of Applied Behavior Analysis, 18,* 343–351.

Tremblay, R. E., Vitaro, F., Bertrand, L., LeBlanc, M., Beauchesne, H., Boileau, H., et al. (1992). Parent and child training to prevent early onset of delinquency: The Montréal Longitudinal–Experimental Study. In J. McCord & R. E. Tremblay (Eds.), *Preventing antisocial behavior: Interventions from birth through adolescence* (pp. 117–138). New York: Guilford Press.

Upadhyaya, H. P., Rose, K., Wang, W., O'Rourke, K., Sullivan, B., Deas, D., et al. (2005). Attention-deficit/hyperactivity disorder, medication treatment, and substance use patterns among adolescents and young adults. *Journal of Child and Adolescent Psychopharmacology, 15*(5), 799–809.

Valera, E. M., Faraone, S. V., Murray, K. E., & Seidman, L. J. (2007).

Meta-analysis of structural imaging findings in attention-deficit/hyperactivity disorder. *Biological Psychiatry, 61*, 1361–1369.

Valo, S., & Tannock, R. (2010). Diagnostic instability of DSM-IV ADHD subtypes: Effects of informant source, instrumentation, and methods for combining symptom reports. *Journal of Clinical Child and Adolescent Psychology, 39*, 749–760.

Van der Oord, E. J. C. G., Boomsa, D. I., & Verhulst, F. C. (1994). A study of problem behaviors in 10- to 15-year-old biologically related and unrelated international adoptees. *Behavior Genetics, 24*, 193–205.

Van der Oord, S., Prins, P. J. M., Oosterlaan, J., & Emmelkamp, P. M. G. (2008). Efficacy of methylphenidate, psychosocial treatments and their combination in school-aged children with ADHD: A meta-analysis. *Clinical Psychology Review, 28*, 783–800.

Vaughn, A. J., & Hoza, B. (2013). The incremental utility of behavioral rating scales and a structured diagnostic interview in the assessment of attention-deficit/hyperactivity disorder. *Journal of Emotional and Behavioral Disorders, 21*, 227–239.

Verbruggen, F., Logan, G. D., & Stevens, M. A. (2008). STOP-IT: Windows executable software for the stop-signal paradigm. *Behavior Research Methods, 40*, 479–483.

Vile Junod, R., DuPaul, G. J., Jitendra, A. K., Volpe, R. J., & Lorah, K. S. (2006). Classroom observations of students with and without ADHD: Differences across types of engagement. *Journal of School Psychology, 44*, 87–104.

Volkow, N. D., & Swanson, J. M. (2008). Does childhood treatment of ADHD with stimulant medication affect substance abuse in adulthood? *American Journal of Psychiatry, 165*, 553–555.

Volpe, R. J., DuPaul, G. J., Jitendra, A. K., & Tresco, K. E. (2009). Consultation-based academic interventions for children with attention deficit hyperactivitiy disorder: Effects on reading and mathematics outcomes at 1–year follow-up. *School Psychology Review, 38*(1), 5–13.

Volpe, R. J., & Fabiano, G. A. (2013). *Daily behavior report cards: An evidence-based system of assessment and intervention.* New York: Guilford Press.

Volpe, R. J., Heick, P. F., & Gureasko-Moore, D. (2005). An agile behavioral model for monitoring the effects of stimulant medication in school settings. *Psychology in the Schools, 42*, 509–523.

Vyse, S. A., & Rapport, M. D. (1989). The effects of methylphenidate on learning in children with ADDH: The stimulus equivalence paradigm. *Journal of Consulting and Clinical Psychology, 57*, 425–435.

Waldman, I. D., & Gizer, I. R. (2006). The genetics of attention deficit hyperactivity disorder. *Clinical Psychology Review, 26*, 396–432.

Walker, H. M., Block-Pedego, A., Todis, B., & Severson, H. (1998). *School archival records search (SARS): User's guide and technical manual.* Longmont, CO: Sopris-West.

Wallander, J. L., Schroeder, S. R., Michelli, J. A., & Gualtieri, C. T. (1987). Classroom social interactions of attention deficit disorder with hyperactivity children as a function of stimulant medication. *Journal of Pediatric Psychology, 12*, 61–76.

Watson, T. S., & Steege, M. W. (2003). *Conducting school-based functional behavioral assessment: A practitioner's guide*. New York: Guilford Press.

Webster-Stratton, C. (1996). *The parents and children series: A comprehensive course divided into four programs*. Seattle, WA: Author.

Webster-Stratton, C., & Reid, J. M. (2014). Tailoring the Incredible Years parent, teacher, and child interventions for young children with ADHD. In J. K. Ghuman & H. S. Ghuman (Eds.), *ADHD in preschool children: Assessment and treatment* (pp. 113–131). New York: Oxford University Press.

Webster-Stratton, C., Reid, J. M., & Hammond, M. (2001). Preventing conduct problems, promoting social competence: A parent and teacher training partnership in Head Start. *Journal of Clinical Child Psychology, 30*, 283–302.

Wechsler, D. (2003). *Wechsler Intelligence Scale for Children* (4th ed.). San Antonio, TX: Psychological Corporation.

Weiss, G., & Hechtman, L. T. (1986). *Hyperactive children grown up: Empirical findings and theoretical considerations*. New York: Guilford Press.

Weiss, G., & Hechtman, L. T. (1993). *Hyperactive children grown up: ADHD in children, adolescents, and adults* (2nd ed.). New York: Guilford Press.

Weiss, G., Kruger, E., Danielson, U., & Elman, M. (1975). Effects of long-term treatment of hyperactive children with methylphenidate. *Canadian Medical Association Journal, 112*, 159–165.

Werry, J. S., Elkind, G. S., & Reeves, J. C. (1987). Attention deficit, conduct, oppositional, and anxiety disorders in children: III. Laboratory differences. *Journal of Abnormal Child Psychology, 15*, 409–428.

Werry, J. S., Sprague, R. L., & Cohen, M. N. (1975). Conners' Teacher Rating Scale for use in drug studies with children: An empirical study. *Journal of Abnormal Child Psychology, 3*, 217–229.

Weyandt, L. (2007). *An ADHD primer* (2nd ed.) Mahwah, NJ: Erlbaum.

Weyandt, L. L., & DuPaul, G. J. (2013). *College students with ADHD: Current issues and future directions*. New York: Springer.

Weyandt, L. L., Linterman, I., & Rice, J. A. (1995). Reported prevalence of attentional difficulties in a general sample of college students. *Journal of Psychopathology and Behavioral Assessment, 17*(3), 293–304.

Whalen, C. K., Collins, B. E., Henker, B., Alkus, S. R., Adams, D., & Stapp, J. (1978). Behavior observations of hyperactive children and methylphenidate (Ritalin) effects in systematically structured classroom environments: Now you see them, now you don't. *Journal of Pediatric Psychology, 3*, 177–187.

Whalen, C. K., Henker, B., Collins, B. E., Finck, D., & Dotemoto, S. (1979). A social ecology of hyperactive boys: Medication effects in structured classroom environments. *Journal of Applied Behavior Analysis, 12*, 65–81.

Whalen, C. K., Jamner, L. D., Henker, B., Delfino, R. J., & Lozano, J. M. (2002). The ADHD spectrum and everyday life: Experience sampling of adolescent moods, activities, smoking, and drinking. *Child Development, 73*(1), 209–227.

White, M. A. (1975). Natural rates of teacher approval and disapproval in the classroom. *Journal of Applied Behavior Analysis, 8*, 367–372.

Wierson, M., & Forehand, R. (1994). Parental behavioral training for child noncompliance: Rationale, concepts, and effectiveness. *Current Directions in Psychological Science, 3*, 146–150.

Wigal, S. B., Childress, A. C., Belden, H. W., & Berry, S. A. (2013). NWP06, an extended-release oral suspension of methylphenidate, improved attention-deficit/hyperactivity disorder symptoms compared with placebo in a laboratory classroom study. *Journal of Child and Adolescent Psychopharmacology, 23*, 3–10.

Wigal, S. B., Wigal, T., Schuck, S., Brams, M., Williamson, D., Armstrong, R. B., et al. (2011). Academic, behavioral, and cognitive effects of OROS® methylphenidate on older children with attention-deficit/hyperactivity disorder. *Journal of Child and Adolescent Psychopharmacology, 21*, 121–131.

Wigal, T., Greenhill, L., Chuang, S., McGough, J., Vitiello, B., Skrobala, A., et al. (2006). Safety and tolerability of methylphenidate in preschool children with ADHD. *Journal of the American Academy of Child and Adolescent Psychiatry, 45*, 1294–1303.

Willcutt, E. G., Nigg, J. T., Pennington, B. F., Solanto, M. V., Rohde, L. A., Tannock, R., et al. (2012). Validity of DSM-IV attention-deficit/hyperactivity disorder symptom dimensions and subtypes. *Journal of Abnormal Psychology, 121*, 991–1010.

Willcutt, E. G., Pennington, B. F., Chhabildas, N. A., Friedman, M. C., & Alexander, J. (1999). Psychiatric comorbidity associated with DSM-IV ADHD in a nonreferred sample of twins. *Journal of the American Academy of Child and Adolescent Psychiatry, 38*, 1355–1362.

Wilson, L. J., & Jennings, J. N. (1996). Parents' acceptability of alternative treatments for attention-deficit hyperactivity disorder. *Journal of Attention Disorders, 1*, 114–121.

Witt, J. C., Daly, E. M., & Noell, G. (2000). *Functional assessments: A step-by-step guide to solving academic and behavior problems.* Longmont, CO: Sopris-West.

Witt, J. C., & Elliott, S. N. (1985). Acceptability of classroom management strategies. In T. R. Kratochwill (Ed.), *Advances in school psychology* (Vol. 4, pp. 251–288). Hillsdale, NJ: Erlbaum.

Wixon, K. K. (1986). Vocabulary instruction and children's comprehension of basal stories. *Reading Research Quarterly, 21*, 317–329.

Wolf, L. E. (2001). College students with ADHD and other hidden disabilities: Outcomes and interventions. In J. Wasserstein, L. E. Wolf, & F. F. LeFever (Eds.), *Adult attention deficit disorder: Brain mechanisms and life outcomes* (pp. 385–395) New York: New York Academy of Sciences.

Wolf, L. E., Simkowitz, P., & Carlson, H. (2009). College students with attention-deficit/hyperactivity disorder. *Current Psychiatry Reports, 11*(5), 415–421.

Wolraich, M. L. (2006). Attention-deficit/hyperactivity disorder: Can it be recognized and treated in children younger than 5 years? *Infants and Young Children, 19*, 86–93.

Wolraich, M. L., Lambert, E. W., Bickman, L., Simmons, T., Doffing, M. A., & Worley, K. A. (2004). Assessing the impact of parent and teacher agreement on diagnosing attention-deficit hyperactivity disorder. *Developmental and Behavioral Pediatrics, 25*, 41–47.

Yildiz, O., Sismanlar, S. G., Memik, N. C., Karakaya, I., & Agaoglu, B. (2011). Atomoxetine and methylphenidate treatment in children with ADHD: The efficacy, tolerability, and effects on executive functions. *Child Psychiatry and Human Development, 42,* 257–269.

Zentall, S. S. (1989). Attentional cuing in spelling tasks for hyperactive and comparison regular classroom children. *Journal of Special Education, 23,* 83–93.

Zentall, S. S., & Leib, S. L. (1985). Structured tasks: Effects on activity and performance of hyperactive and comparison children. *Journal of Educational Research, 79,* 91–95.

Zirkel, P. A. (2013). ADHD checklist for identification under the IDEA and Section 504/ADA. *West's Education Law Reporter, 293,* 13–27.

Zirkel, P. A., & Aleman, S. R. (2000). *Section 504, the ADA and the schools* (2nd ed.). Horsham, PA: LRP.

Zito, J. M., Safer, D. J., de Jong-van den Berg, L. T. W., Janhsen, K., Fegert, J. M., Gardner, J. M., et al. (2008). A three-country comparison of psychotropic medication prevalence in youth. *Child and Adolescent Psychiatry and Mental Health, 2,* Article 26.

Zito, J. M., Safer, D. J., dos Reis, S., Gardner, J. F., Boles, M., & Lynch, F. (2000). Trends in the prescribing of psychotropic medications to preschoolers. *Journal of the American Medical Association, 283,* 1025–1030.

Index

355

Index